Heart Diseases & Disorders
Sourcebook, 2nd Edition

Household Safety Sourcebook

Immune System Disorders Sourcebook

Infant & Toddler Health Sourcebook

Injury & Trauma Sourcebook

Kidney & Urinary Tract Diseases &
Disorders Sourcebook

Learning Disabilities Sourcebook,
2nd Edition

Leukemia Sourcebook

Liver Disorders Sourcebook

Lung Disorders Sourcebook

Medical Tests Sourcebook, 2nd Edition

Men's Health Concerns Sourcebook,
2nd Edition

Mental Health Disorders Sourcebook,
2nd Edition

Mental Retardation Sourcebook

Movement Disorders Sourcebook

Obesity Sourcebook

Osteoporosis Sourcebook

Pain Sourcebook, 2nd Edition

Pediatric Cancer Sourcebook

Physical & Mental Issues in Aging
Sourcebook

Podiatry Sourcebook

Pregnancy & Birth Sourcebook,
2nd Edition

Prostate Cancer

Public Health Sourcebook

Reconstructive & Cosmetic Surgery
Sourcebook

Rehabilitation Sourcebook

Respiratory Diseases & Disorders
Sourcebook

Sexually Transmitted Diseases
Sourcebook, 2nd Edition

Skin Disorders Sourcebook

Sleep Disorders Sourcebook

Sports Injuries Sourcebook, 2nd Edition

Stress-Related Disorders Sourcebook

Stroke Sourcebook

Substance Abuse Sourcebook

Surgery Sourcebook

Transplantation Sourcebook

Traveler's Health Sourcebook

Vegetarian Sourcebook

Women's Health Concerns Sourcebook,
2nd Edition

Workplace Health & Safety Sourcebook

Worldwide Health Sourcebook

Teen Health Series

Cancer Information for Teens

Diet Information for Teens

Drug Information for Teens

Mental Health Information
for Teens

Sexual Health Information
for Teens

Skin Health Information
for Teens

Sports Injuries Information
for Teens

DATE DUE

NOV 2 9 2004	

BRODART.   Cat. No. 23-221

Health Reference Series

First Edition

Healthy Children SOURCEBOOK

*Basic Consumer Health Information about the
Physical and Mental Development of Children between
the Ages of 3 and 12, Including Routine Health Care,
Preventative Health Services, Safety and First Aid,
Healthy Sleep, Dental Care, Nutrition, and Fitness, and
Featuring Parenting Tips on Such Topics as Bedwetting,
Choosing Day Care, Monitoring TV and Other Media,
and Establishing a Foundation for
Substance Abuse Prevention*

*Along with a Glossary of Commonly Used
Pediatric Terms and Resources for Additional
Help and Information*

Edited by
Chad T. Kimball

Omnigraphics

615 Griswold Street • Detroit, MI 48226

Bibliographic Note

Because this page cannot legibly accommodate all the copyright notices, the Bibliographic Note portion of the Preface constitutes an extension of the copyright notice.

Edited by Chad T. Kimball

Health Reference Series

Karen Bellenir, *Managing Editor*
David A. Cooke, MD, *Medical Consultant*
Elizabeth Barbour, *Permissions Associate*
Dawn Matthews, *Verification Assistant*
Laura Pleva Nielsen, *Index Editor*
EdIndex, Services for Publishers, *Indexers*

* * *

Omnigraphics, Inc.

Matthew P. Barbour, *Senior Vice President*
Kay Gill, *Vice President—Directories*
Kevin Hayes, *Operations Manager*
Leif Gruenberg, *Development Manager*
David P. Bianco, *Marketing Consultant*

* * *

Peter E. Ruffner, *Publisher*

Frederick G. Ruffner, Jr., *Chairman*

Library of Congress Cataloging-in-Publication Data

Healthy children sourcebook : basic consumer health information about the physical and mental development of children between the ages of 3 and 12, including routine health care, preventative health services, safety and first aid, healthy sleep, dental care, nutrition, and fitness, and featuring parenting tips on such topics as bedwetting, choosing day care, monitoring TV and other media, and establishing a foundation for substance abuse prevention; along with a glossary of commonly used pediatric terms and resources for additional help and information / edited by Chad T. Kimball.-- 1st ed.
    p. cm. -- (Health reference series)
ISBN 0-7808-0247-0 (lib. bdg. : alk. paper)
    1. Children--Health and hygiene. 2. Child development. 3. Consumer education. 4. Parent and child. 5. Health promotion. I. Kimball, Chad T. II. Health reference series (Unnumbered)

RJ61.H36 2003
613'.0432-dc22

2003058486

Table of Contents

Part II: Physical and Mental Development

Part III: Education

Part IV: Childhood Emergencies: Prevention and First Aid

Part V: Food, Nutrition, and Exercise

Part VI: Other Common Parenting Concerns

Part VII: Additional Help and Information

Preface

About This Book

According to indicators used to measure child health, including assessments of physical, mental, and social well-being, most children are healthy. In fact, the 2000 National Health Interview Survey conducted by the Centers for Disease Control and Prevention's National Center for Health Statistics found that 82 percent were in "very good" or "excellent" health. Numerous advances made over the past several decades have helped achieve these results:

- More than three quarters of the nation's children are currently immunized against diseases such as diphtheria, tetanus, *Haemophilus influenzae* type b, measles, mumps, rubella, polio, and varicella (chickenpox).

- Poverty, which has an impact on child health, has lessened. In 1993, 22 percent of U.S. children lived in families below the poverty threshold. By 2000, the number had fallen to 16 percent. Additionally, the health gap between children in poverty and those living at or above the poverty level decreased slightly.

- The percentage of young children who regularly eat a healthy diet has increased.

Areas of concern still exist, however, and many of the improvements yet to be accomplished are related to choices made by children and their parents regarding safety, diet, fitness, and substance use. Because these kinds of lifelong habits are often developed in childhood, the pre-adolescent years are especially crucial in a child's journey to healthy adulthood.

This *Sourcebook* provides parents and caregivers with information regarding the physical, mental, and emotional development of healthy pre-adolescent children. It offers facts about preventative health care, including check-ups, recommended screening tests, vaccine schedules, eye care, and dental hygiene, along with suggestions for helping children learn to make healthy choices regarding food, fitness, and substance use. It provides parents with practical suggestions for coping with such issues as childhood emergencies and media-related questions, and it offers information regarding other common parenting concerns, including child care, education, bedwetting, healthy sleep, and youth violence. A glossary, suggestions for additional reading, and directories of resources for further help and information are also provided.

How to Use This Book

This book is divided into parts and chapters. Parts focus on broad areas of interest. Chapters are devoted to single topics within a part.

Part I: Basic Preventative Care summarizes facts about general health maintenance. It includes information about routine medical check-ups, eye care, dental care, recommended screening tests, and immunization schedules.

Part II: Physical and Mental Development provides information about patterns of growth and developmental milestones in early and middle childhood, including speech and language acquisition and the evaluation and treatment of delayed development. Mental health in children and symptoms of childhood mental disorders are also described.

Part III: Education explains steps parents can take to help their children prepare for and succeed in school. It offers suggestions for helping students improve reading ability and complete homework assignments. It explains learning disabilities and offers a checklist of common warning signs. Facts about attention deficit hyperactivity disorder and special education services are also included.

Part IV: Childhood Emergencies: Prevention and First Aid offers facts about the causes, consequences, and treatment of injuries in children.

It includes safety information about some of the most common sources of injury at home and on the playground. It provides safety suggestions for biking, sports participation, and water recreation. It also discusses motor vehicle safety for young passengers and pedestrians.

Part V: Food, Nutrition, and Exercise explains the important links between diet, fitness, and health. It offers suggestions for helping children make food choices and develop exercise habits that will promote lifetime wellness.

Part VI: Other Common Parenting Concerns includes facts about such topics as administering medications, treating urinary and stool incontinence, developing healthy sleep habits, and choosing child care. It also provides suggestions for dealing with media-related concerns, including television and the internet, preventing substance abuse, and stopping youth violence.

Part VII: Additional Help and Information offers a glossary of terms related to child health, suggestions for additional reading, and directories of resources for drug abuse prevention, education concerns, and other parenting topics.

Bibliographic Note

This volume contains documents and excerpts from publications issued by the following U.S. government agencies: Administration for Children and Families; Agency for Healthcare Research and Quality (AHRQ); Center for Nutrition Policy and Promotion; Centers for Disease Control and Prevention (CDC); Educational Resources Information Center (ERIC) Clearinghouse on Urban Education; Federal Bureau of Investigation (FBI); Federal Highway Administration; National Center for Chronic Disease Prevention and Health Promotion; National Heart, Lung, and Blood Institute (NHLBI); National Highway Traffic Safety Administration (NHTSA); National Institute for Children and Youth with Disabilities (NICHCY); National Institute for Dental and Craniofacial Research (NIDCR); National Institute of Arthritis and Musculoskeletal and Skin Diseases (NIAMS); National Institute of Child Health and Human Development (NICHD); National Institute of Diabetes and Digestive and Kidney Diseases (NIDDK); National Institute of Mental Health (NIMH); National Institute on Alcohol Abuse and Alcoholism (NIAAA); National Institute on Deafness and Other Communication Disorders (NIDCD); National Kidney and Urologic Diseases Information Clearinghouse; National Parent

Information Network; Office on Women's Health; President's Council on Physical Fitness and Sports; SafeUSA™; Substance Abuse and Mental Health Services Administration (SAMHSA); U.S. Consumer Product Safety Commission (CPSC); U.S. Department of Agriculture (USDA); U.S. Department of Education; U.S. Department of Health and Human Services (DHHS); U.S. Department of Housing and Urban Development (HUD); U.S. Department of Justice; U.S. Department of the Interior; U.S. Department of Transportation; U.S. Environmental Protection Agency (EPA); and the U.S. Food and Drug Administration (FDA).

In addition, this volume contains copyrighted documents from the following organizations and individuals: A.D.A.M., Inc.; American Academy of Family Physicians; American Association of Endodontists; American College of Emergency Physicians; American Dental Association; American Optometric Association; American Speech-Language-Hearing Association; Bright Futures Project; Children's Hospital of Palmetto Health (Columbia, SC); Karen DeBord; Emergency Medical Services for Children; Human Growth Foundation; Immunization Action Coalition; International Dyslexia Association; Kids Sports Network; Kidsmeds, Inc.; Lippincott Williams and Wilkins; Medical College of Wisconsin, Healthlink; Michigan Department of Consumer and Industry Affairs; National Association for the Education of Young Children (NAEYC); National Center for Children Exposed to Violence; National Center for Learning Disabilities; National Eating Disorders Association; National Network for Child Care (NNCC); Nemours Foundation (KidsHealth.org); Oregon Department of Agriculture; Pediatric Development and Behavior; Prevent Blindness America; Self Help for Hard of Hearing People (SHHH); Beth Shortridge, MD; Smiles4Ever.com; STOP (Safe Tables Our Priority); University of Iowa, Virtual Children's Hospital; and the University of Rochester.

Full citation information is provided on the first page of each chapter. Every effort has been made to secure all necessary rights to reprint the copyrighted material. If any omissions have been made, please contact Omnigraphics to make corrections for future editions.

Acknowledgements

Thanks go to the organizations, agencies, and individuals who have contributed materials for this *Sourcebook*. Many other people also played a vital role in its completion, including medical consultant Dr. David Cooke, verification assistant Dawn Matthews, and document engineer Bruce Bellenir. Permissions associate Liz Barbour and editorial assistants Michael Bellenir, Buffy Bellenir, and Nancy Gable Lucas also deserve special thanks for providing support and steadfast dedication to this project.

Note from the Editor

This book is part of Omnigraphics' *Health Reference Series*. The *Series* provides basic information about a broad range of medical concerns. It is not intended to serve as a tool for diagnosing illness, in prescribing treatments, or as a substitute for the physician/patient relationship. All persons concerned about medical symptoms or the possibility of disease are encouraged to seek professional care from an appropriate health care provider.

Our Advisory Board

The *Health Reference Series* is reviewed by an Advisory Board comprised of librarians from public, academic, and medical libraries. We would like to thank the following board members for providing guidance to the development of this *Series*:

Dr. Lynda Baker,
Associate Professor of Library and Information Science,
Wayne State University, Detroit, MI

Nancy Bulgarelli,
William Beaumont Hospital Library, Royal Oak, MI

Karen Imarisio,
Bloomfield Township Public Library, Bloomfield Township, MI

Karen Morgan,
Mardigian Library, University of Michigan-Dearborn,
Dearborn, MI

Rosemary Orlando,
St. Clair Shores Public Library, St. Clair Shores, MI

Medical Consultant

Medical consultation services are provided to the *Health Reference Series* editors by David A. Cooke, MD. Dr. Cooke is a graduate of Brandeis University, and he received his M.D. degree from the University of Michigan. He completed residency training at the University of Wisconsin Hospital and Clinics. He is board-certified in Internal

Medicine. Dr. Cooke currently works as part of the University of Michigan Health System and practices in Brighton, MI. In his free time, he enjoys writing, science fiction, and spending time with his family.

Health Reference Series *Update Policy*

The inaugural book in the *Health Reference Series* was the first edition of *Cancer Sourcebook* published in 1989. Since then, the *Series* has been enthusiastically received by librarians and in the medical community. In order to maintain the standard of providing high-quality health information for the layperson the editorial staff at Omnigraphics felt it was necessary to implement a policy of updating volumes when warranted.

Medical researchers have been making tremendous strides, and it is the purpose of the *Health Reference Series* to stay current with the most recent advances. Each decision to update a volume will be made on an individual basis. Some of the considerations will include how much new information is available and the feedback we receive from people who use the books. If there is a topic you would like to see added to the update list, or an area of medical concern you feel has not been adequately addressed, please write to:

Editor
Health Reference Series
Omnigraphics, Inc.
615 Griswold Street
Detroit, MI 48226
E-mail: editorial@omnigraphics.com

Part One

Basic Preventative Care

Chapter 1

How to Find a Pediatrician

Choosing the right doctor for your child is extremely important. A large part of a pediatrician's job is to educate you about your child's health and to help you deal with behavioral issues that may have little to do with illness. From the time your baby is born until he or she becomes an adolescent, your child's pediatrician will be one of the most important people in your life. That's why the time to carefully choose a pediatrician is before the baby arrives.

So where Do You Begin?

About three months before you're due, start compiling a list of potential pediatricians. Ask your obstetrician or primary care physician for a referral and tell them the qualities you are interested in. Ask other parents, friends, relatives or neighbors.

The American Academy of Pediatrics (AAP) can give you a list of member doctors in your area. A pediatrician must meet certain criteria to become a Fellow of the AAP. Visit the AAP website (www.aap.org) or write to the Pediatrician Referral Department, AAP, PO Box 927, Elk Grove Village, IL 60009-0927. Be sure to include a self-addressed, stamped envelope and the name of the city and state you are interested in.

"Finding a Pediatrician or Specialist," © 1995 Children's Hospital of Palmetto Health, Columbia, South Carolina; reprinted with permission. Despite the older date of this document, the guidelines provided are still applicable.

3

If you belong to a managed care plan, it also is important to find out what pediatricians are affiliated with it. Let your primary care physician pick out a few names from the list.

Schedule Interviews

Now that you have a list, you need to decide what things are important to you and schedule interviews with the pediatricians that make the short list. You certainly want someone with expertise and experience in children's health and development, good credentials and hospital privileges. Just as important, though, is someone you can trust and feel comfortable with. That is something that you will only be able to determine from an in-person visit.

Most doctors' offices will accommodate your request for an interview with the doctor. You'll want to start the process about two months before you're due.

Questions to Ask

Try to understand that the doctor is busy treating other people's children. You wouldn't want your child ignored because the doctor was tied up in an interview for an hour, would you? Try to keep the interview around fifteen minutes. The goal of this meeting is to get to know the doctor's philosophy and personality. Discuss family medical history and issues important to you like breast-feeding, nutrition, sleeping habits, and circumcision. Ask about office hours, scheduling procedures, phone inquiries, and emergencies.

Here are some specific questions to consider:

- How long have you practiced?
- Do you have any sub-specialties?
- What kind of parents do you work best with?
- Do you encourage parents to call for routine questions?
- Will you discuss behavioral and developmental issues?
- Will I get reminders about immunizations in the mail?
- Are there separate appointment times or waiting rooms for sick and well children?

Other Considerations

Knowing when you have met "Dr. Right" is really a gut reaction. Were you seen within a reasonable time of your appointment? Was the office staff courteous and helpful? Did the doctor ask probing questions and listen to answers? Is the doctor well-informed about preventive health measures? Was the office clean? Was it conveniently located?

Also, pay attention to the doctor's style. Do you want a pediatrician who offers you choices and lets you decide, or do you want one who gives a lot of direction? Do you want a warm doctor with a sense of humor, or would you prefer someone very clinical and straightforward? Two of the most important qualities you should keep in mind are competence and compassion.

If you feel uneasy at any point after your initial interview or visit, don't hesitate to talk to other pediatricians until you find one you feel comfortable with. After all, the pediatrician is going to be a partner in your child's health and development for many years to come.

Chapter 2

Check-Ups and Screening Tests

Working with the doctor, nurse, or other health care provider to keep your child well is as important as getting treatment when he or she is sick. Easy-to-use records help you keep track of preventive care for each child and know when shots and other services are needed. This chapter briefly explains preventive care for children—such as check-up visits, immunizations, and tests and exams—and provides guidance on related issues.

To get the most from your child's health care:

- Be an active member of your child's health care team. Ask your health care provider any questions that you may have.

- Order a print copy "Put Prevention into Practice: Child Health Guide," Publication No. APPIP 98-0026, from the Agency for Healthcare Research and Quality Publications Clearinghouse (800-358-9295) and use the records to keep track of the immunizations (shots), tests, exams, and other types of health care that your child receives. Use these records to remind you when your child needs to be seen next.

"Put Prevention into Practice: Child Health Guide," Agency for Healthcare Research and Quality (AHRQ), Rockville, MD; Publication No. APPIP 98-0026, revised 2000, current as of January 2003. Available online at http://www.ahrq. gov/ppip/ppchild.htm. Single print copies are available free from the AHRQ Publications Clearinghouse; call toll free 800-358-9295.

- Keep the "Child Health Guide" and records in a safe place. Check it often to make sure your child is getting the preventive care that he or she needs. Keep the "Child Health Guide" records up-to-date.

- Bring the "Child Health Guide" every time your child goes to a health care provider.

Check-Up Visits

Check-up visits are important because they allow your health care provider to review your child's growth and development, perform tests, or give shots. To help your provider get a complete picture of your child's health status, bring your child's health record (such as the "Child Health Guide") and a list of any medications your child is taking to each visit.

Check-up visits are a time for parents to ask questions. Bring a list of concerns you have. For example:

- My child is not sleeping through the night yet.

- I don't think my child is eating enough.

- My child seems uncoordinated and is always walking into things.

Some authorities recommend check-up visits at ages 2–4 weeks; 2, 4, 6, 9, 12, 15, and 18 months; 2, 3, 4, 5, 6, 8, 10, 12, 14, 16, and 18 years. Some children may need to be seen more often, others less. Ask your clinician how often your child will need to be seen.

Immunizations

Note: The information on immunizations is based on recommendations issued by the Advisory Committee on Immunization Practices, the American Academy of Pediatrics, and the American Academy of Family Physicians.

Your child needs immunizations. Immunizations (shots) protect your child from many serious diseases. Below is a list of immunizations and the ages when your child should receive them. Immunizations should be given at the recommended ages—even if your child has a cold or illness at the time. Ask your health care provider when your child should receive these important shots. Ask also if your child needs other immunizations.

- Polio (inactivated poliovirus vaccine [IPV]): At 2 months, 4 months, 6–18 months, and 4–6 years.

- Diphtheria-tetanus-pertussis (DTaP): At 2 months, 4 months, 6 months, 15–18 months, and 4–6 years.

- Tetanus-diphtheria (Td) at 11–16 years.

- Measles-mumps-rubella (MMR): At 12–15 months and 4–6 years or as soon thereafter as possible.

- *Haemophilus influenzae* type b (Hib): At 2 months, 4 months, 6 months, and 12–15 months; or 2 months, 4 months, and 12–15 months, depending on the vaccine type.

- Hepatitis B: At birth–2 months, 1–4 months, and 6–18 months. If missed, get 3 doses starting at age 11 years.

- Chickenpox (varicella): At 12–18 months or under 13 years.

- Hepatitis A (in selected areas): At 24 months–18 years; second dose 6–12 months after first dose.

- Pneumococcal disease (Prevnar™): At 2 months, 4 months, 6 months, and 12–15 months. If missed, talk to your health care provider.

- Influenza (children at high risk for chronic diseases): At 6 months–18 years. Two doses at least 1 month apart for children aged 6 months–under 9 years who receive influenza vaccine for the first time.

Periodically, the recommended timing for immunizations changes. For the latest immunization schedule, contact Every Child By Two at (202) 783-7034 or visit their website at http://www.ecbt.org/immsche. htm.

Tests and Exams for Children

Blood Pressure

Your child should have blood pressure measurements regularly, starting at around 3 years of age. High blood pressure in children needs medical attention. It may be a sign of underlying disease and, if not treated, may lead to serious illness. Check with your child's health care provider about blood pressure measurements.

Lead

Lead can harm your child, slowing physical and mental growth and damaging many parts of the body. The most common way children get lead poisoning is by being around old house paint that is chipping or peeling.

If you answer "yes" answers to any of the questions below, your child may need to be tested for lead. Has your child:

- lived in or regularly visited a house built before 1950? (This could include a day care center, preschool, the home of a baby-sitter or relative, etc.)

- lived in or regularly visited a house built before 1978 (the year lead-based paint was banned for residential use) with recent, ongoing, or planned renovation or remodeling?

- had a brother or sister, housemate, or playmate followed or treated for lead poisoning?

Vision and Hearing

Your child's vision should be tested before starting school, at about 3 or 4 years of age. Your child may also need vision tests as he or she grows. Some authorities also recommend hearing testing beginning at 3 to 4 years of age.

If at any age your child has any of the vision or hearing warning signs listed below, be sure to talk with your health care provider.

Vision Warning Signs

- Eyes turning inward (crossing) or outward
- Squinting
- Headaches
- Not doing as well in school work as before
- Blurred or double vision

Hearing Warning Signs

- Poor response to noise or voice
- Slow language and speech development
- Abnormal sounding speech

Special Warning: Listening to very loud music, especially with earphones, can permanently damage your child's hearing.

Additional Tests

Your child may need other tests to prevent health problems. Some common tests are:

Anemia (Blood) Test: Your child may need to be tested for anemia ("low blood") when he or she is still a baby (usually around the first birthday). Children may also need this test as they get older. Some children are more likely to get anemia than others. Ask your health care provider about anemia testing.

Tuberculosis (TB) Skin Test: Children may need this test if they have had close contact with a person who has TB, live in an area where TB is more common than average (such as a Native American reservation, a homeless shelter, or an institution) or have recently moved from Asia, Africa, Central America, South America, the Caribbean, or the Pacific Islands.

Health Guidance

Development

Children grow and develop at different rates. Your child's health care provider will measure your child's height and weight regularly. These measurements will help you and your health care provider know if your child is growing properly.

The information below shows the ages by which most children develop certain abilities. It is normal for a child to do some of these things later than the ages noted here. If your child fails to do many of these at the ages given, or you have questions about his or her development, talk with your child's health care provider.

3 Years

- Knows age, helps button clothing, washes and dries hands.
- Throws ball overhand, rides tricycle.

4 Years

- Knows first and last name, tells a story, counts four objects.

11

- Balances on one foot, uses children's scissors.

5 Years

- Names 4 colors, counts 10 objects.
- Hops on one foot, dresses self.

Nutrition

What your child eats is very important for his or her health. Follow the nutrition guidelines below.

Guidelines for a Healthy Diet—2 Years and Older

- Provide a variety of foods, including plenty of fruits, vegetables, and whole grains.
- Use salt (sodium) and sugars in moderation.
- Encourage a diet low in fat, saturated fat, and cholesterol.
- Help your child maintain a healthy weight by providing proper foods and encouraging regular exercise.

Dental/Oral Health

Your child needs regular dental care starting at an early age. Good oral health requires good daily care. Follow these guidelines.

- Talk with your dentist about dental sealants. They can help prevent cavities in permanent teeth.
- Use dental floss to help prevent gum disease. Talk with your dentist about when to start.
- Do not permit your child to smoke or chew tobacco. Set a good example: don't use tobacco products yourself.
- If a permanent tooth is knocked out, rinse it gently and put it back into the socket or in a glass of cold milk or water. See a dentist immediately.

Physical Activity

Your child needs regular physical activity through play and sports to stay fit. Good physical activity habits learned early can help your child become an active and healthy adult. Adults who are physically active are less likely to be overweight or to have heart disease, high blood pressure, and other diseases. Adults and children should try to get at least 30 minutes of physical activity most days of the week.

- Encourage your child to participate in physical activities, including sports.

- Encourage involvement in activities that can be enjoyed into adulthood (walking, running, swimming, basketball, tennis, golf, dancing, and bicycle riding).

- Plan physical activities with family or friends; exercise is more fun with others.

- Limit the time your child spends watching TV to less than 2 hours per day. Encourage going out to the playground, park, gym, or swimming pool instead.

- Physical activity should be fun. Don't make winning the only goal.

- Many communities and schools offer exercise or sports programs—find out what is available for your child.

Tobacco Use

Using tobacco in any form is harmful to you and can harm your child's health. Tobacco use—smoking and/or chewing tobacco—causes cancer, heart disease, and other serious illnesses. Children exposed to tobacco smoke are more likely to get infections of the ears, sinuses, and lungs. Smoking in the home may also cause lung cancer in family members who do not smoke.

Discourage your child from using tobacco (in any form). If you smoke, ask your health care provider about getting help to quit.

Safety

More children die from injuries than any other cause. The good news is that most injuries can be prevented by following simple safety guidelines. Talk with your health care provider about ways to protect your child from injuries.

Read the lists below. Work on those guidelines you don't already follow.

Table 2.1. Clinical Preventive Services for Normal-Risk Children (Birth to 18 Years) Recommended by Most U. S. Authorities (continued on next page)

Immunizations

Type	Age
Hepatitis B (3 doses)	Birth–2 months 1–4 months 6–18 months **or** 3 doses at 11 years if missed previous doses
Polio (IPV) (4 doses)*	2 months 4 months 6–18 months 4–6 years
Haemophilus influenzae type B (Hib) (4 doses)*	2 months 4 months 6 months 12–15 months
Diphtheria, tetanus, pertussis (DTaP, Td) (5 doses)	2 months 4 months 6 months 15–18 months 4–6 years
Tetanus (Td) (1 dose)	11–16 years
Measles, mumps, rubella (MMR) (2 doses)	12–15 months 4–6 years **or** as soon thereafter as possible
Chickenpox (varicella) (1 dose)	12–18 months **or** under 13 years
Hepatitis A (in selected areas)	24 months–18 years; second dose 6–12 months after first dose
Pneumococcal disease (Prevnar™) (4 doses)	2 months 4 months 6 months 12–15 months
Influenza (children at high risk for chronic diseases)	6 months–18 years 2 doses at least 1 month apart for children 6 months–under 9 years who receive influenza vaccine for the first time

Table 2.1. Clinical Preventive Services for Normal-Risk Children (Birth to 18 Years) Recommended by Most U. S. Authorities (continued from previous page)

Screening

Age	Screening Test	How Often
Newborn	Newborn screening (PKU, sickle cell, hemoglobinopathies, hypothyroidism)	Once
Newborn	Hearing	Once
Birth–2 months	Head circumference	Periodically
Birth–18 years	Height and weight	Periodically
1 year	Lead	Once
3–4 years	Eye screening	Once
3–18 years	Blood pressure	Periodically
3–18 years	Dental	Periodically
11–18 years	Alcohol use	Periodically

Counseling

As your child grows, your health care provider should take time to talk to you (and/or your child) about the following topics:

- Development
- Nutrition
- Physical activity
- Safety
- Unintentional injuries and poisonings
- Violent behaviors and firearms
- Sexually transmitted diseases and HIV
- Family planning
- Tobacco use
- Drug use

Source: Child Health Guide, Put Prevention Into Practice, Agency for Healthcare Quality and Research; current as of January 2003.

Safety Guidelines—All Ages

- Use smoke detectors in your home. Change the batteries every year and check once a month to see that they work.

- If you have a gun in your home, make sure that the gun and ammunition are locked up separately and kept out of children's reach.

- Never drive after drinking alcohol.

- Use car safety belts at all times.

- Teach your child traffic safety. Children under 9 years of age need supervision when crossing streets.

- Teach your children how and when to call 911.

- Learn basic life-saving skills (for example, CPR).

- Keep a bottle of ipecac at home to treat poisoning. Talk with a doctor or the local Poison Control Center before using it. Post the number of the Poison Control Center number near your telephone and write it in the space under Important Information. Also, be sure to check the expiration date on the bottle of ipecac to make sure it is still good.

Safety Guidelines—Infants and Young Children

- Use a car safety seat at all times until your child weighs at least 40 pounds.

- Car seats must be properly secured in the back seat, preferably in the middle.

- Keep medicines, cleaning solutions, and other dangerous substances in childproof containers, locked up and out of reach of children.

- Use safety gates across stairways (top and bottom) and guards on windows above the first floor.

- Keep hot water heater temperatures below 120° Fahrenheit.

- Keep unused electrical outlets covered with plastic guards.

- Provide constant supervision for babies using a baby walker. Block the access to stairways and to objects that can fall (such as lamps) or cause burns (such as stoves).

- Keep objects and foods that can cause choking away from your child. This includes things like coins, balloons, small toy parts, hot dogs (unmashed), peanuts, and hard candies.

- Use fences that go all the way around pools and keep gates to pools locked.

Safety Guidelines—Older Children

- Use car safety belts at all times.

- Until children are tall enough so that the lap belt stays on their hips and the shoulder belt crosses their shoulder, they should use a car booster seat.

- Make sure your child wears a helmet while riding on a bicycle or motorcycle.

- Make sure your child uses protective equipment for in-line skating and skateboarding (helmet, wrist and knee pads).

- Warn your child of the dangers of using alcohol and drugs. Many driving and sports-related injuries are caused by the use of alcohol and drugs.

Child Abuse

Child abuse is a hidden, serious problem. It can happen in any family. The scars, both physical and emotional, can last a lifetime. Because children can't protect themselves, we must protect them.

Ways to Prevent Child Abuse

- Teach your child not to let anyone touch his or her private parts.

- Tell your child to say "No" and run away from sexual touches.

- Take any reports by your child of physical or sexual abuse seriously.

- Report any abuse to your local or state child protection agency.

- Local Hotline: Know your local hotline number.

- If you feel angry and out of control, leave the room, take a walk, take deep breaths, or count to 100. Don't drink alcohol or take drugs. These can make your anger harder to control. If you are afraid you might harm your child, get help NOW. Call someone and ask for help. Talk with a friend or relative, other parents, your clergy, or your health care provider. Take time for yourself. Share child care between parents, trade babysitting with friends, or use day care.

As Your Child Grows Up

As your child grows up, he or she will face many other important health issues, such as alcohol use, drugs, sexuality, sexually transmitted diseases (STDs), and birth control. Talk to your health care provider about these important issues—even while your child is still young.

Start early to teach your child to make responsible choices—irresponsible choices can have a lifelong effect. Your child needs you. Take the time to "be there" for your child—listening, advising, and supporting. The rewards will be well worth the effort.

Chapter 3

Immunizations

Chapter Contents

Section 3.1

How Do Vaccines Work?

National Vaccine Program Office, Centers for Disease Control and Prevention (CDC), updated May 2001. For more information from CDC's National Immunization Program, visit the website at http://www.cdc.gov/nip.

Parents are constantly concerned about the health and safety of their children and they take many steps to protect them. These preventive measures range from childproof door latches to child safety seats. In the same respect, vaccines work to safeguard children from illnesses and death caused by infectious diseases. Vaccines protect children by helping prepare their bodies to fight deadly diseases.

How Do Vaccines Work?

There are a series of steps that a person's body goes through in learning how to fight off a vaccine-preventable disease:

- **First:** A vaccine is given by a shot or liquid by mouth. An alternative needle-free route is the use of inhalation by aerosol and powder. Most vaccines contain a weakened or dead disease germ or part of a disease germ. Other vaccines use inactivated toxins. Some of the bacteria that cause disease do so by producing toxins that invade the bloodstream.

- **Next:** The body makes antibodies against the weakened or dead germs in the vaccine.

- **Then:** These antibodies can fight the real disease germs—which can be lurking all around—if they invade the child's body. The antibodies will know how to destroy them and the child will not become ill. Most vaccines don't cause the diseases that are usually caused by viruses and bacteria.

- **Finally:** Protective antibodies stay on guard in the child's body to safeguard it from the real disease germs.

After exposure to a live, weakened, or dead germ, the antibodies or memory cells fight infectious diseases and usually stay in a person's immune system for a lifetime. This protects a person from getting sick again. This protection is called immunity.

Why Are Vaccines Important?

It is true that newborn babies are immune to many diseases because they have antibodies they got from their mothers. However, this immunity only lasts about a year. Further, most young children do not have maternal immunity from diphtheria, whooping cough, polio, tetanus, hepatitis B, or *Haemophilus influenzae* type b.

Immunizing individual children also helps to protect the health of our community. People who are sick will be less likely to be exposed to disease germs that can be passed around by unvaccinated children. Immunization also slows down or stops disease outbreaks.

If a child is not vaccinated and is exposed to a disease germ, the child's body may not be strong enough to fight the disease. Before vaccines, many children died of diseases vaccines prevent, like whooping cough, measles, and polio. Those same germs exist today, but babies are now protected by vaccines and so we do not see these diseases as often.

Section 3.2

Vaccine-Preventable Childhood Diseases

National Vaccine Program Office, Centers for Disease Control and Prevention (CDC), updated August 2001. For more information from CDC's National Immunization Program, visit the website at http://www.cdc.gov/nip.

Polio

- Polio is a disease of the lymphatic and nervous systems that is spread by contact with an infected person.

- Polio virus causes fever, sore throat, nausea, headaches, and stomach aches and may also cause stiffness in the neck, back and legs.

- Polio virus may cause paralysis that can lead to permanent disability and death.

- Polio vaccine (inactivated poliovirus vaccine [IPV]) can prevent this disease.

Diphtheria

- Diphtheria is a respiratory disease caused by bacteria and spread by coughing and sneezing.

- It is marked by the gradual onset of sore throat and low-grade fever.

- Airway obstruction, coma, and death can result if the disease is not treated.

- Diphtheria toxoid (contained in DTP, DTaP, DT and Td vaccines) can prevent this disease.

Tetanus (lockjaw)

- Tetanus is a disease of the nervous system caused by a bacteria that enters the body through a break in the skin.

- Early symptoms include lockjaw, stiffness in the neck and abdomen, and difficulty swallowing.

- Later symptoms include fever, elevated blood pressure, and severe muscle spasms.

- One-third of the cases are fatal, especially in people over age 50.

- Tetanus toxoid (contained in DTP, DT, DTaP and Td vaccines) can prevent this disease.

Pertussis (whooping cough)

- Pertussis is a highly contagious respiratory disease caused by bacteria and spread by coughing and sneezing.

- Symptoms include severe spasms of coughing that can interfere with eating, drinking, and breathing.

- Severe cases result in pneumonia, encephalitis (swelling of the lining of the brain) due to lack of oxygen, and possibly death, especially in infants.

- Pertussis vaccine (contained in DTP and DTaP) can prevent this disease.

Measles

- Measles is a highly contagious respiratory disease caused by a virus and spread by coughing and sneezing.

- Measles virus causes rash, high fever, cough, runny nose, and red, watery eyes, lasting about a week.

- More severe symptoms include diarrhea, ear infections, pneumonia, encephalitis (swelling of the lining of the brain), seizures, and death.

- Measles vaccine (contained in MMR, MR, and measles vaccines) can prevent this disease.

Mumps

- Mumps is a disease of the salivary glands caused by a virus and spread by coughing and sneezing.

- Symptoms include fever, headache, muscle ache, and swelling of the salivary glands close to the jaw.

- Other symptoms include meningitis, inflammation of the testicles or ovaries, inflammation of the pancreas, and deafness, usually permanent.
- Mumps vaccine (contained in MMR) can prevent this disease.

Rubella (German measles)

- Rubella is a respiratory disease caused by bacteria and spread by coughing and sneezing.
- Symptoms in children and young adults include rash and fever for 2 to 3 days.
- Causes devastating birth defects if acquired by a pregnant woman; there is at least a 20 percent chance of damage to the fetus if a woman is infected early in pregnancy.
- Birth defects include deafness, cataracts, heart defects, mental retardation, and liver and spleen damage.
- Rubella vaccine (contained in MMR vaccine) can prevent this disease.

Haemophilus influenzae type b (Hib)

- *Haemophilus influenzae* type b causes meningitis, pneumonia, sepsis, arthritis, and skin and throat infections.
- Spread by coughing and sneezing.
- More serious in children under age 1; after age 5, there is little risk of getting the disease.
- One out of 20 children who get Hib meningitis will die and 10 percent to 30 percent of survivors will have permanent brain damage.
- Hib vaccine can prevent this disease.

Varicella (chickenpox)

- Varicella-zoster is a virus of the herpes family.
- Highly contagious and is spread through coughing and sneezing.
- Causes a skin rash of a few or hundreds of blister-like lesions, usually on the face, scalp, or trunk.

- Usually more severe in older children (13 or older) and adults.
- Complications include bacterial infection of the skin, swelling of the brain, and pneumonia.
- Often leads to children to missing school and parents to missing work.
- Varicella vaccine can prevent this disease.

Hepatitis A

- Hepatitis A is a disease of the liver caused by hepatitis A virus.
- The virus is spread by the fecal-oral route, usually from person to person by putting something in the mouth that has been contaminated with the stool of a person with hepatitis A. Less often, the virus is spread by swallowing food or water that contains the virus.
- The younger a person is, the less likely he or she will have symptoms. If symptoms occur, they are similar to the other types of hepatitis and may include yellow skin or eyes, tiredness, stomach ache, loss of appetite, or nausea.
- Since young children may not have symptoms, disease is not often recognized until the child's caregiver becomes ill with hepatitis A.
- Hepatitis A vaccine can prevent this disease.

Hepatitis B

- Hepatitis B is a disease of the liver caused by hepatitis B virus.
- The virus is spread through contact with the blood of an infected person or by having sex with an infected person.
- The younger a person is, the less likely he or she will have symptoms when first infected. If symptoms do occur, they may include yellow skin or eyes, tiredness, stomach ache, loss of appetite, nausea, or joint pain.
- The younger a person is, the more likely he or she will stay infected with the virus and have life-long liver problems, such as scarring of the liver and liver cancer.
- Hepatitis B vaccine can prevent this disease.

Figure 3.1. Recommended Childhood and Adolescent Immunization Schedule—United States, 2003.

Vaccine ▼ / Age ►	Birth	1 mo	2 mos	4 mos	6 mos	12 mos	15 mos	18 mos	24 mos	4-6 yrs	11-12 yrs	13-18 yrs
Hepatitis B[1]	HepB #1	HepB #2 (only if mother HBsAg (-))				HepB #3					HepB series	
Diphtheria, Tetanus, Pertussis[2]			DTaP	DTaP	DTaP		DTaP	DTaP		DTaP	Td	
Haemophilus influenzae Type b[3]			Hib	Hib	Hib	Hib						
Inactivated Polio			IPV	IPV		IPV				IPV		
Measles, Mumps, Rubella[4]						MMR #1				MMR #2	MMR #2	
Varicella[5]						Varicella				Varicella		
Pneumococcal[6]			PCV	PCV	PCV	PCV	PCV		PCV / PPV			
Hepatitis A[7]									Hepatitis A series			
Influenza[8]						Influenza (yearly)						

range of recommended ages — catch-up vaccination — preadolescent assessment

Vaccines below this line are for selected populations

This schedule indicates the recommended ages for routine administration of currently licensed childhood vaccines, as of December 1, 2002, for children through age 18 years. Any dose not given at the recommended age should be given at any subsequent visit when indicated and feasible. Indicates age groups that warrant special effort to administer those vaccines not previously given. Additional vaccines may be licensed and recommended during the year. Licensed combination vaccines may be used whenever any components of the combination are indicated and the vaccine's other components are not contraindicated. Providers should consult the manufacturers' package inserts for detailed recommendations.

1. Hepatitis B vaccine (HepB). All infants should receive the first dose of hepatitis B vaccine soon after birth and before hospital discharge; the first dose may also be given by age 2 months if the infant's mother is HBsAg-negative. Only monovalent HepB can be used for the birth dose. Monovalent or combination vaccine containing HepB may be used to complete the series. Four doses of vaccine may be administered when a birth dose is given. The second dose should be given at least 4 weeks after the first dose, except for combination vaccines which cannot be administered before age 6 weeks. The third dose should be given at least 16 weeks after the first dose and at least 8 weeks after the second dose. The last dose in the vaccination series (third or fourth dose) should not be administered before age 6 months.

Infants born to HBsAg-positive mothers should receive HepB and 0.5 mL Hepatitis B Immune Globulin (HBIG) within 12 hours of birth at separate sites. The second dose is recommended at age 1-2 months. The last dose in the vaccination series should not be administered before age 6 months. These infants should be tested for HBsAg and anti-HBs at 9-15 months of age.

Infants born to mothers whose HBsAg status is unknown should receive the first dose of the HepB series within 12 hours of birth. Maternal blood should be drawn as soon as possible to determine the mother's HBsAg status; if the HBsAg test is positive, the infant should receive HBIG as soon as possible (no later than age 1 week). The second dose is recommended at age 1-2 months. The last dose in the vaccination series should not be administered before age 6 months.

2. Diphtheria and tetanus toxoids and acellular pertussis vaccine (DTaP). The fourth dose of DTaP may be administered as early as age 12 months, provided 6 months have elapsed since the third dose and the child is unlikely to return at age 15-18 months. **Tetanus and diphtheria toxoids (Td)** is recommended at age 11-12 years if at least 5 years have elapsed since the last dose of tetanus and diphtheria toxoid-containing vaccine. Subsequent routine Td boosters are recommended every 10 years.

3. Haemophilus influenzae type b (Hib) conjugate vaccine. Three Hib conjugate vaccines are licensed for infant use. If PRP-OMP (PedvaxHIB® or ComVax® [Merck]) is administered at ages 2 and 4 months, a dose at age 6 months is not required. DTaP/Hib combination products should not be used for primary immunization in infants at ages 2, 4 or 6 months, but can be used as boosters following any Hib vaccine.

4. Measles, mumps, and rubella vaccine (MMR). The second dose of MMR is recommended routinely at age 4-6 years but may be administered during any visit, provided at least 4 weeks have elapsed since the first dose and that both doses are administered beginning at or after age 12 months. Those who have not previously received the second dose should complete the schedule by the 11-12 year old visit.

5. Varicella vaccine. Varicella vaccine is recommended at any visit at or after age 12 months for susceptible children, i.e. those who lack a reliable history of chickenpox. Susceptible persons aged ≥13 years should receive two doses, given at least 4 weeks apart.

6. Pneumococcal vaccine. The heptavalent **pneumococcal conjugate vaccine (PCV)** is recommended for all children age 2-23 months. It is also recommended for certain children age 24-59 months. **Pneumococcal polysaccharide vaccine (PPV)** is recommended in addition to PCV for certain high-risk groups. See *MMWR* 2000;49(RR-9);1-38.

7. Hepatitis A vaccine. Hepatitis A vaccine is recommended for children and adolescents in selected states and regions, and for certain high-risk groups; consult your local public health authority. Children and adolescents in these states, regions, and high risk groups who have not been immunized against hepatitis A can begin the hepatitis A vaccination series during any visit. The two doses in the series should be administered at least 6 months apart. See *MMWR* 1999;48(RR-12);1-37.

8. Influenza vaccine. Influenza vaccine is recommended annually for children age ≥6 months with certain risk factors (including but not limited to asthma, cardiac disease, sickle cell disease, HIV, diabetes, and household members of persons in groups at high risk; see *MMWR* 2002;51(RR-3);1-31), and can be administered to all others wishing to obtain immunity. In addition, healthy children age 6-23 months are encouraged to receive influenza vaccine if feasible because children in this age group are at substantially increased risk for influenza-related hospitalizations. Children aged ≤12 years should receive vaccine in a dosage appropriate for their age (0.25 mL if age 6-35 months or 0.5 mL if aged ≥3 years). Children aged ≤8 years who are receiving influenza vaccine for the first time should receive two doses separated by at least 4 weeks.

For additional information about vaccines, including precautions and contraindications for immunization and vaccine shortages, please visit the National Immunization Program Website at www.cdc.gov/nip or call the National Immunization Information Hotline at 800-232-2522 (English) or 800-232-0233 (Spanish).

Approved by the Advisory Committee on Immunization Practices (www.cdc.gov/nip/acip), the American Academy of Pediatrics (www.aap.org), and the American Academy of Family Physicians (www.aafp.org).

Section 3.3

Recommended Childhood Immunization Schedule

National Vaccine Program Office, Centers for Disease Control and Prevention (CDC), updated August 2001. For more information from CDC's National Immunization Program, visit the website at http://www.cdc.gov/nip.

Every year, the National Immunization Program (NIP), along with the American Academy of Pediatrics (AAP) and the American Academy of Family Physicians (AAFP), issues a recommended childhood immunization schedule. This schedule tells parents and health care providers which vaccines children need to receive, and when children need to receive those vaccines. The currently recommended vaccines protect all children against 11 common infectious diseases.

Highlights

- A child's best defense against many dangerous childhood diseases is to be immunized on time.

- Immunizations protect children against: hepatitis B, polio. Measles, mumps, rubella (German measles), pertussis (whooping cough), diphtheria, tetanus (lockjaw), *Haemophilus influenzae* type b (causes a type of meningitis), pneumococcal disease (also causes meningitis), and chicken pox. All of these immunizations need to be given before children are two years old in order for them to be protected during their most vulnerable period.

- Each year, the Centers for Disease Control and Prevention's (CDC) Advisory Committee on Immunization Practices (ACIP) reviews the recommended childhood immunization schedule to address changes in the use of both previously and newly licensed vaccines.

- The schedule is updated every January.

Recent Updates to the Childhood Schedule

The immunization schedule was last published in January 2001. The ACIP, AAP, and AAFP have made the following changes:

- Pneumococcal conjugate vaccine, which was licensed in February 2000, has been added to the schedule. It is routinely recommended for all children aged 2–23 months, and for certain children aged 24–59 months.

- Recommendations for hepatitis A vaccine have been expanded to include adolescents through age 18 years and persons in certain high-risk groups.

Section 3.4

What to Do If Your Child Has Discomfort after a Shot

Excerpted from "After the Shots...What to Do If Your Child Has Discomfort," Immunization Action Coalition, http://www.immunize.org/nslt.d/n17/p4015.htm, August 1999. Reprinted with permission.

Your child may need extra love and care after getting immunized. Many of the shots that protect children from serious diseases can also cause discomfort for a while. Here are answers to questions many parents have about the fussiness, fever, and pain their children may experience after they have been immunized. If you don't find the answers to your questions, call the clinic.

My child has been fussy since he/she was immunized. What should I do?

After immunization, children may be fussy due to pain and/or fever. You may want to give your child acetaminophen, a medicine that helps to reduce pain and fever. Some examples of acetaminophen are

Tylenol, Panadol, and Tempra. DO NOT GIVE ASPIRIN. If the fussiness lasts for more than 24 hours, you should call the clinic.

My child's arm (or leg) is swollen, hot, and red. What should I do?

- A clean, cool washcloth may be applied over the sore area as needed for comfort.
- If there is increasing redness or tenderness after 24 hours, call the clinic.
- For pain, give acetaminophen. DO NOT GIVE ASPIRIN.

I think my child has a fever. What should I do?

Check your child's temperature to find out if there is a fever. The most accurate way to do this is by taking a rectal temperature. (Be sure to use a lubricant, such as petroleum jelly, when doing so.) If your child's fever is 105° F (Fahrenheit) or higher by rectum, you need to call the clinic.

If you take the temperature by mouth (for an older child) or under the arm, these temperatures are generally lower and may be less accurate. Call your clinic if you are concerned about these temperatures.

Here are some things you can do to reduce fever:

- Give your child plenty to drink.
- Clothe your child lightly. Do <u>not</u> cover or wrap your child tightly.
- Give your child acetaminophen. DO NOT USE ASPIRIN.
- Sponge your child in a few inches of lukewarm (not cold) bath water.

My child seems really sick. Should I call the doctor?

If you are worried AT ALL about how your child looks or feels, please call the clinic.

Overview: When to Call Your Child's Doctor

Call the clinic if you answer "yes" to any of the following questions:

- Does your child have a rectal temperature of 105° F or higher? (Remember, a temperature taken under the arm or by mouth usually registers lower than a rectal temperature. You should call the clinic if you are concerned about these temperatures.)

- Is your child pale or limp?

- Has your child been crying for over 3 hours and just won't quit?

- Does your child have a strange cry that isn't normal (a high-pitched cry)?

- Is your child's body shaking, twitching, or jerking?

Section 3.5

Questions and Answers about the Smallpox Vaccine

Excerpted from "Smallpox Questions and Answers: The Disease and The Vaccine," Centers for Disease Control and Prevention, March 2003.

What should I know about smallpox?

Smallpox is an acute, contagious, and sometimes fatal disease caused by the variola virus (an orthopoxvirus), and marked by fever and a distinctive progressive skin rash. In 1980, the disease was declared eradicated following worldwide vaccination programs. However, in the aftermath of the events of September and October 2001, the U.S. government is taking precautions to be ready to deal with a bioterrorist attack using smallpox as a weapon. As a result of these efforts: 1) There is a detailed nationwide smallpox preparedness program to protect Americans against smallpox as a biological weapon. This program includes the creation of preparedness teams that are ready to respond to a smallpox attack on the United States. Members of these teams—health care and public health workers—are being vaccinated so that they might safely protect others in the event of a smallpox outbreak. 2) There is enough smallpox vaccine to vaccinate everyone who would need it in the event of an emergency.

What is the smallpox vaccine, and is it still required?

The smallpox vaccine is the only way to prevent smallpox. The vaccine is made from a virus called *vaccinia,* which is another "pox"-type virus related to smallpox but cannot cause smallpox. The vaccine helps the body develop immunity to smallpox. It was successfully used to eradicate smallpox from the human population.

Routine vaccination of the American public against smallpox stopped in 1972 after the disease was eradicated in the United States. Until recently, the U.S. government provided the smallpox vaccine only to a few hundred scientists and medical professionals who work with smallpox and similar viruses in a research setting. After the events of September and October 2001, however, the U.S. government took further actions to improve its level of preparedness against terrorism. For smallpox, this included updating a response plan and ordering enough smallpox vaccine to immunize the American public in the event of a smallpox outbreak. The plans are in place, and there is sufficient vaccine available to immunize everyone who might need it in the event of an emergency. In addition, in December of 2002, the Bush Administration announced a plan to better protect the American people against the threat of smallpox attack by hostile groups or governments. This plan includes the creation of smallpox healthcare teams that would respond to a smallpox emergency. Members of these teams are being vaccinated against smallpox. The plan also included vaccination of certain military and civilian personnel who are or may be deployed in high threat areas.

Should I get vaccinated against smallpox?

The smallpox vaccine is not available to the public at this time.

Many vaccinations are required. Why don't people have to get the smallpox vaccine?

The last case of smallpox in the United States was in 1949. The last naturally occurring case in the world was in Somalia in 1977. After the disease was eliminated from the world, routine vaccination against smallpox among the general public was stopped because it was no longer necessary for prevention.

If someone is exposed to smallpox, is it too late to get a vaccination?

Vaccination within 3 days of exposure will completely prevent or significantly modify smallpox in the vast majority of persons. Vaccination

4 to 7 days after exposure likely offers some protection from disease or may modify the severity of disease.

How long does a smallpox vaccination last?

Past experience indicates that the first dose of the vaccine offers protection from smallpox for 3 to 5 years, with decreasing immunity thereafter. If a person is vaccinated again later, immunity lasts longer.

Is the vaccine safe for children?

Children younger than 12 months of age should not get the vaccine. Also, the Advisory Committee on Immunization Practices (ACIP) advises against non-emergency use of smallpox vaccine in children younger than 18 years of age.

Vaccinated parents of young children need to be careful not to inadvertently spread the virus to their children. They should follow site care instructions that are essential to minimizing the risk of contact transmission of vaccinia. These precautions include covering the vaccination site, wearing a sleeved shirt, and careful hand washing anytime after touching the vaccination site or anything that might be contaminated with virus from the vaccination site. If these precautions are followed, the risk for children is very low. Individuals who do not believe that they can adhere to such instructions should err on the side of caution and not be vaccinated at this time.

Pregnant women should NOT be vaccinated in the absence of a smallpox outbreak because of risk of fetal infection. Inadvertent transmission of vaccinia virus to a pregnant woman could also put the fetus at risk. Vaccinated persons must be very cautious to prevent transmission of the vaccine virus to pregnant women or other contacts.

Chapter 4

Caring for Young Eyes

Chapter Contents

Section 4.1

Your Children's Eyes

This section includes text from "Protect Your Child's Sight," Reprinted with permission from Prevent Blindness America. Copyright 1998, "Play It Safe With Your Eyes!" and "Safe Toys Checklist," Reprinted with permission from Prevent Blindness America. Copyright 2000. For additional information, call the Prevent Blindness America toll-free information line at 800-331-2020, or visit their website at www.preventblindness.org. Information about online vision screening tests for children is available at www.preventblindness.org/children/children_eye_tests.html.

Protect Your Child's Sight

Most eye problems can be corrected if they are detected and treated early. Appropriate eye care is essential for maintaining good vision. Some problems, if left untreated—even for a short period—can result in permanent vision loss.

The eyes of newborn infants should be evaluated in the hospital nursery. This examination can help detect several congenital eye problems, some of which can be very serious.

Between six months and one year of age, infants should be checked for good eye health by a doctor or other appropriately trained health care provider during routine well-baby care or other doctor's office visits.

Similarly, children's vision should be tested between 3 and 4, either during a well-child visit to the doctor, a visit to an eye doctor, or at a vision screening conducted by trained personnel such as those performed by Prevent Blindness America. The more you learn about children's eyes, the better you can help protect them.

Play It Safe with Your Eyes

The frequency and severity of at least 90 percent of all eye injuries to children can be reduced by understanding the dangers, identifying and correcting hazards and using greater care when supervising children. The most common causes of eye injuries to children include:

- Misuse of toys or altering toys.

- Falls involving home furnishings and fixtures such as beds, stairs, tables, and toys.

- Misuse of everyday objects like home repair and yard care products, personal-use items, kitchen utensils, silverware, pens and pencils.

- Accidental exposure to harmful household and cleaning products such as detergents, paints, pesticides, glues and adhesives.

- Automobile accidents (which are the leading cause of death and serious injuries, including eye injuries, to young children).

Recognizing Eye Injuries

Any of the following symptoms may indicate a serious eye injury. Get immediate medical attention for:

- Obvious pain or vision problems.

- Cut or torn eyelid.

- One eye that does not move as completely as the other.

- One eye that sticks out in comparison to the other.

- Abnormal pupil size or shape.

- Blood in the clear portion of the eye.

- Something in the eye or under the eyelid that cannot be easily removed.

Regular eye exams are recommended to make sure that both eyes are healthy. A child's eyes should be examined shortly after birth, at six months of age, again before the age of four or five and periodically throughout the school years.

Safe Toys Checklist

Young children are often described as "accidents waiting to happen." Too often, accidents do occur and may result in eye injuries. Hospital emergency rooms treat an estimated 290,000 product-related eye injuries each year. Children under five years of age make up 10 percent of that number, with most product-related injuries occurring in or around the home and at play.

Toy Selection Guidelines

- Read all warnings and instructions.

- Consider a child's ability rather than age when purchasing toys; age warnings on toys are not guarantees of safety.

- Avoid toys with sharp or rigid points, spikes, rods and dangerous edges.

- Inspect toys for safe, sturdy construction.

- Repair or replace damaged or defective toys.

- Store toys properly after play to avoid trips and falls.

- Supervise children's craft projects; scissors and glue are among the products most dangerous to a youngster's eyesight.

- Check the lenses and frames of children's sunglasses before buying them; many (particularly the inexpensive, novelty type) can break and cause injuries.

- Stay away from flying toys and projectile-firing toys.

- BB guns are not toys and should not be given to children too young to handle them safely.

- Keep older children's toys away from younger children.

- Children should wear appropriate eye protection for sports (face shields, helmets).

For more information on selecting safe toys and gifts, contact Prevent Blindness America or the Prevent Blindness affiliate near you. Visit www.preventblindness.org for more information.

Section 4.2

Children Need a Complete Eye Exam

After an initial eye examination by an optometrist at age 6 months, children should have another thorough exam at age three to determine how their vision is developing and to rule out any serious problems, says an optometrist who specializes in pediatrics.

The exam at age three is much more than a routine screening," says Valerie Kattouf, O.D., an optometrist in private practice and on the faculty at Illinois College of Optometry in Chicago. "At this point we can check the child's ability to focus, to see clearly at all distances, and to use both eyes together as a team. We measure their depth perception and color vision, and we test for nearsightedness, farsightedness, astigmatism, and eye muscle problems, such as crossed-eyes and lazy eye."

Parents should take their child before the three-year point, however, if they suspect problems. "There are a number of behaviors and signs in children ages 2 to 6 that will key parents that something may be wrong," says Dr. Kattouf, who lectured on pediatric vision at the American Optometric Association's annual meeting, June 23–27, 1999, in San Antonio, Texas.

Behaviors that may be a cause for concern include:

- Squinting

- Sitting very close to the television

- Avoiding reading or looking at picture books

- Covering one eye when looking at something up close

- Complaints about headaches (In school children, note if these only occur at the end of school days and not on weekends.)

A physical sign that is a cause for concern is when one or both eyes appear to be crossed, turning either in, out, up or down.

Parents should not be alarmed at these signs but they should visit an optometrist to have them checked. Most problems detected at these young ages are correctable. But early detection and treatment of vision problems is important.

"A very low percentage of young children in this country who see an eye care professional have serious conditions," Dr. Kattouf says. "Some may have to wear glasses or contact lenses."

If a child does need a vision correction, stylish frames that fit well are now made especially for children and even the very young can be fitted with contacts. Parents, of course, need to help with contact lens care.

Family optometrists who are accustomed to working with children use kid-friendly tools and techniques when it comes to conducting these exams. Their eye charts have pictures instead of letters, and since most of the tests are based on the doctor's observations, these visits often seem more like playing games for the children.

Dr. Kattouf uses glow worms, puppets, and stickers on her nose to see how children use their eyes up close. To check their distance vision, she runs cartoon videos for them, which she says work like a charm. She never wears a doctor's lab coat, and always lets the child sit on the parent's lap.

Her advice for making children's visits easier:

- Bring them in when they are rested; morning is usually best.

- Talk to them ahead of time; assure them that they won't get shots or be poked and prodded.

- Make a game of it; tell them they will be looking at pictures and having fun.

- Practice dropping a few artificial tears (over-the-counter) in their eyes a day or so before the visit, so the dilating drops won't seem scary to them.

- Relax and your child will most likely be relaxed too.

If the optometrist finds no problems at this three-year checkup, the child will not need to be examined again until just before entering school. Thereafter, the American Optometric Association recommends eye exams every two years throughout the school years.

Section 4.3

Glasses and Sunglasses for Children

This section includes "How to Encourage Children to Wear Their Glasses," and "Sunglasses for Children" undated fact sheets © American Optometric Association (www.aoa.org), accessed online through www.healthtouch.com, April 2003; reprinted with permission.

How to Encourage Children to Wear Their Glasses

Thanks to fashionable, durable frames, many children who need prescription glasses today willingly wear them but, if your child is not among these happy wearers, there are things you can do to bring about change.

Start by giving your child some say in selecting the frame. Take along a friend or two and involve them in the selection process. Your child may be more apt to wear the glasses if he or she knows that friends approve.

Also point out eyeglass-wearing role models to your child. For very young children, "being just like Mommy or Daddy" may be what counts. Older children may be impressed by a favorite sports or entertainment star who wears glasses. For young children, ask your optometrist or librarian for books about children wearing glasses. There are several good ones available.

Make teachers aware of your child's prescribed wearing schedule so that they can report to you if it is not being followed. To help overcome peer pressure that may be inhibiting wear, ask your child's teacher to have a class session on eye care that includes pointing out how important glasses are in helping people to see well. Your optometrist may be willing to present such a program for your child's class or school.

If your child is in middle school, junior high, or high school and has an aversion to wearing glasses, ask your optometrist about contact lenses. They are a good choice for children and teens who have the maturity to follow wear and care instructions properly.

Sunglasses for Children

Space-age protection from the sun's rays is what children's eyes need today but finding the right sunglasses can be tricky. Recent studies show that the earlier children start wearing sunglasses outdoors the better their chances of avoiding major eye health problems later in life. The sun's ultraviolet (UV) radiation is the culprit. It contributes to potentially blinding conditions like cataract and macular degeneration, that plague significant numbers of today's older adults.

Children's eyes get exposed to more UV radiation than adults because they usually spend more time outdoors and their young eyes let more UV rays inside. They also live at a time when loss of some of the ozone layer lets more UV rays reach the earth. Bonnets and wide-brimmed hats can keep about 50 percent of UV radiation from reaching the eyes but that's not enough.

Children need to wear sunglasses that block 99 to 100 percent of both UV-A and UV-B radiation. Such sunglasses are available for children but studies show many sunglass labels are misleading. Parents should ask their optometrist's advice, look for sunglasses with the American Optometric Association's Seal of Acceptance or buy sunglasses where equipment is available to check the lenses' UV protection capabilities. Parents should also consider polycarbonate lenses, which are the most impact-resistant lenses available.

Section 4.4

Virtual Reality Games and Children's Vision

Virtual reality (VR) games are among the newest "high tech" computer games to gain popularity. While they are novel and exciting to play, children (and adults) need to understand the potential impact these games may have on vision.

VR games involve wearing a headset which is designed to exclude one's perception of the outside world as much as possible. The headset provides sound through earphones, images via a miniature video display screen with focusing lenses placed in front of each eye, and feedback to the game's computer about the user's eye and body movements. The images seen change in response to the user's body movements. The games generally involve motion (for example, flying an airplane or rocket-ship, running down a tunnel, or moving through a maze).

Sometimes users of VR games experience problems due to sensory overload. Visual and perceptual problems can arise because of the nature and design of the headset and the visual environment which is created:

- The video display screen is located very close to the user's eye, but to see the screen clearly, the eyes must focus as if the screen were many feet away. This can cause the eyes' focusing and alignment mechanisms to become fatigued leading to discomfort.

- The small focusing lenses must be adjusted properly in order for the user to see the screen clearly and comfortably. The separation of the lenses must be placed to match the distance between the user's eyes (interpupillary distance). If not properly adjusted, the eyes will have difficulty maintaining alignment, further increasing eyestrain.

43

Not all VR games have headsets which provide the range of adjustment or quality of focusing lenses needed to provide clear, distortion-free images. Some people, especially those who wear glasses, may find it difficult or impossible to adjust the headsets for clear, comfortable vision.

Some users of VR games may also experience problems of motion sickness, dizziness and disorientation. For some persons, these symptoms may be severe enough to prevent them from using the games; others may overcome them with time.

Children who use VR games and their parents need to be knowledgeable about the potential effects of their use in order to minimize risks while maximizing the fun. More research and experience with VR games is needed to determine their impact on vision. However, here are some suggestions from the American Optometric Association when playing VR games:

- Make sure your vision is up to the task. Have regular vision examinations, tell your doctor of optometry that you like to play VR or other video games, and follow his or her recommendations for vision care.

- Learn how to properly set up, adjust and maintain the VR headset. When buying a VR game set, look for an adjustable headset that allows the user to see the video display screen clearly and comfortably. Get a demonstration or trial of the headset before you buy it.

- Limit the amount of VR game sessions to about 15 minutes at a time, with sufficient breaks or rest periods to recover equilibrium and orientation. If motion sickness, eyestrain, headache or other symptoms occur, reduce the time or stop playing entirely.

VR and other video or computer-based games can be interesting and fun to play. It is important for children and parents to use these games wisely in order to ensure maximum safety and enjoyment. If you have questions about VR games, talk to your family optometrist or contact the American Optometric Association:

American Optometric Association

243 North Lindbergh Blvd.
St. Louis, MO 63141
Phone: 314-911-4100
Website: www.aoa.org

Chapter 5

Caring for Young Ears

Chapter Contents

Section 5.1

Advocating Hearing Evaluation in Children

"Hearing Screening in Schools," *Hearing Loss*, May–June 1999. © 1999 Self-Help for Hard of Hearing People, Inc. Reprinted with permission.

A hearing loss is not only a frequent occurrence in school children, but can have more severe consequences than are generally realized. As reported in the *Journal of the American Medical Association,* the incidence of unilateral or bilateral hearing loss among children from 6 to 19 years of age was found to be almost 15 percent using a criterion of 16 dB or more in either the high or the low frequencies (Niskar et al., 1998). Depending upon the nature and extent of the hearing loss, it may be responsible for deficient or delayed speech and language skills, poorer academic accomplishments, and more problematical psychosocial adjustment.

These effects not only occur with children who have moderate, severe, or profound hearing loss, but may also be present in children with unilateral, minimal, and fluctuating conductive problems as well. Because individual children with lesser degrees of hearing losses may not overtly display any apparent communication or academic problems (that is, they apparently hear and respond appropriately in face-to-face situations), the academic and linguistic "risk" status of such children tends to be overlooked. It is only when group performance is considered, or when a detailed evaluation is conducted on a specific child, that deficiencies in a number of areas become apparent.

This is clearly shown in a study conducted by Bess, Dodd-Murphy, & Parker (1998). The primary focus of the study was the academic achievement and functional status of children with minimal sensorineural hearing loss (MSHL); secondarily, the overall incidence of hearing loss in a public school setting was also determined. The investigators took great pains to ensure a representative sample of children in their study, and it is likely that their results would be applicable to school systems throughout the country.

The overall prevalence rate of a hearing loss in their study population was 11.3 percent, of which 5.4 percent of the children exhibited MSHL. The other children had conductive and mixed hearing losses. Three categories of children with MSHL were identified: (1) unilateral hearing loss (one ear normal); (2) bilateral losses averaging between 20 and 40 dB; and (3) a hearing loss of 25 dB or more in either ear at frequencies above 2000 Hz (high frequency hearing loss). When they compared the academic and functional status of the MSHL children to their hearing peers, they found that 37 percent of them failed at least one grade, compared to a 2 percent failure rate by their normally hearing peers.

Other academic achievement problems were noted as well, particularly for the children in the lower grades. For the MSHL children in the higher grades, functional comparisons revealed poorer ratings for stress, self-esteem, and social support than those observed with the normally hearing children. It is important to stress that these results are not unique. There are many other studies that show the negative impact of unilateral and mild hearing losses upon school-age children (the Bess study contains extensive references to them).

These findings should send an unequivocal signal that a hearing loss, of whatever degree, is not an inconsequential event. They demonstrate the crucial role that audition plays in learning. Hearing is the key avenue with which children become acculturated into our society and learn its language. Moreover, it is through this auditory-based language that children can most effectively approach the reading process. It is important to emphasize this latter point: children normally learn how to read by associating the language learned through audition with the written word. Reading skills, in other words, are initially and most efficiently grounded in the sense of hearing. It is because congenitally and profoundly deaf children do not possess an auditory-based linguistic system that they have such difficulty reading at grade level.

Children in regular schools, and this applies to normally hearing children as well as to those with minimal hearing losses, must hear in order to learn, and the more they hear, the more they are likely to learn. They must be able to hear the teacher as he/she moves around the room, faces the blackboard, and during the noise of normal classroom activities. They must be able to hear the comments and questions of the other children in the class. Since even a 10 dB reduction from normal thresholds will reduce the subjective loudness sensation of a speech signal by half, no degree of hearing loss can be considered "acceptable." Hearing the teacher at half or quarter (a 20 dB hearing loss) of the loudness sensation enjoyed by other children may permit comprehension of most of the teacher's message most of the time, but at a cost of increased fatigue, "tuning out" or "acting out," and an uncertain grasp of many of the grammatical features of speech (particularly those conveyed by weak final consonants). Children have enough hurdles to overcome during the learning process without the added problem of an undetected and untreated hearing loss.

The need to identify children with hearing loss in schools was recognized more than 70 years ago (Roush, 1992). Many states now mandate some sort of hearing screening program, but others make no such provision. In some states, the authority for the hearing-screening program rests with the state department of health, while in others the department of education takes on this responsibility. When a state does not require a hearing-screening program, the local school authorities may or may not fill the gap. Some states mandate that kindergarten children entering school have their hearing examined, and then follow through with a hearing-screening program at later times.

For other children, however, this kindergarten "certification" may be the last time in their school career that the status of their hearing is examined. In some locales, newly enrolled children, those with special needs, or children with known hearing losses are examined every year, while other jurisdictions have different or no such provisions at all. Some states and districts provide guidelines that incorporate specific testing procedures, including tympanometry and otoscopic examination, as well as required follow-up procedures, while others leave the details to the local authorities. When a state or district does offer a hearing-screening program for the children, rarely are children in private or parochial schools included. In short, the national status of hearing screening programs for school-age children is a disorganized mess, varying from nonexistent or incomplete, to excellent in a few places.

Self-Help for Hard of Hearing People (SHHH) believes that the hearing of school children is too important to be left to chance. We believe that it is essential that all school-age children in all our schools have their hearing screened at regular intervals. Moreover, it is our recommendation that the hearing screening activity itself be integrated with, and a component of, an overall hearing conservation program in which the implications of each child's hearing loss are explicitly addressed. Our experiences over the past number of years have shown that it is not reasonable to expect each state independently to conduct an effective hearing-screening program in schools. SHHH, therefore, recommends that the U.S. Department of Education develop and enforce specific guidelines for a nationwide hearing-screening program. We recommend that these guidelines be established by a task force composed of representatives from state and national health and education agencies, as well as those from the medical and audiological professions.

Furthermore, SHHH believes that, at a minimum, the following elements must be included in the guidelines:

- All children in the lower grades and some of the upper grades in all schools in our country (public and private) should have their hearing screened.

- Tympanometry should be a routine part of the program for the children at the lower elementary levels.

- Only specially trained personnel should conduct the program, under the general supervision of a certified audiologist.

- If a child does not pass the entire screening process, parents must be notified and encouraged to have their children's ears examined by a physician.

- All children who do not pass the screening must be carefully followed up, both with the parents (to ensure compliance) and in the school (to ensure appropriate educational management).

- Children with permanent hearing loss and conductive hearing losses not responsive to medical/surgical treatment should receive comprehensive audiological, speech and language, educational, and psychosocial evaluations.

- Private and parochial schools, as well as public schools, should be included in a nationally mandated hearing screening program. Given the inclusion of these elements in a hearing screening (conservation) program, it should be possible to minimize the potential impact of a hearing loss upon the academic achievement and psychosocial adjustment of school children. Moreover, the very fact that such a national program is implemented can, in itself, send a message to all segments of our society regarding the crucial importance of hearing to learning. It will help remove hearing loss from society's "back-burner" and truly make it an "issue of national concern."

References

Bess, F. H., Dodd-Murphy, J. and Parker, R. A. (1998). "Children with Minimal Sensorineural Hearing Loss: Prevalence, Educational Performance, and Functional Status." *Ear and Hearing,* 19(5), 339–354.

Niskar, A. S., Kieszak, S. M., Holmes, A., Esteban, E., Rubin, C., and Brody, D. B. (1998). "Prevalence of Hearing Loss Among Children 6 to 19 Years of Age." *Journal of the American Medical Association,* 279(14), 1071–1075.

Roush, J. (1992). "Screening the School-Age Child." In *Screening Children for Auditory Function* (F. Bess and J. Hall, eds.), Nashville, TN: Bill Wilkerson Center Press.

Section 5.2

Children and Ear Wax

Ear Wax (Cerumen)

Where is ear wax?

It is in the ear canal ("outer ear," medically), outside of the ear drum. It is not behind the ear drum. The lining of the ear canal is simply skin and needs to be kept clean like skin. The problem is, it is difficult to keep clean since it tunnels into the head.

What is ear wax?

Ear wax is made up of dead skin cells and secretions from glands in the lining of the ear canal. Mother nature has a way to get rid of this debris by gradually moving it towards the outside hole (meatus).

Does ear wax cause "ear infections?"

No. Usually, an "ear infection" is a middle ear or ear drum infection. These infections result from infected mucus behind the ear drum (towards the nose). This occurs on the other side of the ear drum from where the wax is. Dirty water can cause an outer ear infection or "swimmer's ear." This usually occurs when the head is immersed in contaminated such as a pond or improperly chlorinated swimming pool. (Sometimes too much wax allows the dirty water to stay in the ear canal longer).

How can I help keep my child's ear canal free of wax?

You cannot prevent the skin in the ear canal from making wax, but you can try to keep the passage clean and open so that the wax can get out and won't build up inside the canal. Although proper cleansing of the ear canal helps prevent wax build-up, some people inherit a tendency towards wax build-up because they produce thicker, stickier or, sometimes, simply more, ear wax.

At the beginning of every bath, when the water is clean, gently cleanse the outside of the ear canal with a washcloth. A corner of the washcloth may be twisted to cleanse the outside of the hole (meatus). Plain water is best for younger infants. Warm soapy water is okay for older infants and children. Keeping the meatus clean and free of wax and dirt allows the wax to move from the inner part of the canal to the outside. (In most children this amount of wax is too small to see on a daily basis.)

Never stick anything, especially a Q-Tip, into the canal. This pushes the wax further in, delaying the time for the wax to move out, and it can compress the wax, making it harder to move out naturally. It is safe to use Q-Tips to clean the folds in the outer ear (pinna) and around the meatus. For children who take showers, the same technique can be used.

Won't water hurt my child's ear?

Small amounts of clean water are not harmful to healthy ear canals and ear drums. If the child has an eardrum (middle ear) infection, it is safe to clean the outside ear and rinse the ear canal, as long as the child is not in discomfort. If your child has ear tubes, a history of holes in the ear drum, or swimmer's ear (an infection of the ear canal), check with the doctor regarding a safe regimen for cleaning the ears.

My child has an ear wax problem, what do I do?

Sometimes, even though good ear canal hygiene is used, and neither the child nor caretakers use Q-Tips in the ear canal, the ear wax becomes stuck or "impacted".

In the doctor's office:

The doctor may use a special instrument, an ear curette, to scoop the cerumen out. Because this is a plastic or metal loop or spoon, this does not push the wax back in as a Q-Tip might. Never attempt to scoop out ear wax yourself.

or

The doctor may use a special large metal ear syringe, and mix up half-strength peroxide to flush the ear wax out. This takes 10–20 minutes and usually requires a separate appointment.

At home:

Commercial products are available over-the-counter and have convenient dispensing bottles. They are basically fancy hydrogen peroxide. Some physicians feel these products only make the wax goopy. With time and good hygiene, these products can work. These cost about $20–$25. Murine and Debrox ear wax removal systems provide an irrigation bulb in addition to drops.

A homemade hydrogen peroxide remedy is cheaper and offers more flexible dosing. Follow these simple instructions to mix your own remedy to use at bath or shower time:

Mix one part plain hydrogen peroxide with one part hot water in a plastic cup (no glass in the bathroom).

Make sure the temperature of the solution is skin temperature. Hydrogen peroxide is cold, and flushing ear canals with cold liquids is very uncomfortable.

Draw up the solution with a bulb syringe.

Lay the tip of the syringe against the hole of the ear with impacted (or "stuck") wax, but do not seal up the hole.

Gently pull the ear away from the head and upwards.

Flush (squirt) the affected canal(s) until the syringe is empty.

Continue drawing up about 8–12 oz of solution to flush the ear.

Repeat 3 times/week for 2–4 weeks, then once every 1–2 weeks.

Note: All hydrogen peroxide solutions are alkaline, and flushing the ears more often than recommended can damage the hairs and skin lining the canal.

Section 5.3

Ear Infections: Facts for Parents

"Ear Infections: Facts for Parents about Otitis Media," National Institute on Deafness and Other Communication Disorders (NIDCD), NIH Pub. No. 00-4216. Updated February 2002.

What is otitis media?

Otitis media is an ear infection. Three out of four children experience otitis media by the time they are 3 years old. In fact, ear infections are the most common illnesses in babies and young children.

Are there different types of otitis media?

Yes. There are two main types. The first type is called acute otitis media (AOM). This means that parts of the ear are infected and swollen. It also means that fluid and mucus are trapped inside the ear. AOM can be painful.

The second type is called otitis media with effusion (fluid), or OME. This means fluid and mucus stay trapped in the ear after the infection is over. OME makes it harder for the ear to fight new infections. This fluid can also affect your child's hearing.

How does otitis media happen?

Otitis media usually happens when viruses and/or bacteria get inside the ear and cause an infection. It often happens as a result of another illness, such as a cold. If your child gets sick, it might affect his or her ears.

It is harder for children to fight illness than it is for adults, so children develop ear infections more often. Some researchers believe that other factors, such as being around cigarette smoke, can contribute to ear infections.

What's happening inside the ear when my child has an ear infection?

When the ears are infected the eustachian tubes become inflamed and swollen. The adenoids can also become infected.

53

- The eustachian tubes are inside the ear. They keep air pressure stable in the ear. These tubes also help supply the ears with fresh air.

- The adenoids are located near the eustachian tubes. Adenoids are clumps of cells that fight infections.

Swollen and inflamed eustachian tubes often get clogged with fluid and mucus from a cold. If the fluids plug the openings of the eustachian tubes, air and fluid get trapped inside the ear. These tubes are smaller and straighter in children than they are in adults. This makes it harder for fluid to drain out of the ear and is one reason that children get more ear infections than adults. The infections are usually painful.

Adenoids are located in the throat, near the eustachian tubes. Adenoids can become infected and swollen. They can also block the openings of the eustachian tubes, trapping air and fluid. Just like the eustachian tubes, the adenoids are different in children than in adults. In children, the adenoids are larger, so they can more easily block the opening of the eustachian tube.

Can otitis media affect my child's hearing?

Yes. An ear infection can cause temporary hearing problems. Temporary speech and language problems can happen, too. If left untreated, these problems can become more serious.

An ear infection affects important parts in the ear that help us hear. Sounds around us are collected by the outer ear. Then sound travels to the middle ear, which has three tiny bones and is filled with air. After that, sound moves on to the inner ear. The inner ear is where sounds are turned into electrical signals and sent to the brain. An ear infection affects the whole ear, but especially the middle and inner ear. Hearing is affected because sound cannot get through an ear that is filled with fluid.

How do I know if my child has otitis media?

It is not always easy to know if your child has an ear infection. Sometimes you have to watch carefully. Your child may get an ear infection before he or she has learned how to talk. If your child is not old enough to say "My ear hurts," you need to look for other signals that there is a problem.

Here are a few signs your child might show you if he or she has otitis media:

- Does she tug or pull at her ears?
- Does he cry more than usual?
- Do you see fluid draining out of her ears?
- Does he have trouble sleeping?
- Can she keep her balance?
- Does he have trouble hearing?
- Does she seem not to respond to quiet sounds?

A child with an ear infection may show you any of these signs. If you see any of them, call a doctor.

What will a doctor do?

Your doctor will examine your child's ear. The doctor can tell you for sure if your child has an ear infection. The doctor may also give your child medicine. Medicines called antibiotics are sometimes given for ear infections. It is important to know how they work. Antibiotics only work against organisms called bacteria, which can cause illness. Antibiotics are not effective against viruses, such as those associated with a cold. In order to be effective, antibiotics must be taken until they are finished. A few days after the medicine starts working, your child may stop pulling on his or her ear and appear to be feeling better. This does not mean the infection is gone. The medicine must still be taken. If not, the bacteria can come back. You need to follow the doctor's directions exactly.

Your doctor may also give your child pain relievers, such as acetaminophen. Medicines such as antihistamines and decongestants do not help in the prevention or treatment of otitis media.

How can I be sure I am giving the medicine correctly?

If your doctor gives you a prescription for medicine for your child, make sure you understand the directions completely before you leave his or her office. Here are a few suggestions about giving medicine to your child.

1. **Read.** Make sure the pharmacy has given you printed information about the medicine and clear instructions about how to give it to your child. Read the information that comes with the medicine. If you have any problems understanding the information, ask the pharmacist, your doctor, or a nurse. You should know the answers to the following questions:

- Does the medicine need to be refrigerated?

- How many times a day will I be giving my child this medicine?

- How many days will my child take this medicine?

- Should it be given with food or without food?

2. **Plan.** Sometimes it is hard to remember when you have given your child a dose of medicine. Before you give the first dose, make a written plan or chart to cover all of the days of the medication. Some children may require 10 to 14 days of treatment. Put a chart on the refrigerator so you can check off the doses at every meal. Be sure to measure carefully. Use a measuring spoon or special medicine-measuring cup if one comes with the medicine. Do not use spoons that come with tableware sets because they are not always a standard size.

3. **Follow through.** Be sure to give all of the medicine to your child. Make sure it is given at the right times. If your doctor asks you to bring your child back for a "recheck", do it on schedule. Your doctor wants to know if the ears are clear of fluid and if the infection has stopped. Write down and ask the doctor any questions you have before you leave his or her office.

Will my child need surgery?

Some children with otitis media need surgery. The most common surgical treatment involves having small tubes placed inside the ear. This surgery is called a myringotomy. It is recommended when fluids from an ear infection stay in the ear for several months. At that stage, fluid may cause hearing loss and speech problems. A doctor called an otolaryngologist (ear, nose, and throat surgeon) will help you through this process if your child needs an operation. The operation will require anesthesia.

In a myringotomy, a surgeon makes a small opening in the ear drum. Then a tube is placed in the opening. The tube works to relieve pressure in the clogged ear so that the child can hear again. Fluid cannot build up in the ear if the tube is venting it with fresh air.

After a few months, the tubes will fall out on their own. In rare cases, a child may need to have a myringotomy more than once.

Another kind of surgery removes the adenoids. This is called an adenoidectomy. Removing the adenoids has been shown to help some children with otitis media who are between the ages of 4 and 8. We know less about whether this can help children under age 4.

What about children in daycare, pre-school, or school?

Even before your child has an ear infection or needs to take medicine, ask the daycare program or school about their medication policy. Sometimes you will need a note from your doctor for the staff at the school. The note can tell the people at your child's school how and when to give your child medicine if it is needed during school hours. Some schools will not give children medicine. If this is the case at your child's school, ask your doctor how to schedule your child's medicine.

What else can I do for my child?

Here are a few things you can do to lower your child's risk of getting otitis media. The best thing you can do is to **pay attention** to your child. Know the warning signs of ear infections and be on the lookout if your child gets a cold. If you think your child has an ear infection, call the doctor.

Do not smoke around your child. Smoke is not good for the delicate parts inside your child's ear.

Chapter 6

Routine Dental Care for Children

Chapter Contents

Section 6.1

How to Find a Dentist

Excerpted from "Frequently Asked Questions: Access to Dental Care." Reprinted with permission of the American Dental Association. © 2002 American Dental Association. For additional information, visit www. ada.org.

Tips for Choosing a Dentist

How do you find a dentist?

The American Dental Association (ADA) offers these suggestions:

- Ask family, friends, neighbors, or coworkers for recommendations.
- Ask your family physician or local pharmacist.
- If you're moving, your current dentist may be able to make a recommendation.
- Call or write your local or state dental society. Your local and state dental societies also may be listed in the telephone directory under "dentists" or "associations."
- Use ADA.org's ADA Member Directory at www.ada.org/public/ disclaimer.html to search for dentists in your area.

You may want to call or visit more than one dentist before making your decision. Dental care is a very personalized service that requires a good relationship between the dentist and the patient.

What should I look for when choosing a dentist?

You may wish to consider several dentists before making your decision. During your first visit, you should be able to determine if this is the right dentist for you. Consider the following:

- Is the appointment schedule convenient for you?

- Is the office easy to get to from your home or job?

- Does the office appear to be clean, neat, and orderly?

- Was your medical and dental history recorded and placed in a permanent file?

- Does the dentist explain techniques that will help you prevent dental health problems? Is dental health instruction provided?

- Are special arrangements made for handling emergencies outside of office hours? (Most dentists make arrangements with a colleague or emergency referral service if they are unable to tend to emergencies.)

- Is information provided about fees and payment plans before treatment is scheduled?

You and your dentist are partners in maintaining your oral health. Take time to ask questions and take notes if that will help you remember your dentist's advice.

What is the difference between a DDS and a DMD?

The DDS (Doctor of Dental Surgery) and DMD (Doctor of Dental Medicine) are the same degrees. The difference is a matter of semantics. The majority of dental schools award the DDS degree; however, some award a DMD degree. The education and degrees are the same.

Section 6.2

Dental Hygiene

From "Prevention Information." This information is reprinted with permission of Richard M. Weledniger, DDS, PC. For more information visit www.smiles4ever.com/prevention.htm; © 2001.

Brushing

One of the best ways to ensure healthy teeth and gums is with a good home care program. Proper brushing and flossing is the one way you can make sure you are doing what you can to protect your mouth. Proper brushing consists of about three to five minutes of concentrated brushing. A quick brush may make your mouth feel fresh, but will do very little to remove the plaque that normally develops during the course of the day. Be sure to cover all areas of the teeth, inside, outside on the biting surfaces, and along the gum line as well. Since plaque is the substance responsible for tooth decay, a good brushing at least twice a day will help to prevent tooth decay. Plaque also has germs, which irritate the gums. Because plaque forms every 12 hours, brushing twice a day is very important in order to prevent the plaque from turning into an even more irritating substance known as tartar.

Once tartar has formed on the teeth your dentist can only remove it. A soft round bristled toothbrush is the best to use because it won't scrub away the enamel on your teeth nor irritate the gums. Gently massage your gums while brushing, this helps to clean them as well as increasing circulation in the area, which is helpful in the prevention of gum disease. A good home care program that consists of brushing and flossing upon rising, before going to bed, and after every meal, along with regular visits to your family dentist for a check up and cleaning will certainly help you in keeping your teeth and gums healthy.

Flossing

One of the major causes of tooth loss today is due to periodontal disease, or gingivitis, as it is commonly called. Gum disease is caused by tartar. Tartar is what plaque turns into when it is not removed.

One of the most difficult areas from which to remove plaque is in between the teeth. Because plaque turns into tartar literally overnight it is very important to floss twice a day in order to maintain healthy teeth and gums. Unfortunately, because flossing seems tedious and time consuming few people floss as often as they should. A good time to floss is while watching TV. Once you get the hang of flossing, you don't need a mirror to se what you are doing.

When flossing be careful not to snap the floss up through the teeth as you can cut your gums that way. Use a gentle sawing motion to work the floss between the teeth, when you reach the gum line, curve the floss against the wall of the tooth to remove the plaque. If your gums bleed initially do not be alarmed. If you have not been flossing regularly the gums need to be conditioned. Tenderness after flossing the first several times is normal as well. Warm saltwater rinses will help to relieve this tenderness. Bleeding and tender gums are an indication of gum disease, if these symptoms persist after one week of daily flossing, be sure to contact your dentist for proper treatment. Periodontal disease will not go away by itself and can cause serious problems in the mouth due to bone loss and result in loss of teeth. A good home care program along with routine dental visits will certainly do much to ensure a lifelong healthy smile.

Bad Breath

Nothing can defeat a first impression easier than bad breath. Most of the time, you don't even know you have a problem until someone tells you, making it even more embarrassing. Some people tend to think that using the right mouthwash will solve their troubles. But generally speaking, a mouthwash will only sweeten your breath for just a short time. The real problem behind recurring bad breath is the presence of plaque on your teeth. The plaque contains bacteria, a key factor in bad breath. If you have a problem with your breath, you may not be doing the proper oral hygiene at home. At least twice a day, your teeth require a 2½–3-minute brushing. Flossing should be done as well to loosen the plaque between your teeth. If your gums bleed when you brush or floss, it could be a sign of gum disease. Gums that bleed are not normal. Regular dental examinations allow for early detection of dental problems.

Mouthwash to Prevent Tooth Decay?

Mouthwash does not prevent tooth decay. A fluoride rinse however is a good addition to a thorough brushing and flossing routine. Plaque reacts with sugars and starches to form an acid, which breaks down the minerals in the enamel of the teeth, thereby causing a cavity. Your saliva contains minerals that can replace the minerals destroyed by the acids. Fluoride acts together with these minerals to help this re-mineralization process. Mouthwashes with fluorides in them will work together with your saliva to help your teeth ward off cavities. Adding a fluoride rinse to a to a thorough brushing routine, along with the fluoride treatments your dentist can provide, will help keep your teeth healthy.

Fluoride

Fluoride is a nutrient, which our bodies need for growth and development. Fluoride also helps to reduce dental decay. When fluoride is taken internally during the time that the teeth are being formed, it is incorporated into the enamel of the teeth thereby helping to make the teeth less prone to decay. Once teeth are formed in the mouth, however, fluoride taken internally no longer has any effects on the tooth structure. At this point fluoridated toothpastes and rinses will work with your saliva on the enamel of the teeth, helping to re-mineralize any enamel that has been broken down. Plaque and sugars work with each other to create an acid that causes decay.

Using fluoridated toothpaste together with limiting sugary foods will also help to prevent decay. Fluoride is also effective in decreasing sensitivity of teeth. A fluoride toothpaste or rinse can be used at home as a remedy for sensitive teeth. Your dentist can also administer fluoride in a stronger form. This treatment is also effective for teeth that are sensitive at the gum line. Fluoride has been a big help in reducing dental decay. Together with regular visits to your dentist, you can work towards a lifelong healthy and happy smile.

Plaque

Plaque is a sticky, soft invisible film that forms on exposed surfaces of your teeth. The bacteria, which make up the plaque, react with sugars and starches in foods to produce an acid. It's the acid that dissolves tooth enamel and begins the decaying process. After repeated acid attacks, and if plaque is not removed daily, the enamel eventually breaks down and decays—thus a cavity is formed.

The irritants in plaque also cause inflammation of the gums making them tender and prone to bleeding. This is the first stage of periodontal disease. If you don't remove the soft plaque, it will mix with saliva and harden. Once this takes place, brushing will not take the film off your teeth and your dentist or dental hygienist must remove the tartar. To keep plaque under control, brush and floss at least twice a day. Visiting your dentist for regular examinations also play a large role in prevention.

Sensitive Teeth

If occasionally you experience discomfort due to either hot or cold foods, or cold air hitting the teeth you may or may not have a dental problem. Some people have very thin enamel or have worn away enamel due to improper brushing. Using a brush that is not hard will help in preventing the erosion of enamel. If, however, your teeth are very sensitive let your dentist know so they can be properly treated.

Concerns Regarding Tongue Piercing

Tongue piercing is becoming more common. Like other forms of body piercing, it carries serious risks during the procedure itself. These include the risk of local or systemic infection. Local infection can occur because the mouth is hard to sterilize and many places that pierce tongues do not always maintain a sterile environment.

Systemic infection is always a possibility and includes the risk of hepatitis and AIDS. The rinsing with mouthwash may not take care of an infection, if it is serious. It is important to remember that piercing establishments are not regulated by law nor are the operators licensed. The operators' experience and competence can vary and are not guaranteed. Like other forms of body piercing, tongue piercing also can result in an allergy if the metals used are not of the highest quality. Many times, the stated price of the piercing does not include the jewelry to be placed.

Unlike other forms of piercing, the tongue also caries the increased risk of bleeding problems. The tongue has major blood vessels within it and many operators are not aware of this. The jewelry may also be swallowed, if loosened, and result in choking.

In addition, unlike other forms of body piercing, tongue piercing also carries the risk of damage to the surrounding teeth. The hard jewelry can chip and break the enamel or fillings of the teeth as one talks and eats. This damage can also result in the death of the tooth's inner pulp, if the trauma to the tooth is chronic. This tooth damage may result in the need for expensive crowns to restore a smile or even a root canal to keep the tooth. These are important matters to consider before undergoing tongue piercing. If there is a problem after tongue piercing, it is important not only to contact the piercing establishment, but your physician and dentist as needed. Your smile and your health are important in the long run.

> —*section by Margaret J. Fehrenbach, RDH,*
> *MS Educational Consultant*

Choice of Foods to Prevent Cavities

Plaque, which is a sticky film that coats our teeth during the day, has thousands of bacteria that interact with the foods we eat and cause cavities. By limiting the diet of certain types of foods which are the biggest causes of decay you can help to limit the number of cavities you may get. The bacteria in plaque feed on the sugars and starch we eat to form an acid, which breaks down the enamel of the teeth and forms cavities. Since dental healthy foods also contain sugars it is impossible to remove all sugar and starch from the diet. Sugars and starches should be eaten with a main meal, after which a thorough brushing will remove any leftover food particles. If a place to brush is not handy, rinse the mouth with water, this too will help to remove some of the sugars and food particles.

An important key to dental health is calcium. Children and teenagers need more calcium than adults to help in the formation of strong, healthy teeth and bones. Pregnant women also require extra calcium in order for their baby's teeth and bones to form properly. Milk products are very high in calcium as is spinach and canned salmon. Children are just as prone to cavities as adults. It is not good to allow your child to nurse on a bottle with milk or fruit juice for extended periods of time because the sugars will decay the teeth. Keep snacking at a minimum and definitely clean your teeth afterwards. A good diet along with regular visits to the dentist will help to keep your teeth healthy.

Healthy Food for Teeth

Foods recommended for dental health are high in nutrients and low in sugar. In other words, you should try to eat the foods that will do the most for your teeth and body. For better dental health stick to the foods that are high in nutritional value. Whether these foods are chosen as part of a meal or an between-meal snack, these types of foods will contribute greatly to your daily nutritional needs.

Eat properly and use the traffic light system with go, caution, and stop foods. Some of the go foods include milk, eggs, yogurt, Melba toast, peanuts, and cheese. Milk acts as an acid inhibitor when combined with starches such as cereal and works against the potential acid production of the cereal. If milk is used to wash away sweets they will not have as harmful an effect. Certain cheeses, such as cheddar, are a good preventive food because their sharpness increases salivary flow.

Caution foods are not recommended for dental health because they are high in sugar but do have nutritional value. Some of these foods include ice cream, raisins, dried fruits, and unsweetened juices, if taken frequently. Other foods in this category are foods that are nutritionally poor but dentally acceptable. These types of food include pretzels, popcorn, and potato chips. The last group of foods is the stop group. These foods are both dentally and nutritionally unacceptable. Chocolate, candies, gum, jellies, and beverages high in sugars. Avoid these foods whenever possible.

Snacks that save smiles include meat, seafood, hard-boiled eggs, milk, cheese, raw vegetables, plain popcorn, seeds, and nuts. Snacks that are not good for a healthy smile include candy, cookies, cakes, pastries, presweetened cereals, marshmallows, granola bars, fast foods; and sugar-sweetened gum and soda. Eat sensibly, brush and floss your teeth, visit your dentist regularly, and you will be on your way to better dental health.

Orthodontics and Oral Hygiene

The level of cooperation between the patient and the orthodontist determines the rate of success of orthodontic treatment. It is important to remember that, although orthodontic appliances do not cause cavities, they can contribute to them if the mouth is not properly maintained.

Because bands and appliances act as traps for food particles and bacteria the teeth underneath are more susceptible to decay. It is for this reason that a thorough brushing routine be established and maintained. Routine visits to your regular dentist for check-ups and cleanings will aid in preventing major problems or destruction of the teeth under the bands or appliances. Because good success is guaranteed by the teamwork between orthodontist and patient, it is important to keep regularly scheduled appointments and follow the instructions given by your orthodontist.

Although the wearing of rubber bands, headgear or appliances may not be pleasant, the degree of cooperation will determine the rate of success. Broken appliances, brackets, or wires need to be repaired immediately—be sure to call your orthodontist as soon as possible. Remember you have made an investment in your smile—cooperation between you and your orthodontist will guarantee that investment.

Section 6.3

Dental Sealants

"Frequently Asked Questions: Dental Sealants," National Center for Chronic Disease Prevention and Health Promotion, Centers for Disease Control and Prevention, Fall 2001.

What are dental sealants?

Dental sealants are thin plastic coatings which are applied to the chewing surfaces of the molars (back teeth). Most tooth decay in children and teens occurs in these surfaces. Sealants cover the chewing surfaces to prevent decay.

Which teeth are suitable for sealants?

Permanent molars are the most likely to benefit from sealant application. First molars usually come into the mouth when a child is about 6 years of age. Second molars appear at about age 12. It is best if the sealant is applied soon after the molars have erupted, before the teeth have a chance to decay. For that reason, children between the ages of 5 and 15 benefit most from sealants.

How are sealants applied?

Applying sealants does not require drilling or removing tooth structure. It is an easy three-step process: A dentist or dental hygienist cleans the tooth with a special toothpaste. A special cleansing liquid, on a tiny piece of cotton, is rubbed gently on the tooth and is washed off. Finally, the sealant is painted on the tooth. It takes about a minute for the sealant to form a protective shield.

Are sealants visible?

Upon close examination sealants can be seen. Sealants can be clear, white, or slightly tinted. Because they are used only on the back teeth, sealants cannot be seen when a child talks or smiles.

Will sealants make teeth feel different?

Like anything new that is placed in the mouth, a child may feel the sealant with the tongue. Sealants, however, are very thin and only fill the pits and grooves on molar teeth.

How long will sealants last?

One sealant application can last for as long as 5 to 10 years. Sealants should be checked regularly, and reapplied if they are no longer in place.

Will sealants replace fluoride?

No. fluorides, such as those used in community water, toothpaste, and mouthrinse also help to prevent decay. Fluoride works best on the smooth surfaces of teeth. The chewing surfaces on the back teeth, however, have tiny grooves where decay often begins. Sealants keep germs out of the grooves by covering them with a safe plastic coating. Sealants and fluorides work together to prevent tooth decay.

How do sealants fit into a preventive dentistry program?

Sealants should be used as part of a child's total preventive dental care. A complete preventive dental program includes use of sealants, fluoride, plaque removal, careful food choices, and regular dental care.

Why is sealing a tooth better than waiting for decay and filling the cavity?

Sealants help maintain sound, intact teeth. Decay destroys the structure of the tooth. Each time a tooth is filled or a filling is replaced, additional tooth structure is lost. Fillings last an average of 6 to 8 years before they need to be replaced. Appropriate use of sealants can save time, money, and the discomfort associated with dental treatment procedures.

69

Section 6.4

Fluoride Facts

This section includes text from "Using Fluoride to Prevent and Control Dental Caries in the United States," August 2001 and "Dietary Fluoride Supplement Schedule," February 2002. Both fact sheets are from the National Center for Chronic Disease Prevention and Health Promotion, Centers for Disease Control and Prevention (CDC).

Using Fluoride to Prevent and Control Dental Caries

The Centers for Disease Control and Prevention (CDC) has issued new recommendations on using fluoride to prevent dental caries (tooth decay). The recommendations provide guidance to health care providers, public health officials, policymakers, and the general public on how to achieve maximum dental decay protection while efficiently using dental care resources and minimizing any cosmetic concerns. In 1999, CDC profiled the widespread practice of fluoridating community drinking water to prevent dental decay as one of 10 great public health achievements of the twentieth century.

Fluoride Facts

- Fluorine, from which fluoride is derived, is the thirteenth most abundant element and is released into the environment naturally in both water and air.

- Fluoride is naturally present in all water. Community water fluoridation is the addition of fluoride to adjust the natural fluoride concentration of a community's water supply to the level recommended for optimal dental health, approximately 1.0 ppm (parts per million). One ppm is the equivalent of 1 mg/L (comparable to 1 inch in 16 miles).

- Community water fluoridation is an effective, safe, and inexpensive way to prevent tooth decay. Fluoridation benefits Americans of all ages and socioeconomic status.

- Children and adults who are at low risk of dental decay can stay cavity-free through frequent exposure to small amounts of fluoride. This is best gained by drinking fluoridated water and using a fluoride toothpaste twice daily.

- Children and adults at high risk of dental decay may benefit from using additional fluoride products, including dietary supplements (for children who do not have adequate levels of fluoride in their drinking water), mouthrinses, and professionally applied gels and varnishes.

- Good scientific evidence supports the use of community water fluoridation and the use of fluoride dental products for preventing tooth decay for both children and adults.

- Fluoride was first used purposefully to prevent tooth decay in Grand Rapids, Michigan, in 1945 by adjusting the level of fluoride in drinking water. Fluoridation of drinking water has been used successfully in the United States for more than 50 years.

- Fluoridation of community water has been credited with reducing tooth decay by 50–60 percent in the United States since World War II. More recent estimates of this effect show decay reduction at 18–40 percent, which reflects that even in communities that are not optimally fluoridated, people are receiving some benefits from other sources (for example, bottled beverages, toothpaste).

- Fluoride's main effect occurs after the tooth has erupted above the gum. This topical effect happens when small amounts of fluoride are maintained in the mouth in saliva and dental plaque (the film that adheres to tooth enamel).

- Fluoride works by stopping or even reversing the tooth decay process. It keeps the tooth enamel strong and solid by preventing the loss of (and enhancing the reattachment of) important minerals from the tooth enamel.

- Of the 50 largest cities in the United States, 43 have community water fluoridation. Fluoridation reaches 62 percent of the population on public water supplies—more than 144 million people.

- Water fluoridation costs, on average, 72 cents per person per year in U.S. communities (1999 dollars).

- Consumption of fluids—water, soft drinks, and juice—accounts for approximately 75 percent of fluoride intake in the United States.

- Children aged 6 years or less may develop enamel fluorosis if they ingest more fluoride than needed. Enamel fluorosis is a chalk-like discoloration (white spots) of tooth enamel. A common source of extra fluoride is unsupervised use of toothpaste in very young children.

• Fluoride also benefits adults, decreasing the risk of cavities at the root surface as well as the enamel crown. Use of fluoridated water and fluoride dental products will help people maintain oral health and keep more permanent teeth.

Dietary Fluoride Supplement Schedule

It is suggested that only children living in non-fluoridated areas use dietary fluoride supplements between the ages of 6 months to 16 years. Your physician or dentist can prescribe the correct dosage for your child based on the following considerations.

Level of fluoride in your drinking water. If the fluoride level is not known, it should be tested first. State and local health departments can provide information on testing drinking water for fluoride levels.

A complete fluoride history should include all the your child's sources of fluoride. Don't forget all water sources, or the amount and frequency of fluoridated toothpaste used when toothbrushing.

If your child is to benefit from the cavity protection that dietary fluoride supplements can provide, long-term use on a daily basis is needed.

Table 6.1 Fluoride ion level in drinking water (ppm)*. Approved by the American Dental Association, the American Academy of Pediatrics, and the American Academy of Pediatric Dentistry.

Age	less than 0.3 ppm	0.3–0.6 ppm	greater than 0.6 ppm
Birth–6 months	None	None	None
6 months–3 years	0.25 mg/day**	None	None
3–6 years	0.50 mg/day	0.25 mg/day	None
6–16 years	1.0 mg/day	0.50 mg/day	None

*1 part per million (ppm) = 1 milligram/liter (mg/L)

**2.2 mg sodium fluoride contains 1 mg fluoride ion.

Data Sources

American Dental Association, Council on Access Prevention and Interprofessional Relations. Caries diagnosis and risk assessment: a review of preventive strategies and management. *J Am Dent Assoc* 1995;126(Suppl).

Special Issue: Reference Manual, 1994–1995. Academy of Pediatric Dentistry. *Pediatric Dentistry* 1994–1995; 16(7):1–96.

Committee on Nutrition, American Academy of Pediatrics. Fluoride supplementation for children: interim policy recommendations. *Pediatrics* 1995, 95(5):777.

Section 6.5

Orthodontics

From "Information about Orthodontics." This information is reprinted with permission of Richard M. Weledniger, DDS, PC. For more information visit www.smiles4ever.com/prevention.htm; © 2001.

Orthodontics

Why braces? Why orthodontics? If you have teeth that are in poor alignment you may face a functional or cosmetic problem.

Orthodontics (braces) can eliminate that problem for you. One of the first things people notice about you when they see you is your smile and how your teeth look. You don't have to be a dentist to see poorly positioned crooked teeth.

In today's culture, crooked teeth are not regarded as being attractive or desirable, and when given a chance to express an opinion, most of us state that they would like to have straight teeth. Straight teeth and white teeth are the cosmetic dental improvements patients most request.

If you are lucky, the need for orthodontics is discovered when you are young. A dentist will have a good indication of whether or not teeth will be straight when he sees a child 6–8 years old. Most treatment may not begin until the patient is 8, although in some instances it can be started earlier.

It is easier to direct the movement of teeth in a child. Early tooth guidance is a very important phase of orthodontic care. This guidance takes place even though all the permanent teeth are not yet in place. Certain problems are much easier to correct at this stage of a "mixed (baby and permanent teeth) dentition."

If more treatment than the early tooth guidance is required, an average case can last from 18–24 months. Most adult cases take this long to complete. You are never too old to begin orthodontics. The number of adults seeking orthodontic treatment has been rising dramatically during the past decades, and as long as you have healthy bone support for the teeth, you can have braces to make your teeth look better.

After the active phase of orthodontic treatment, when the braces are removed, it is usually necessary to have a retainer made. This retainer will maintain the new tooth alignment until the teeth have had a chance to become firmly set in their new position. This retainer may be either removable or fixed in place.

Braces may also be suggested to correct a specific dental problem that only affects one or several teeth. This is not a cosmetic tooth repositioning, but rather a necessary functional tooth movement. Occasionally, in order to properly finish an orthodontic case, the orthodontist may ask the dentist to adjust the enamel of some teeth or bond a resin to some teeth to improve an occlusion (bite alignment) or a cosmetic problem that cannot be successfully treated by orthodontics alone.

While the orthodontics is in its active phase, that is, the braces are on your teeth, you must be very diligent about keeping your teeth clean. If you think it is difficult to clean your teeth properly without braces, imagine what it will be like with the braces in place. It is suggested that you have your teeth cleaned professionally by the dental hygienist at least every 3 months while the braces are on. Sometimes the use of dental floss threaders and oral irrigation devices to flush out debris may prove to help maintain optimum oral health during the orthodontic treatment phase.

Important Things to Remember about Orthodontic Care

- You are never too old to begin.

- It may be easier (and less expensive) to be treated at a young age—around the age of 8.

- You MUST brush your teeth each night.

- Have your teeth cleaned professionally by a dental hygienist every 3 months to reduce the chance of decay and gum disease

- Brush and floss properly every day.

- Depending upon your individual situation, dental floss threaders to help you clean under the orthodontic wires, other periodontal aids, a powered toothbrush like the Rota Dent™ (if you have problems with manual brushing), and a Waterpik™ irrigator help remove loose debris.

- If you have any questions, please feel comfortable in asking your dentist, dental hygienist or orthodontist.

- Orthodontics can make a dramatic improvement in your appearance, your life, and how you feel about yourself.

Part Two

Physical and Mental Development

Chapter 7

Physical Growth

Chapter Contents

Section 7.1

Growth Charts for Stature and Body Mass

This section includes text excerpted from "CDC Growth Charts: United States," Centers for Disease Control and Prevention (CDC), reviewed June 2002, and "Frequently Asked Questions about the 2000 CDC Growth Charts," CDC, reviewed October 2002.

Introduction

Growth charts consist of a series of percentile curves that illustrate the distribution of selected body measurements in U.S. children. Pediatric growth charts have been used by pediatricians, nurses, and parents to track the growth of infants, children, and adolescents in the United States since 1977. The 1977 growth charts were developed by the National Center for Health Statistics (NCHS) as a clinical tool for health professionals to determine if the growth of a child is adequate. The 1977 charts were also adopted by the World Health Organization for international use.

When the 1977 NCHS growth charts were first developed, NCHS recommended that they be revised periodically as necessary. With more recent and comprehensive national data now available, along with improved statistical procedures, the 1977 growth charts were revised and updated to make them a more valuable clinical tool for health professionals. The 2000 Centers for Disease Control and Prevention (CDC) growth charts represent the revised version of the 1977 NCHS growth charts. Most of the data used to construct these charts come from the National Health and Nutrition Examination Survey (NHANES), which has periodically collected height and weight and other health information on the American population since the early 1960s.

Growth charts are not intended to be used as a sole diagnostic instrument. Instead, growth charts are tools that contribute to forming an overall clinical impression for the child being measured. The revised growth charts provide an improved tool for evaluating the growth of children in clinical and research settings.

The 2000 CDC Growth Charts and the New Body Mass Index-for-Age Charts

The revised growth charts consist of 16 charts (8 for boys and 8 for girls). These charts represent revisions to the 14 previous charts, as well as the introduction of two new body mass index-for-age (BMI-for-age) charts for boys and for girls, ages 2 to 20 years.

Most of the specific differences between the revised charts and the original charts occur in the charts for infants, where national data were previously lacking. The revised head circumference charts also show some noticeable differences when compared to the earlier charts. Compared to the original infant charts that were based on primarily formula-fed infants, the revised growth charts for infants contain a better mix of both breast- and formula-fed infants in the U. S. population. (On average, since 1970 approximately one-half of children born in the United States are reported to have been breast fed at some point, and about one-third have been breast fed for 3 months or more.) The addition of the BMI charts is probably the single most significant new feature of the revised growth charts.

These BMI-for-age charts were created for use in place of the 1977 weight-for-stature charts. BMI (wt/ht^2) is calculated from weight and height measurements and is used to judge whether an individual's weight is appropriate for their height. BMI is the most commonly used approach to determine if adults are overweight or obese and is also the recommended measure to determine if children are overweight. The new BMI growth charts can be used clinically beginning at 2 years of age, when an accurate stature can be obtained.

In recent years, BMI has received increased attention for pediatric use. In 1994, an expert committee charged with developing guidelines for overweight in adolescent preventive services (ages 11–21 years) recommended that BMI be used routinely to screen for overweight adolescents. In addition, in 1997 an expert committee on the assessment and treatment of childhood obesity concluded that BMI should be used to screen for overweight children, ages 2 years and older, using the BMI curves from the revised growth charts. BMI can also be used to characterize underweight (though no expert guidelines exist for the classification of underweight based on BMI).

Further information about the revision process can be found on the growth charts website at www.cdc.gov/growthcharts.

Figure 7.1

2 to 20 years: Boys
Stature-for-age and Weight-for-age percentiles

NAME _____

RECORD # _____

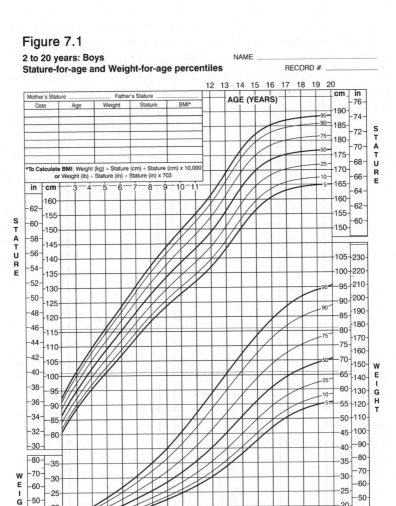

Published May 30, 2000 (modified 11/21/00).
SOURCE: Developed by the National Center for Health Statistics in collaboration with
the National Center for Chronic Disease Prevention and Health Promotion (2000).
http://www.cdc.gov/growthcharts

SAFER · HEALTHIER · PEOPLE™

Figure 7.2

2 to 20 years: Girls
Stature-for-age and Weight-for-age percentiles

NAME _____

RECORD # _____

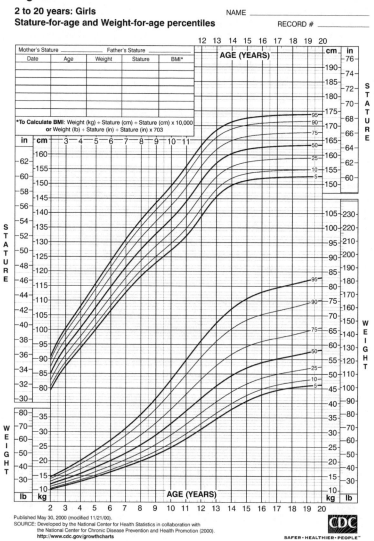

Published May 30, 2000 (modified 11/21/00).
SOURCE: Developed by the National Center for Health Statistics in collaboration with
the National Center for Chronic Disease Prevention and Health Promotion (2000).
http://www.cdc.gov/growthcharts

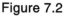

SAFER·HEALTHIER·PEOPLE™

Figure 7.3

2 to 20 years: Boys
Body mass index-for-age percentiles

NAME _____

RECORD # _____

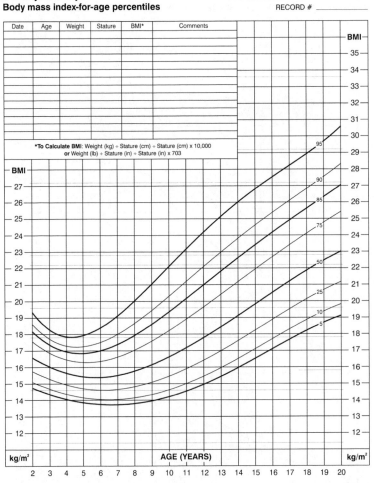

*To Calculate BMI: Weight (kg) ÷ Stature (cm) ÷ Stature (cm) x 10,000
or Weight (lb) ÷ Stature (in) ÷ Stature (in) x 703

Published May 30, 2000 (modified 10/16/00).
SOURCE: Developed by the National Center for Health Statistics in collaboration with
the National Center for Chronic Disease Prevention and Health Promotion (2000).
http://www.cdc.gov/growthcharts

SAFER · HEALTHIER · PEOPLE™

Figure 7.4

2 to 20 years: Girls
Body mass index-for-age percentiles

NAME _____

RECORD # _____

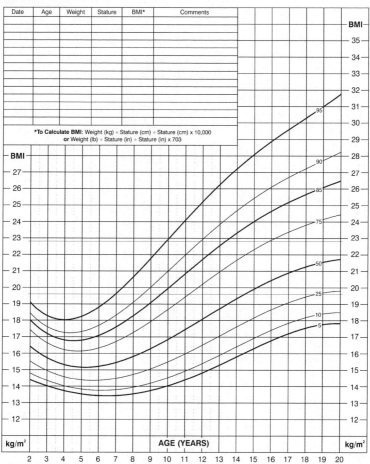

Date	Age	Weight	Stature	BMI*	Comments

*To Calculate BMI: Weight (kg) ÷ Stature (cm) ÷ Stature (cm) x 10,000
or Weight (lb) ÷ Stature (in) ÷ Stature (in) x 703

Published May 30, 2000 (modified 10/16/00).
SOURCE: Developed by the National Center for Health Statistics in collaboration with
the National Center for Chronic Disease Prevention and Health Promotion (2000).
http://www.cdc.gov/growthcharts

SAFER·HEALTHIER·PEOPLE™

Figure 7.5

Weight-for-stature percentiles: Boys

NAME _____

RECORD # _____

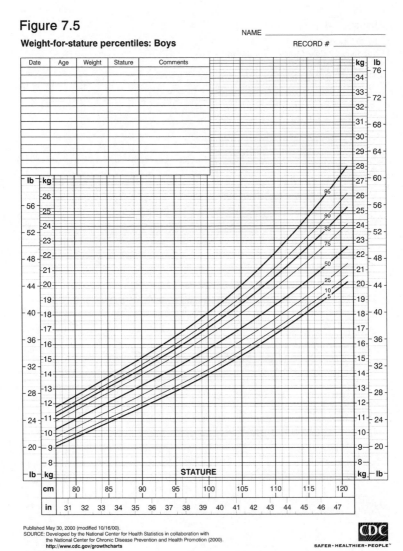

Published May 30, 2000 (modified 10/16/00).
SOURCE: Developed by the National Center for Health Statistics in collaboration with
the National Center for Chronic Disease Prevention and Health Promotion (2000).
http://www.cdc.gov/growthcharts

CDC
SAFER·HEALTHIER·PEOPLE™

Figure 7.6

NAME _____

Weight-for-stature percentiles: Girls

RECORD # _____

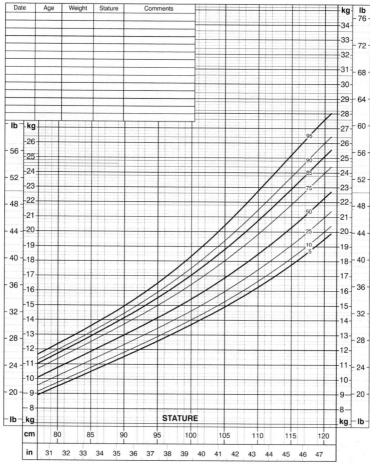

Date	Age	Weight	Stature	Comments

STATURE

Published May 30, 2000 (modified 10/16/00).
SOURCE: Developed by the National Center for Health Statistics in collaboration with
the National Center for Chronic Disease Prevention and Health Promotion (2000).
http://www.cdc.gov/growthcharts

CDC
SAFER · HEALTHIER · PEOPLE™

Frequently Asked Questions about the 2000 CDC Growth Charts

How can I get copies of the growth charts?

The charts are available on the NHANES Growth Charts Web (www.cdc.gov/growthcharts) and can be downloaded and copied. For your convenience, charts for boys and girls between the ages of 2 and 20 are included in this chapter.

What is a percentile?

Percentiles are the most commonly used clinical indicator to assess the size and growth patterns of individual children in the United States. Percentiles rank the position of an individual by indicating what percent of the reference population the individual would equal or exceed. For example, on the weight-for-age growth charts, a 5-year-old girl whose weight is at the 25th percentile, weighs the same or more than 25 percent of the reference population of 5-year-old girls, and weighs less than 75 percent of the 5-year-old girls in the reference population.

What is a z-score?

A z-score is the deviation of the value for an individual from the mean value of the reference population divided by the standard deviation for the reference population. Because z-scores have a direct relationship with percentiles, a conversion can occur in either direction using a standard normal distribution table. Therefore, for every z-score there is a corresponding percentile and vice versa.

My child is at the 5th percentile on a chart, what should I do?

In you are concerned about your child's growth, talk with your child's health care provider.

Are these charts appropriate for exclusively breast-fed babies?

The 2000 CDC growth charts can be used to assess the growth of exclusively breast-fed infants, however when interpreting the growth pattern one must take into account that mode of infant feeding can influence infant growth. In general, exclusively breast-fed infants tend to gain weight more rapidly in the first 2 to 3 months. From 6 to 12 months breast-fed infants tend to weigh less than formula-fed infants.

The 2000 CDC Growth Chart reference population includes data for both formula-fed and breast-fed infants, proportional to the distribution of breast- and formula-fed infants in the population. During the past two decades, approximately one-half of all infants in the United States received some breast milk and approximately one-third were breast-fed for three months or more. A Working Group of the World Health Organization is collecting data at seven international study centers to develop a new set of international growth charts for infants and preschoolers through age 5 years. These charts will be based on the growth of exclusively or predominantly breast-fed children.

Section 7.2

Patterns of Growth

"Patterns of Growth," by Patricia A. Rinser, Family Nurse Practitioner, from original text by Robert M. Blizzard, MD, © 2001 Human Growth Foundation. All rights reserved; reprinted with permission. For more information from the Human Growth Foundation visit their website at www.hgfound.org or call 800-451-6434.

Introduction

"How tall will my 2-year-old be when he grows up?"

"Doctor, my 12-year-old daughter is already 5 feet, 10 inches tall. Is there anything I can do to keep her from growing over 6 feet tall?"

"My child has a cartilage problem and is very short. Will my other children also be short?"

These are questions often asked by parents when the growth of a child seems unusual. What determines how a child grows? How is height inherited? How does one recognize a growth problem? How are growth problems treated? Children may ask parents why they are not as tall as their playmates; parents ask doctors, and doctors ask endocrine (hormone) specialists and geneticists.

This section will explain normal and abnormal patterns of growth and answer some of the questions about growth that parents find puzzling.

Normal Growth

Let's discuss the process of normal growth before we talk about its variations and abnormalities. While we all start out about the same size at birth, some of us end up tall and some end up short. Most of us wind up with about the same build as our parents—the characteristics a child inherits will reflect those of the parents.

A baby is about 20 inches long at birth (give or take an inch) and will grow another 10 inches over the first year to reach about 30 inches by 1 year of age. During the second year of life, growth is half this fast, so at 2 years of age, the child will be about 35 inches tall. From 2 years until about 12 years of age, the child will grow at a steady rate of 2 to 2½ inches a year. The growth spurt that goes along with adolescence begins at about age 11 in girls and 13 in boys. This pubertal growth spurt usually lasts 2 years and is accompanied by sexual development. Growth ceases between 16 and 18 years of age, when the growing ends of the bones fuse. A person's adult height is determined by many factors, including the heights of his or her parents, the age at which puberty begins and the length and vigor of the pubertal growth spurt. An x-ray of the hand or knee allows the doctor to assess the maturity of the bones (bone age) and estimate how much growth potential remains.

Normal But Unusual Growth Patterns

Variations from the usual pattern of growth may occur and still be within the range of normal. Some children are taller than expected at a given age, and some are shorter. Parents are more often concerned when their children are shorter than their age-mates than when they are taller, although most short children fall within the normal range of height.

Many children are short because they have inherited shortness from their parents. Even though the American population is taller than in previous generations, there will always be healthy individuals whose height will be in the low part of the normal range. This is called familial short stature.

A common variant of the usual growth pattern occurs when a child is shorter than average for most of his or her life, then is late entering puberty. This condition is called constitutional growth delay with delayed adolescence or delayed maturation. More boys than girls seek medical attention for this condition, although it is not known whether it is really more common in boys. These children generally are the shortest among their age-mates. A 10-year-old child with this condition may be about the size of a 7-year-old; their bone age and growth potential will also be more like that of a 7-year-old. Typical children with constitutional growth delay have been behind their age-mates in height since very early in childhood, but have continued to grow at a slow normal rate. They will enter puberty 2, 3 or even 4 years later than other children their age, but will have a normal growth spurt and end up about as tall as their parents. It is not unusual for this type of growth pattern to run in families—often a father remembers that he didn't have his growth spurt or begin shaving until much later than other boys his age or a mother remembers being late starting her periods.

This type of growth delay may create stress for a child. Nature's timetable can be speeded up by giving a low dose of sex hormone (testosterone or estrogen), although there is a small risk that this will speed up closure of the growth plates, resulting in a slightly shorter adult height. Studies are being done to determine the physical and psychological effects of growth hormone treatment in children with severe constitutional growth delay; the results of these studies are not yet known.

A second type of normal, but unusual, growth pattern is that of the very tall girl. It comes as no surprise to very tall parents that their children grow rapidly and are taller than other children. Some girls feel uncomfortable being five or six inches taller than their friends. This is an individual matter; some girls feel it is an advantage and enjoy their tallness, while others slouch and try to hide it. Adult height can be predicted on the basis of a bone age x-ray and height measurement. If a height prediction made before age 12 indicates that a girl will be very tall, she can be treated with a high dose of female hormones. These hormones will push the girl into puberty and speed up closure of the growth plates of the bones, so that the girl will end up shorter than she would have been otherwise. These hormones may have undesirable side effects, however, and doctors disagree about the safety and effectiveness of this treatment.

Abnormal Growth Patterns

Poor Nutrition and Systemic Diseases

These are many diseases and disorders that can cause short stature and growth failure. Nutritional deficiencies will cause poor growth eventually—a balanced diet with adequate calories and protein is essential for growth. There are a number of intestinal disorders which may lead to poor absorption of food. Failure to absorb nutrients and energy from food then leads to growth failure. Children with these conditions may have complaints that involve the stomach or intestines (bowels) and may have bowel movements that are unusual in pattern, appearance, and odor. Treatment of these conditions often involves a special diet. Normal growth usually resumes after the condition has been treated.

Diseases of the kidneys, lungs, and heart may lead to growth failure as a result of inadequate intake of nutrients or buildup of waste products and undesirable substances in the body. Children with diabetes, or "high sugar," may grow slowly, particularly when their blood sugar is not kept near the normal range.

Any disease that is severe, untreated, or poorly controlled can have an adverse effect on growth. Severe stress or emotional trauma can also cause growth failure.

Bone Disorders

One form of extreme short stature is caused by abnormal formation and growth of cartilage and bone. Children with a skeletal dysplasia, or chondrodystrophy, are short and have abnormal body proportions; intelligence is normal. Some chondrodystrophies are inherited, others are not. The underlying causes of most of these skeletal dysplasia are not known, although researchers are working to identify the genetic and biochemical mechanisms that are involved. The chances of parents having a second child with the same problem cannot be estimated until the specific type of skeletal dysplasia is identified from physical examination and bone x-rays.

Children who will be very short as adults and adults with short stature may benefit from social contact with others having similar growth problems and with short adults who are living full and happy lives. The Little People of America is an organization that provides opportunities for such contact.

Intrauterine Growth Retardation

Some infants are small at birth. When pregnancy ends earlier than usual, the baby is premature. These babies are small, but usually are normal size given their gestational age (length of time in the womb). However, some infants are shorter and weigh less than they should at birth. In other words, they had a chance to grow in the womb, but did not reach the length and weight they should have for their gestational age. This failure to grow normally in the womb is called intrauterine growth retardation.

This condition may result from a problem with the placenta, the organ in the mother's womb that supplies nutrients and oxygen to the baby. A viral infection, such as German measles, during pregnancy may affect the placenta and infant and cause intrauterine growth retardation. Sometimes the cause of this condition cannot be identified. Some of these children will remain small throughout life, while others may reach normal size. Because there are so many different causes of intrauterine growth retardation, no single treatment is effective in increasing the height of these individuals. Studies are underway to see if growth hormone is effective in increasing the growth rate and adult height of these children; the results are not yet known.

Turner Syndrome

Short stature in girls may be caused by a genetic condition that affects the X chromosome. Chromosomes are small thread-like bodies in the nucleus of each cell; they contain the genetic material that determines the characteristics we inherit. Two of these chromosomes determine sexual development—the X and Y chromosomes. Boys have one X and one Y chromosome, and girls have two X chromosomes. In girls with Turner Syndrome, one of the X chromosomes is misshapen or missing in many or all body cells. Because of this, affected girls are short—they seldom reach 5 feet in height—and may have undeveloped ovaries (female sex glands that produce eggs and female hormones). Intelligence is normal. Turner Syndrome may be suspected because of the presence of certain physical features, but poor growth is sometimes the only sign. This condition is diagnosed by doing a special blood test (karyotype) to look for damaged or missing sex chromosomes. Replacement of the missing ovarian hormones enables these girls to develop normal female sexual characteristics. Treatment with biosynthetic growth hormone appears to be effective in increasing adult height in many of these young women, although long-term studies are still underway.

Precocious Puberty

One type of unusual growth pattern is caused by the early onset of adolescence. This pattern occurs more frequently in girls than boys.

The term sexual precocity is used to describe this condition, which includes early development of adult sexual characteristics. Children with sexual precocity grow rapidly and are tall for their age initially, but their bones also mature rapidly, so they stop growing at an early age and may be short as adults. A recently developed synthetic hormone (LHRH) is useful in halting this type of early sexual development and allowing additional growth. Studies are underway to determine if the addition of growth hormone to this regimen increases adult height of children with sexual precocity.

Sometimes a tumor or disease of the ovaries, adrenal glands, pituitary gland, or brain will cause premature sexual development. In these cases, removal of the tumor or treatment of the disease may interrupt the rapid sexual development and result in increased adult height.

Thyroid Hormone Deficiency

Hormone deficiencies may cause growth failure in addition to other problems. A child with thyroid hormone deficiency has slow growth and is physically and mentally sluggish. Hypothyroidism, or lack of thyroid hormone, may be present at birth or develop anytime during childhood or later in life. It is very important to treat hypothyroidism promptly, especially if it occurs during the rapid growth period of infancy. Untreated hypothyroidism during this time can cause permanent damage to sensitive, rapidly growing brain cells. Thyroid hormone deficiency is easy to diagnose with a simple blood test and easy to treat with a daily pill that replaces the missing thyroid hormone. With early diagnosis and continuous treatment, these children grow and develop normally.

Growth Hormone Deficiency

Although many hormones work together to stimulate normal growth, growth hormone is one of the most important. It is produced by a bean-sized gland called the pituitary, which is located beneath a special part of the brain (hypothalamus) in the middle of the skull. The pituitary gland makes other hormones that stimulate other glands, so it is sometimes called the master gland. Pituitary abnormalities can cause a number of problems that result in poor growth: hypothyroidism, discussed earlier, may result from a pituitary malfunction, as may hypercortisolism (excess stress hormone). Growth hormone deficiency may result from abnormal formation of the pituitary gland or hypothalamus, or damage to one of these areas occurring during or after birth.

Children with growth hormone deficiency grow slowly, but have normal body proportions. Without treatment, few would reach 5 feet in height as adults. A variety of tests may be necessary to diagnose this condition. A child with growth hormone deficiency also may be missing other pituitary hormones, (thyroid, adrenal or stress hormones, sex hormones). All hormones must be present in the proper balance for normal growth to occur, so these hormones must be replaced if they are missing. Biosynthetic human growth hormone, produced by recombinant DNA technology, is available for the treatment of growth hormone deficiency. Children who are diagnosed promptly and respond well to treatment can expect to reach normal adult height.

Abnormal Tall Stature

Most tall children have tall parents and are healthy and normal, but there are some medical conditions that cause abnormal tall stature and rapid growth. A small tumor in the pituitary gland may cause too much growth hormone to be secreted, resulting in unusually fast growth and tall stature. Growth hormone excess (also called acromegaly) may be treated with medication or with surgical removal of the tumor. Some genetic conditions cause abnormal tall stature; Marfan's syndrome and Klinefelter's syndrome are two examples. These syndromes are associated with distinctive physical traits in addition to tall stature. Precocious puberty, discussed earlier, results in tall stature during childhood, although early closure of the growth plates results in short adult height.

Tall children, like short children, may stand out from their classmates and experience stress and teasing because of their size. They often look older than they are, so adults may expect too much of them. It is important for parents and teachers to be aware of the stress these children may experience as a result of looking different from their peers.

Summary

These are many causes of slow growth. Some are temporary and merely variations of normal growth patterns, and others are inherited or associated with other physical problems. These require evaluation by a doctor who can differentiate among various types of growth problems. A rule of thumb for parents who suspect a growth problem in their child is that any child who grows less than two inches a year after their second birthday should be seen by a physician. One of the most important things a parent can do to safeguard a child's growth and general health is to have the child examined and measured regularly by a pediatrician, family doctor, or other qualified health care provider.

Many of the conditions associated with short stature or abnormal growth can be treated. Researchers are working on developing better methods of diagnosing and treating many types of growth problems. Even though no treatment exists for some of these conditions, there are many ways a child and family may benefit from thorough evaluation of the situation. Doctors, nurses, psychologists, social workers and other professionals can work together to assist children with growth problems and their families in setting and attaining appropriate physical, emotional, and educational goals.

Chapter 8

An Overview of Physical and Mental Developmental Stages

Chapter Contents

Section 8.1

Early Childhood

Excerpted and reprinted with permission from: Green M, Palfrey JS, eds. 2002. *Bright Futures: Guidelines for Health Supervision of Infants, Children, and Adolescents*, (2nd ed., rev.) Arlington Va.: National Center for Education in Material and Child Health. This version of the text was reviewed and updated in November 2002 by Dr. David A. Cooke, MD, Diplomate, American Board of Internal Medicine.

The one-year-old who is well cared for has a secure sense of attachment to his important caregivers, is developing an expanded capacity to communicate through sounds and gestures, and can navigate by cruising, perhaps by taking a few steps alone or, if necessary, by dropping to all fours and crawling with great speed.

At the beginning of this developmental period, a child's understanding of the world of people and objects is bound by what he can see, hear, feel, and manipulate physically. By the end of early childhood, the process of thinking moves beyond the here and now to incorporate the use of mental symbols and the development of fantasy. For the infant, mobility is a goal to be mastered. For the healthy young child, it is a mechanism for exploration and increasing independence. The one-year-old is beginning to use the art of imitation in his repetition of familiar sounds and physical gestures. The five-year-old has mastered most of the complex rules of his native language, and can communicate thoughts and ideas effectively.

The toddler stands on the threshold of the process of separation and individuation from his primary caregivers who nurtured and protected him during his early months. By the end of early childhood, the well-adjusted child, having internalized the security of early bonds, pursues new relationships outside of the family as an individual in his own right. Understanding and respecting this evolving independence is an important parental challenge.

The healthy toddler has been immunized against diphtheria, tetanus, pertussis, polio, measles, mumps, rubella, *Haemophilus influenza* type B, hepatitis B, and varicella. His growth and development have been monitored, and adequate nutrition has been ensured through dietary supervision and supplemental vitamins, fluoride, and iron when necessary. By the end of early childhood, some children have had to contend with significant disease or disability, and virtually all have experienced the common nonpreventable early childhood illnesses. As a consequence, each child learns the difference between health/well-being and illness/discomfort.

Physical Development

The chubby, pot-bellied infant who tripled his birth weight in the first year of life slows his rate of gain significantly. The active toddler sheds his baby fat and straightens his posture. His physical strength, coordination, and dexterity all improve dramatically. The cautious and tentative walker becomes the reckless runner, climber, and jumper. As a fearless and tireless explorer and experimenter, the toddler is vulnerable to injury, but appropriate adult supervision can ensure an environment that balances safety with the freedom to take controlled risks.

The range of physical abilities among young children during this age period is considerable. Some are endowed with natural grace and agility; others demonstrate less fine tuning in their physical prowess, yet they get the job done.

Parents and other caregivers can encourage young children's independence in eating by serving a nutritionally well-balanced selection of foods and allowing children to choose what and how much to eat. Good oral health is a part of the child's well-being. Early counseling on feeding practice is the essential first step. Regular dental visits, access to fluoride, and healthy nutrition and snacking practices can lead to the prevention of dental decay.

Although parents and other primary caregivers, including providers of child care services, have considerable control over the environment in which a young child is raised, the community also plays an important role. Children with access to safe play areas in a neighborhood free of violence have opportunities for the protected risk taking that is important during this developmental period. For those who grow up in the presence of physical and emotional dangers, the risk for harm is high.

Cognitive and Linguistic Development

Young children learn through play. If the toddler experienced the security of a nurturing and reliable source of protection and attachment during infancy, he now has a strong base from which to explore the world. The egocentricity of the young child is related less to a sense of selfishness than to a cognitive inability to see things from the perspective of others.

Young children live largely in a world of magic in which they often have difficulty differentiating what is real from what is make-believe. Some have imaginary friends. Many engage in elaborate fantasy play. Learning to identify the boundaries between fantasy and reality, and developing an elementary ability to think logically, are among the more important developmental tasks of this age period.

Caregivers need to provide a safe laboratory for these young scientists to conduct their research. Children need access to a variety of tools and experiences. They need opportunities to learn through trial and error, as well as through planned effort. Their seemingly endless string of repetitive questions can test the limits of the most patient parent. These queries, however, must be acknowledged and responded to in a manner that not only provides answers but also validates and reinforces the child's burgeoning curiosity.

Social, Emotional, and Behavioral Development

During the dynamic years from age one to five, children develop an emerging sense of themselves as individuals who live in families, as well as within larger social systems. Building on the secure and trusting relationships established in the first year of life, and venturing beyond the parallel play of toddlers, the maturing young child establishes an expanding network of friends and acquaintances.

The culture of the family and that of the community provide a framework within which the socialization process unfolds. The increasingly self-conscious young child grapples with such complex issues as gender roles, peer and/or sibling competition, and the difference between right and wrong. The temperamental differences that were manifested in the feeding, sleeping, and self-regulatory behaviors of the infant are transformed into the varied styles of coping and adaptation demonstrated by the young child. Some young children appear to think before they act; others are impetuous. Some children are slow to warm up while others operate on a very short fuse. Some accept limits and rules with more equanimity than others. The range of normal behavior is broad and highly dependent upon the match between the child's and the caregiver's styles. Aggression, acting out, excessive risk taking, and antisocial behaviors are common. Caregivers need to respond with a variety of interventions that set constructive limits and help children achieve self-discipline. Ultimately, healthy social and emotional development depend on how children view themselves and the extent to which they feel valued by others.

Healthy Behavior

As young children identify with their parents, caregivers, and other important role models, they internalize a wide range of lifestyle attributes. They can benefit from the exhilaration of regular physical exercise and the joy of laughter shared with family and friends. Meals may be a pleasurable opportunity for nutrition and social interaction, or the focus of family conflict amidst the hurried ingestion of high-fat snacks. Well-monitored, selective television viewing may be an appropriate form of education and entertainment; conversely, television can be a constant source of passive diversion, background noise, and exposure to violence.

When faced with adversity or stress, young children may be taught both healthy and unhealthy coping strategies, ranging from denial or retreat to active mastery. During a period when the power of role models and the process of identification are strong, young children incorporate salient features of the lifestyles of those who are most important in their lives. Good health supervision, a collaborative process that involves parents and professionals, can serve as a significant protective factor. In addition, health supervision can contribute to individual autonomy and a growing sense of personal competence and mastery, while enhancing positive interpersonal interactions and the development of rich human relationships.

Table 8.1. Childhood Developmental Chart (*continued on next page*)

Achievements during Early Childhood

- Regular sleeping habits.
- Independence in eating.
- Completion of toilet training.
- Ability to dress and undress.
- Ability to separate from parents.
- Progression from parallel to interactive play and sharing.
- Warm relationship and good communication with parents and siblings.
- Clear communication of needs and wishes.
- Expression of feelings such as joy, anger, sadness, and frustration.
- Self-comforting behavior.
- Self-discipline.
- Intelligible speech.
- Positive self-image.
- Demonstrates curiosity and initiative.
- Asks frequent questions.
- Demonstrates imaginative, make-believe, and dress-up play

Tasks for the Child in Early Childhood

- Learn good eating habits.
- Practice good dental hygiene.
- Participate in physical games and play.
- Develop autonomy, independence, and assertiveness.
- Respond to limit-setting and discipline.
- Learn self-quieting behaviors and self-discipline.
- Learn appropriate self-care.
- Make friends and meet new people.
- Play with and relate well to siblings and peers.
- Learn to understand and use language to meet needs.
- Listen to stories.
- Limit television viewing.

Table 8.1. Childhood Developmental Chart (*continued*)

Achievements during Middle Childhood

- Responsibility for good health habits.
- Ability to play in groups.
- One or more close friendships.
- Identification with peer groups.
- Competence as member of family, community, and other groups.
- Ability to express feelings.
- Belief in capacity for success.
- Understanding of right and wrong.
- Awareness of safety rules.
- Ability to read, write, and communicate increasingly complex and creative thoughts.
- Responsibility for homework.
- School achievement

Tasks for the Child in Middle Childhood

- Maintain good eating habits.
- Practice good dental hygiene.
- Participate in athletic or exercise programs.
- Maintain appropriate weight.
- Wear bicycle helmet, seat belt, and contact sports mouth guard.
- Avoid alcohol, tobacco, and other drugs.
- Resist peer pressure to engage in risk-taking behaviors.
- Control impulses.
- Resolve conflict and manage anger constructively.
- Assume responsibility for belongings, chores, and good health habits.
- Play with and relate well to siblings and peers.
- Communicate well with parents, teachers, and other adults.
- Be industrious in school

Excerpted and reprinted with permission from: Green M, Palfrey JS, eds. 2002. *Bright Futures: Guidelines for Health Supervision of Infants, Children, and Adolescents*, (2nd ed., rev.) Arlington Va.: National Center for Education in Material and Child Health.

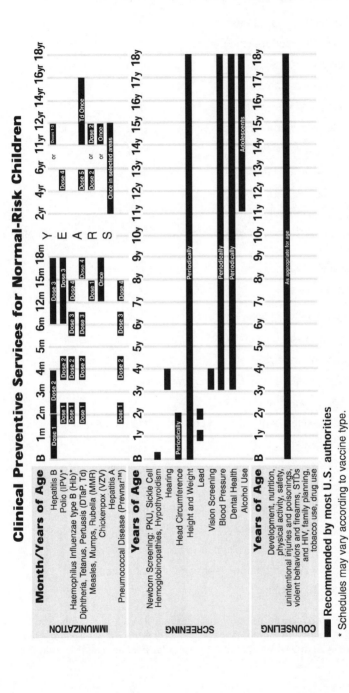

Figure 8.1. *Child Preventive Care Timeline. The information on immunizations is based on recommendations issued by the Advisory Committee on Immunization Practices, the American Academy of Pediatrics, and the American Academy of Family Physicians. (Source: Child Health Guide, Put Prevention Into Practice, Agency for Healthcare Research and Quality, 1998.)*

Section 8.2

Middle Childhood

From "Childhood Years: Ages Six through Twelve," by Karen DeBord, Ph.D., Associate Professor and Extension Child Development Specialist, North Carolina State University. © 1996. Reprinted with permission. Reviewed and updated in November 2002 by Dr. David A. Cooke, MD, Diplomate, American Board of Internal Medicine.

When they start school, children enter middle childhood and remain there until they reach adolescence. This text will help parents and other adults look at the general characteristics of children ages 6–12, consider special concerns of parents and caregivers, and give practical tips.

Overview

Between the ages of 6 and 12, the child's world expands outward from the family as relationships are formed with friends, teachers, coaches, caregivers, and others. Because their experiences are expanding, many factors can alter children's actions and impact how they learn to get along. Some situations can create stress and affect self-esteem. The middle childhood period is a time to prepare for adolescence.

Children develop at various rates. Some children in middle childhood seem very mature while others seem very immature. During this stage, behavior may depend on the child's mood, his or her experience with various types of people, or even what happened that day.

Parental Concerns

Parents with children in middle childhood may begin to re-evaluate what kind of parent they have been up to this point. With children entering school, parents may be wondering if their child has what it takes to make it and succeed. Up to this point, children have always looked up to parents as the source of information, but now children judge parents more and label their actions differently. Parents struggle with how to support their children's independence while understanding the child's new connections with others (friends and teachers). With children's natural curiosity and expanding knowledge, parents often find children question them more, and they are asked to respond in greater detail to larger issues, such as why they must work overtime, why some people act unfairly, or even why there is war. Children continually struggle to understand new information that is difficult to understand.

In middle childhood, children typically spend less time with their families and parents, and families spend less time in caretaking, reading, talking, teaching, and playing. Less monitoring and fewer verbal cues are needed, particularly for routine tasks (such as baths or brushing teeth).

As children get older, behavior can be managed with verbal reasoning, deprivation of privileges, appeals to child's sense of humor, or reminders of the consequences of his or her actions.

In addition to typical development, daily life challenges are normal. For example, most children will attend school. With school comes many transitions. Being afraid of new situations or feeling peer pressure are predictable stressors. Other stressors are not as predictable. Any disruption of what is considered normal for the child causes stress.

Developmental Aspects of Middle Childhood

Social and Emotional Development

- There are signs of growing independence. Children are becoming so worldly that they typically test their growing knowledge with back talk and rebellion.

- Common fears include the unknown, failure, death, family problems, and rejection.

- Friends may live in the same neighborhood and are most commonly the same sex.

- Children average five best friends and at least one enemy, who often changes from day to day.

- Children act nurturing and commanding with younger children but follow and depend on older children.

- Children are beginning to see the point of view of others more clearly.

- Children define themselves in terms of their appearance, possessions, and activities.

- There are fewer angry outbursts and more ability to endure frustration while accepting delays in getting things they want.

- Children often resolve conflict through peer judges who accept or reject their actions.

- Children are self-conscious and feel as if everyone notices even small differences (new haircut, facial hair, a hug in public from a parent).

- Tattling is a common way to attract adult attention in the early years of middle childhood.

- Inner control is being formed and practiced each time decisions are made.

- Around age 6–8, children may still be afraid of monsters and the dark. These are replaced later by fears of school or disaster and confusion over social relationships.

- To win, lead, or to be first is valued. Children try to be the boss and are unhappy if they lose.

- Children often are attached to adults (teacher, club leader, caregiver) other than their parents and will quote their new hero or try to please him or her to gain attention.

- Early in middle childhood, good and bad days are defined as what is approved or disapproved by the family.

- Children's feelings get hurt easily. There are mood swings, and children often don't know how to deal with failure.

Physical Development

- Growth is slower than in preschool years, but steady. Eating may fluctuate with activity level. Some children have growth spurts in the later stages of middle childhood.

- In the later stages of middle childhood, body changes (hips widen, breasts bud, pubic hair appears, testes develop) indicate approaching puberty.

- Children recognize that there are differences between boys and girls.

- Children find difficulty balancing high energy activities and quiet activities.

- Intense activity may bring tiredness. Children need around 10 hours of sleep each night.

- Muscle coordination and control are uneven and incomplete in the early stages, but children become almost as coordinated as adults by the end of middle childhood.

- Small muscles develop rapidly, making playing musical instruments, hammering, or building things more enjoyable.

- Baby teeth will come out and permanent ones will come in.

- Permanent teeth may come in before the mouth has fully grown, causing dental crowding.

- Eyes reach maturity in both size and function.

- The added strain of school work (smaller print, computers, intense writing) often creates eye-tension and leads some children to request eye examinations.

Mental Development

- Children can begin to think about their own behavior and see consequences for actions. In the early stages of concrete thinking, they can group things that belong together (for instance babies, fathers, mothers, aunts are all family members). As children near adolescence, they master sequencing and ordering, which are needed for math skills.

- Children begin to read and write early in middle childhood and should be skillful in reading and writing by the end of this stage.

- They can think through their actions and trace back events that happened to explain situations, such as why they were late to school.

- Children learn best if they are active while they are learning. For example, children will learn more effectively about traffic safety by moving cars, blocks, and toy figures rather than sitting and listening to an adult explain the rules.

- Six- to 8-year-olds can rarely sit for longer than 15–20 minutes for an activity. Attention span gets longer with age.

- Toward the beginning of middle childhood, children may begin projects but finish few. Allow them to explore new materials. Nearing adolescence, children will focus more on completion.

- Teachers set the conditions for social interactions to occur in schools. Understand that children need to experience various friendships while building esteem.

- Children can talk through problems to solve them. This requires more adult time and more sustained attention by children.

- Children can focus attention and take time to search for needed information.

- They can develop a plan to meet a goal.

- There is greater memory capability because many routines (brushing teeth, tying shoes, bathing, etc.) are automatic now.

- Child begins to build a self-image as a worker. If encouraged, this is positive in later development of career choices.

- Many children want to find a way to earn money.

Moral Development

Moral development is more difficult to discuss in terms of developmental milestones. Moral development occurs over time through experience. Research implies that if a child knows what is right, he or she will do what is right. Even as adults, we know that there are often gray areas when it comes to making tough decisions about right and wrong. There are a lot of it depends responses depending on the particular situation.

Most adults agree that they should act in a caring manner and show others they care about them. People want to come into contact with others who will reinforce them for who they are. It is no different for children. To teach responsible and caring behaviors, adults must first model caring behaviors with young children as they do with other adults. While modeling, focus on talking with children. This does not mean talking at children but discussing with them in an open-ended way. Work to create an air of learning and a common search for understanding, empathy, and appreciation. Dialogue can be playful, serious, imaginative, or goal oriented. It can also provide the opportunity to question why. This is the foundation for caring for others.

Next, practice caring for others. Adults need to find ways to increase the capacity to care. Adults generally spend time telling children what to do or teaching facts. There is little time to use the newly developed higher order thinking and to practice caring interactions and deeds.

The last step to complete the cycle of caring is confirmation. Confirmation is encouraging the best in others. A trusted adult who identifies something admirable and encourages the development of that trait can go a long way toward helping children find their place in this world. Love, caring, and positive relations play central roles in ethics and moral education.

Practical Advice for All Adults Working with Children in Middle Childhood

Social and Emotional Development

- Encourage non-competitive games, particularly toward the beginning of middle childhood, and help children set individual goals.

- Give children lots of positive attention and let them help define the rules.

- Talk about self-control and making good decisions. Talk about why it is important to be patient, share, and respect others' rights. Adults must pick battles carefully so there is limited nagging and maximized respect while children build confidence in their ability to make decisions.

- Teach them to learn from criticism. Ask, "how could you do that differently next time?"

- Always be alert to the feelings associated with what children tell you.

- Give children positive feedback for successes.

Physical Development

- It is important to help children feel proud of who they are and what they can do. Avoid stereotyping girls into particular activities and boys into others. Let both genders choose from a range of activities.

- Encourage children to balance their activities between high energy and quiet activity. Children release tension through play. Children may be extremely active when tired. Encourage quiet reading, painting, puzzles, or board games before bedtime.

- Regular dental and physical check-ups are an important part of monitoring a child's growth and development. This allows parents to screen for potential problems. If a child accidentally loses a permanent tooth, finding the tooth and taking it and the child to the dentist may save the permanent tooth.

Mental Development

Rapid mental growth creates many of the positive as well as negative interactions between children and adults during middle childhood. Some of the ways adults can help children continue to develop their thinking skills are:

- Adults can ask "what if..." or "how could we solve this" questions to help children develop problem-solving skills.

- Reading signs, making lists, and counting prices are all exercises to practice sequencing skills.

- Asking children if you can help them think about ways to talk with other children can provide limited guidance as they negotiate social relationships.

- Picking focused times to talk—without distractions—allows adults and children to converse and listen.

Reflections

Each stage in life is a time of growth. Middle childhood is a time to bridge dependence with approaching independence. The time of wonder and spontaneity is fading, replaced by feeling self-conscious and on guard. The new ways children act are ways they are exploring their future potential. Some behaviors will pass, but they must be experienced in order for the child to grow and be ready to face the stage of finding his or her identity during adolescence.

Television

A few cautions about TV: Too little physical activity can affect weight in children. Too many aggressive acts on TV can affect mood and actions, and children can begin to think that what they see on TV is the norm. Limiting the amount of television watched and monitoring what is watched can help parents assure that the TV that is seen relates to their family's values.

Self-Care

There is no magic age at which a child is ready to be left alone. Parents should consider carefully the child's willingness to be left alone, the child's day to day responsibility, the child's ability to anticipate and avoid unsafe situations.

Chores

Children want to feel useful and have a sense that they are contributing to the family. To help children learn household responsibilities, parents might allow children to choose from a list of chores. Paid chores should be in addition to what is generally expected. For example: brushing teeth, taking a bath, and keeping a room clean may be expected. Drying dishes, putting away folded clothes, or emptying trash cans may be chores that earn allowance and contribute to the family.

Money becomes more important since children now understand how it is valued in our society. Earning an allowance is a two-way agreement; children do agreed upon work with little reminders in exchange for agreed upon money or goods. Charts with pictures to check-off chores help children remember what to do. The older children get, the more capable they are, but remember to choose age-appropriate duties.

Chapter 9

Communication Concerns

Chapter Contents

Section 9.1

Speech and Language: Developmental Milestones

National Institute on Deafness and Other Communication Disorders (NIDCD), National Institutes of Health (NIH), NIH Pub. No. 00-4781, http://www.nidcd.nih.gov/health/parents/speechandlanguage.htm, April 2000.

What Are Speech and Language?

Speech and language are tools that humans use to communicate or share thoughts, ideas, and emotions. Language is the set of rules, shared by the individuals who are communicating, that allows them to exchange those thoughts, ideas, or emotions. Speech is talking, one way that a language can be expressed. Language may also be expressed through writing, signing, or even gestures in the case of people who have neurological disorders and may depend upon eye blinks or mouth movements to communicate.

While there are many languages in the world, each includes its own set of rules for phonology (phonemes or speech sounds or, in the case of signed language, handshapes), morphology (word formation), syntax (sentence formation), semantics (word and sentence meaning), prosody (intonation and rhythm of speech), and pragmatics (effective use of language).

How Do Speech and Language Normally Develop?

The most intensive period of speech and language development for humans is during the first three years of life, a period when the brain is developing and maturing. These skills appear to develop best in a world that is rich with sounds, sights, and consistent exposure to the speech and language of others.

There is increasing evidence suggesting that there are "critical periods" for speech and language development in infants and young children. This means that the developing brain is best able to absorb a language, any language, during this period. The ability to learn a

114

language will be more difficult, and perhaps less efficient or effective, if these critical periods are allowed to pass without early exposure to a language. The beginning signs of communication occur during the first few days of life when an infant learns that a cry will bring food, comfort, and companionship. The newborn also begins to recognize important sounds in his or her environment. The sound of a parent's voice can be one important sound. As they grow, infants begin to sort out the speech sounds (phonemes) or building blocks that compose the words of their language. Research has shown that by six months of age, most children recognize the basic sounds of their native language.

As the speech mechanism (jaw, lips, and tongue) and voice mature, an infant is able to make controlled sound. This begins in the first few months of life with "cooing," a quiet, pleasant, repetitive vocalization. By six months of age, an infant usually babbles or produces repetitive syllables such as "ba, ba, ba" or "da, da, da." Babbling soon turns into a type of nonsense speech (jargon) that often has the tone and cadence of human speech but does not contain real words. By the end of their first year, most children have mastered the ability to say a few simple words. Children are most likely unaware of the meaning of their first words, but soon learn the power of those words as others respond to them.

By eighteen months of age, most children can say eight to ten words. By age two, most are putting words together in crude sentences such as "more milk." During this period, children rapidly learn that words symbolize or represent objects, actions, and thoughts. At this age they also engage in representational or pretend play. At ages three, four, and five, a child's vocabulary rapidly increases, and he or she begins to master the rules of language.

What Are Speech and Language Developmental Milestones?

Children vary in their development of speech and language. There is, however, a natural progression or "timetable" for mastery of these skills for each language. The milestones are identifiable skills that can serve as a guide to normal development. Typically, simple skills need to be reached before the more complex skills can be learned. There is a general age and time when most children pass through these periods. These milestones help doctors and other health professionals determine when a child may need extra help to learn to speak or to use language.

How Do I Know If My Child Is Reaching the Milestones?

Here is a checklist that you can follow to determine if your child's speech and language skills are developing on schedule.

Birth to 5 Months

- reacts to loud sounds
- turns head toward a sound source
- watches your face when you speak
- vocalizes pleasure and displeasure sounds (laughs, giggles, cries, or fusses)
- makes noise when talked to

6–11 Months

- understands "no-no"
- babbles (says "ba-ba-ba" or "ma-ma-ma")
- tries to communicate by actions or gestures
- tries to repeat your sounds

12–17 Months

- attends to a book or toy for about two minutes
- follows simple directions accompanied by gestures
- answers simple questions nonverbally
- points to objects, pictures, and family members
- says two to three words to label a person or object (pronunciation may not be clear)
- tries to imitate simple words

18–23 Months

- enjoys being read to
- follows simple commands without gestures
- points to simple body parts such as "nose"

- understands simple verbs such as "eat" and "sleep"
- correctly pronounces most vowels and n, m, p, h, especially in the beginning of syllables and short words. Also begins to use other speech sounds
- says 8 to 10 words (pronunciation may still be unclear)
- asks for common foods by name
- makes animal sounds such as "moo"
- starting to combine words such as "more milk"
- begins to use pronouns such as "mine"

2–3 Years

- knows about 50 words at 24 months
- knows some spatial concepts such as "in" and "on"
- knows pronouns such as "you," "me," and "her"
- knows descriptive words such as "big," "happy"
- says around 40 words at 24 months
- speech is becoming more accurate but may still leave off ending sounds. Strangers may not be able to understand much of what is said.
- answers simple questions
- begins to use more pronouns such as "you" and "I"
- speaks in two to three word phrases
- uses question inflection to ask for something (for example, "My ball?")
- begins to use plurals such as "shoes" or "socks" and regular past tense verbs such as "jumped"

3–4 Years

- groups objects such as foods, clothes, etc.
- identifies colors
- uses most speech sounds but may distort some of the more difficult sounds such as l, r, s, sh, ch, y, v, z, th. These sounds may not be fully mastered until age 7 or 8.

- uses consonants in the beginning, middle, and ends of words. Some of the more difficult consonants may be distorted, but attempts to say them.
- strangers are able to understand much of what is said
- able to describe the use of objects such as "fork," "car," etc.
- has fun with language. Enjoys poems and recognizes language absurdities such as, "Is that an elephant on your head?"
- expresses ideas and feelings rather than just talking about the world around him or her
- uses verbs that end in "ing," such as "walking" and "talking"
- answers simple questions such as "What do you do when you are hungry?"
- repeats sentences

4–5 Years

- understands spatial concepts such as "behind" and "next to"
- understands complex questions
- speech is understandable but makes mistakes pronouncing long, difficult, or complex words such as "hippopotamus"
- says about 200–300 different words
- uses some irregular past tense verbs such as "ran" and "fell"
- describes how to do things such as painting a picture
- defines words
- lists items that belong in a category such as animals, vehicles, etc.
- answers "why" questions

5 Years

- understands more than 2,000 words
- understands time sequences (what happened first, second, third, etc.)
- carries out a series of three directions
- understands rhyming
- engages in conversation

- sentences can be 8 or more words in length
- uses compound and complex sentences
- describes objects
- uses imagination to create stories

What Should I Do If My Child's Speech or Language Appears to Be Delayed?

You should talk to your family doctor if you have any concerns about your child's speech or language development. The above checklist should help you talk about your concerns. Your doctor may decide to refer you to a speech-language pathologist, a health professional trained to evaluate and treat people who have speech, language, voice, or swallowing disorders that affect their ability to communicate. The speech-language pathologist will talk to you about your child's communication and general development. He or she will also evaluate your child with special speech and language tests. A hearing test is often included in the evaluation because a hearing problem can affect speech and language development.

Depending upon the test results, the speech-language pathologist may suggest activities for home to stimulate speech and language development. These activities may include reading to your child regularly; speaking in short sentences using simple words so that your child can successfully imitate you; or repeating what your child says, using correct grammar or pronunciation. For example, if your child says, "Ball baybo" you can respond with, "Yes, the ball is under the table." This allows you to demonstrate more accurate speech and language without actually "correcting" your child which can eventually make speaking unpleasant for him or her.

The speech-language pathologist may also recommend group or individual therapy or suggest further evaluation by other health professionals such as an audiologist, a health care professional who is trained to identify and measure hearing loss, or a developmental psychologist.

What Research Is Being Conducted on Developmental Speech and Language Problems?

Scientists are examining a variety of issues related to speech and language development. Brain imaging studies are defining the relationship between exposure to speech and language, brain development,

119

and communication skills. Genetic studies are investigating the likelihood that at least some speech and language problems may be inherited or passed down from parents to their children. Additional studies are characterizing inherited communication disorders. The effect of frequent ear infections on the development of speech and language is also an area of investigation. Other scientists are distinguishing types of speech and language errors to determine which ones may be overcome by maturation alone and which will need some type of intervention or therapy. Another area of study is the effect of speech and language development on later school performance. Further research is characterizing dialects that belong to certain ethnic or regional groups. This knowledge will help professionals distinguish a language difference or dialect (which should be preserved to help an individual identify with a group) from a language disorder, which may require treatment.

Section 9.2

Evaluation and Treatment of Speech-Language Delays and Disorders

How Is the Evaluation Done?

Evaluation may be formal or informal and include any combination of standardized tests; direct observation of play and interaction with caregivers; report by parent, teacher, or physician; and collection and detailed analysis of spontaneous speech samples. Several sessions as well as ongoing evaluation may be required to obtain enough information to make an accurate diagnosis.

The early identification team may consist of the speech-language pathologist, audiologist, psychologist, neurologist, electrophysiologist, otolaryngologist, pediatrician, nurse, and social worker. Because speech-language delays and disorders may be due to a variety of causes, each professional makes valuable contributions to the evaluation.

What Is Speech-Language Treatment?

From the result of the evaluation, certain services may be recommended. Prevention includes those children who have been identified as at-risk for a communication delay or disorder, for example, due to low birth weight. Services are provided before a specific diagnosis has been made. Remediation increases function in areas identified as delayed or disabling and may serve to prevent other related problems. For example, remediation of a language disorder can help to offset learning difficulties. Compensation enables the child and the family to make adjustments for limitations, as in some cases of cerebral palsy.

Language is taught in a natural setting. It is presented at the child's developmental level; responses are consistently stimulated; and output is rewarded. Play may be used to teach communication, language models or rules of conversation, such as turn taking. Feeding and swallowing treatment may be needed to sustain life. It can also be used to encourage speech-like movements, stimulate sound production, or increase the child's awareness of speech movements.

If you are concerned about a possible speech-language delay or disability, consult a speech-language pathologist.

Questions for Consumers to Ask

- Are all of your speech-language pathologists and audiologists certified and licensed?

- What age groups do you work with?

- Do you work primarily with particular speech, language, or hearing disorders? What are they?

- How soon can I be seen for an evaluation?

- Once I am evaluated, is there a waiting list for treatment? If so, how long is it?

- Do I need to be referred to your program by a particular source such as a community agency?

- Once I have been evaluated, will you be able to anticipate the amount of time needed to treat my problem?

- How much do you charge?

- Will my insurance pay for the evaluation? For some or all of the treatment?

- If you cannot work with me, who would you suggest I contact?

Section 9.3

Stuttering

National Institute on Deafness and Other Communication Disorders (NIDCD), National Institutes of Health (NIH), NIH Pub. No. 97-4232, http://www.nidcd.nih.gov/health/pubs_vsl/stutter.htm, August 1997. Reviewed 2002.

Introduction

Stuttering is a speech disorder in which the normal flow of speech is disrupted by frequent repetitions or prolongations of speech sounds, syllables or words or by an individual's inability to start a word. The speech disruptions may be accompanied by rapid eye blinks, tremors of the lips and/or jaw, or other struggle behaviors of the face or upper body that a person who stutters may use in an attempt to speak. Certain situations, such as speaking before a group of people or talking on the telephone, tend to make stuttering more severe, whereas other situations, such as singing or speaking alone, often improve fluency.

Stuttering may also be referred to as stammering, especially in England, and by a broader term, disfluent speech. Stuttering is different from two additional speech fluency disorders, cluttering (characterized by a rapid, irregular speech) and spasmodic dysphonia, a voice disorder.

How Is Speech Normally Produced?

Speech is normally produced through a series of precisely coordinated muscle movements involving respiration (the breathing mechanism), phonation (the voicing mechanism) and articulation (throat, palate, tongue, lips, and teeth). These muscle movements are initiated, coordinated, and controlled by the brain and monitored through the senses of hearing and touch.

Before speaking, an individual takes a breath and the vocal folds (or vocal cords), which are two bands of muscular tissue located in the voice box directly above the trachea or windpipe, must come together. The air that is held in the lungs is gradually released, passing through the gently closed vocal folds thus causing vibration and producing the voice. The sound of the voice is passed through the throat and is directed into the mouth for most speech sounds, or into the nose for nasal sounds such as "m," "n," and "ng." The palate, tongue, jaw, and lips move in precise ways to modify the sounds in order to make speech sounds.

Who Stutters?

It is estimated that over three million Americans stutter. Stuttering affects individuals of all ages but occurs most frequently in young children between the ages of 2 and 6 who are developing language. Boys are three times more likely to stutter than girls. Most children, however, outgrow their stuttering, and it is estimated that less than 1 percent of adults stutter.

Many individuals who stutter have become successful in careers that require public speaking. The list of individuals includes Winston Churchill, actress Marilyn Monroe, actors James Earl Jones, Bruce Willis, and Jimmy Stewart, and singers Carly Simon and Mel Tillis, to name only a few.

What Causes Stuttering?

Scientists suspect a variety of causes. There is reason to believe that many forms of stuttering are genetically determined. The precise mechanisms causing stuttering are not understood.

The most common form of stuttering is thought to be developmental, that is, it is occurring in children who are in the process of developing speech and language. This relaxed type of stuttering is felt to occur when a child's speech and language abilities are unable to meet his or her verbal demands. Stuttering happens when the child searches for the correct word. Developmental stuttering is usually outgrown.

Another common form of stuttering is neurogenic. Neurogenic disorders arise from signal problems between the brain and nerves or muscles. In neurogenic stuttering, the brain is unable to coordinate adequately the different components of the speech mechanism. Neurogenic stuttering may also occur following a stroke or other type of brain injury.

Other forms of stuttering are classified as psychogenic or originating in the mind or mental activity of the brain such as thought and reasoning. Whereas at one time the major cause of stuttering was thought to be psychogenic, this type of stuttering is now known to account for only a minority of the individuals who stutter. Although individuals who stutter may develop emotional problems such as fear of meeting new people or speaking on the telephone, these problems often result from stuttering rather than causing the stuttering. Psychogenic stuttering occasionally occurs in individuals who have some types of mental illness or individuals who have experienced severe mental stress or anguish.

Scientists and clinicians have long known that stuttering may run in families and that there is a strong possibility that some forms of stuttering are, in fact, hereditary. No gene or genes for stuttering, however, have yet been found.

How Is Stuttering Diagnosed?

Stuttering is generally diagnosed by a speech-language pathologist, a professional who is specially trained to test and treat individuals with voice, speech and language disorders. The diagnosis is usually based on the history of the disorder, such as when it was first noticed and under what circumstances, as well as a complete evaluation of speech and language abilities.

How Is Stuttering Treated?

There are a variety of treatments available for stuttering. Any of the methods may improve stuttering to some degree, but there is at present no cure for stuttering. Stuttering therapy, however, may help prevent developmental stuttering from becoming a life-long problem. Therefore a speech evaluation is recommended for children who stutter for longer than six months or for those whose stuttering is accompanied by struggle behaviors.

Developmental stuttering is often treated by educating parents about restructuring the child's speaking environment to reduce the episodes of stuttering. Parents are often urged to:

- provide a relaxed home environment that provides ample opportunities for the child to speak. Setting aside specific times when the child and parent can speak free of distractions is often helpful.

- refrain from criticizing the child's speech or reacting negatively to the child's dysfluencies. Parents should avoid punishing the child for any dysfluencies or asking the child repeat stuttered words until they are spoken fluently.

- resist encouraging the child to perform verbally for people.

- listen attentively to the child when he or she speaks.

- speak slowly and in a relaxed manner. If a parent speaks this way, the child will often speak in the same slow, relaxed manner.

- wait for the child to say the intended word. Don't try to complete the child's thoughts.

- talk openly to the child about stuttering if he or she brings up the subject.

Many of the currently popular therapy programs for persistent stuttering focus on relearning how to speak or unlearning faulty ways of speaking. The psychological side effects of stuttering that often occur, such as fear of speaking to strangers or in public, are also addressed in most of these programs.

Other forms of therapy utilize interventions such as medications or electronic devices. Medications or drugs which affect brain function often have side effects that make them difficult to use for long-term treatment. Electronic devices which help an individual control fluency may be more of a bother than a help in most speaking situations and are often abandoned by individuals who stutter.

Unconventional methods of stuttering therapy also exist. It is always a good policy to check the credentials, experience, and goals of the person offering treatment. Avoid working with anyone who promises a "cure" for stuttering.

What Research Is Being Done about Stuttering?

Stuttering research is exploring ways to improve the diagnosis and treatment of stuttering as well as to identify its causes. Emphasis is being placed on improving the ability to determine which children will outgrow their stuttering and which children will stutter the rest of their lives. Stuttering characteristics are being examined to help identify groups of individuals who have similar types of stuttering and therefore may have a common cause. Research is also being conducted that will help locate the possible genes for the types of stuttering that tend to run in families. Modern medical tools such as PET (positron emission tomography) scans and functional MRI (magnetic resonance imaging) scans are offering insight into the brain organization of individuals who stutter. The effectiveness of different types of treatment are also being examined, and new treatments are being developed.

Chapter 10

Mental Health in Children

The future of our country depends on the mental health and strength of our young people. However, many children have mental health problems that interfere with normal development and functioning. A 1999 study estimated that almost 21 percent of U.S. children ages 9 to 17 had a diagnosable mental or addictive disorder that caused at least some impairment. When diagnostic criteria were limited to significant functional impairment, the estimate dropped to 11 percent. Moreover, in any given year, it is estimated that fewer than one in five of these youth receives needed treatment. Recent evidence compiled by the World Health Organization indicates that by the year 2020, childhood neuropsychiatric disorders will rise proportionately by over 50 percent, internationally, to become one of the five most common causes of morbidity, mortality, and disability among children. The mental health problems affecting children and adolescents include the following.

Depressive Disorders

Depressive disorders, which include *major depressive disorder, dysthymic disorder,* and *bipolar disorder,* adversely affect mood, energy, interest, sleep, appetite, and overall functioning. In contrast to

"Brief Notes on the Mental Health of Children and Adolescents," National Institute of Mental Health (NIMH), updated October 2002. For more information from NIMH visit their website at http://www.nimh.nih.gov.

the normal emotional experiences of sadness, feelings of loss, or passing mood states, symptoms of depressive disorders are extreme and persistent and can interfere significantly with a young person's ability to function at home, at school, and with peers. Researchers estimate that the prevalence of any form of depression among children and adolescents in the United States is more than 6 percent in a 6-month period, with almost 5 percent having major depressive disorder.

Major depressive disorder (major depression) is characterized by five or more of the following symptoms: persistent sad or irritable mood, loss of interest in activities once enjoyed, significant change in appetite or body weight, difficulty sleeping or oversleeping, psychomotor agitation or slowing, loss of energy, feelings of worthlessness or inappropriate guilt, difficulty concentrating, and recurrent thoughts of death or suicide. *Dysthymic disorder,* a typically less severe but more chronic form of depression, is diagnosed when depressed mood persists for at least 1 year in children and is accompanied by at least two other symptoms of depression (without meeting the criteria for major depression). Youth with dysthymic disorder are at risk for developing major depression.

Although *bipolar disorder* (manic-depressive illness) typically emerges in late adolescence or early adulthood, there is increasing evidence that this illness also can begin in childhood. According to one study, 1 percent of adolescents ages 14–18 were found to have met criteria for bipolar disorder or cyclothymia, a similar but less severe illness, in their lifetime. Bipolar disorder beginning in childhood or early adolescence may be a different, possibly more severe form of the illness than older adolescent- and adult-onset bipolar disorder. Research has revealed that when the illness begins before or soon after puberty, it is often characterized by a continuous, rapid-cycling, irritable, and mixed manic and depressive symptom state that may co-occur with disruptive behavior disorders, particularly attention deficit hyperactivity disorder (ADHD) or conduct disorder (CD), or may have features of these disorders as initial symptoms.

The manic symptoms of bipolar disorder in children and adolescents may include the following: either extremely irritable or overly silly and elated mood; overly inflated self-esteem; exaggerated beliefs about personal talents or abilities; increased energy; decreased need for sleep; increased talking; distractibility; increased sexual thoughts, feelings, behaviors, or use of explicit sexual language; increased goal-directed activity or physical agitation; and excessive involvement in risky behaviors or activities.

There is evidence that depressive disorders emerging early in life often continue into adulthood, and that early-onset depressive disorders may predict more severe illnesses in adult life. Diagnosis and treatment of depressive disorders in children and adolescents are critical for enabling young people with these illnesses to live up to their full potential.

Depressive disorders are associated with an increased risk of suicidal behavior. In 1999, suicide was the third leading cause of death in 15- to 24-year-olds, following unintentional injuries (#1) and homicide (#2), and the fourth leading cause of death among 10- to 14-year-olds. Early identification and treatment of depressive disorders in young people may play an important role in reducing or preventing suicidal behavior.

Both medication and specialized forms of psychotherapy are prescribed to treat depressive disorders in children and adolescents. Recent studies indicate that certain selective serotonin reuptake inhibitor (SSRI) medications are safe and efficacious treatments for major depression in young people. In addition, cognitive-behavioral therapy (CBT) has proven effective for treating depression in adolescents. The ongoing Treatment for Adolescents with Depression Study (TADS), funded by the National Institute of Mental Health (NIMH), is comparing the effectiveness of an SSRI medication, CBT, and their combination to determine the best approach for treating major depression in teenagers. Other studies are evaluating the effectiveness of different individual, family, and group psychotherapies for treating depressive disorders in young people.

At present, the treatment of bipolar disorder in children and adolescents is based mainly on experience with adults, since as yet there are limited data on the safety and efficacy of treatments for this disorder in young people. The essential treatment in adults involves the use of mood-stabilizing medications, typically lithium and/or valproate, which are often very effective for controlling mania and preventing recurrences of manic and depressive episodes. However, because medications may have different effects in children than they do in adults, they should be carefully monitored by a physician. For example, there is some evidence indicating that valproate may cause hormonal problems in teenage girls. Antidepressant medication, if needed, generally must be used together with a mood stabilizer, since antidepressants taken alone may induce manic symptoms or rapid cycling in people with bipolar disorder. Current NIMH-funded studies are attempting to fill the gaps in knowledge about treatments for bipolar disorder in children and adolescents.

129

Anxiety Disorders

Anxiety disorders, as a group, are the most common mental illnesses that occur in children and adolescents. Researchers estimate that the prevalence of any anxiety disorder among children and adolescents in the United States is 13 percent in a 6-month period.

- *Generalized anxiety disorder:* characterized by persistent, exaggerated worry and tension over everyday events.

- *Obsessive-compulsive disorder* (OCD): characterized by intrusive, unwanted, repetitive thoughts and behaviors performed out of a feeling of urgent need.

- *Panic disorder:* characterized by feelings of extreme fear and dread that strike unexpectedly and repeatedly for no apparent reason, often accompanied by intense physical symptoms, such as chest pain, pounding heart, shortness of breath, dizziness, or abdominal distress.

- *Post-traumatic stress disorder* (PTSD): a condition that can occur after exposure to a terrifying event, most often characterized by the repeated re-experience of the ordeal in the form of frightening, intrusive memories; brings on hypervigilance and deadening of normal emotions.

- *Phobias: social phobia*—extreme fear of embarrassment or being scrutinized by others; *specific phobia*—excessive fear of an object or situation, such as dogs, heights, loud sounds, flying, costumed characters, enclosed spaces, etc.

- *Other disorders: separation anxiety*—excessive anxiety concerning separation from the home or from those to whom the person is most attached; and *selective mutism*—persistent failure to speak in specific social situations.

Various forms of psychotherapy, including cognitive-behavioral therapy and family therapy, as well as certain medications, particularly selective serotonin reuptake inhibitors (SSRIs), are used to treat anxiety disorders in children and adolescents. Research on the safety and efficacy of these treatments is ongoing.

ADHD

Attention deficit hyperactivity disorder (ADHD) affects an estimated 4 percent of children and adolescents in the United States in a 6-month period. Its core symptoms include developmentally inappropriate levels of attention, concentration, activity, distractibility, and impulsivity. Children with ADHD usually have impaired functioning in peer relationships and multiple settings including home and school. Untreated ADHD also has been found to have long-term adverse effects on academic performance, vocational success, and social-emotional development.

Psychostimulant medications, including methylphenidate (Ritalin®) and amphetamine (Dexedrine® and Adderall®), are by far the most widely researched and commonly prescribed treatments for ADHD. Numerous short-term studies have established the safety and efficacy of stimulants and psychosocial treatments for alleviating the symptoms of ADHD. A major NIMH-funded study of children with ADHD concluded that the two most effective treatment methods for elementary school-aged children with ADHD are a closely monitored medication treatment and a treatment that combines medication with intensive behavioral interventions. Other research has shown that treating ADHD in children may reduce the likelihood of future drug and alcohol abuse.

Eating Disorders

Eating disorders involve serious disturbances in eating behavior, such as extreme and unhealthy reduction of food intake or severe overeating, as well as feelings of distress or extreme concern about body shape or weight. In the United States, eating disorders are most common among adolescent girls and young adult women; only an estimated 5 to 15 percent of people with *anorexia nervosa* or *bulimia nervosa* and an estimated 35 percent of those with *binge-eating disorder* are male. Eating disorders often co-occur with other illnesses such as depression, substance abuse, and anxiety disorders. In addition, eating disorders are associated with a wide range of other health complications, including serious heart conditions and kidney failure, which may lead to death.

Eating disorders are not due to a failure of will or behavior; rather, they are real, treatable medical illnesses in which certain maladaptive patterns of eating take on a life of their own. Because of their complexity, eating disorders require a comprehensive treatment plan involving medical care and monitoring, psychotherapy, nutritional counseling, and when appropriate, medication management. The treatment plan depends on the type of illness and the specific needs of the individual. Studies are investigating the causes of eating disorders and effectiveness of treatments.

Autism and Other Pervasive Developmental Disorders

Autism and other pervasive developmental disorders (PDDs), including *Asperger's disorder, Rett's disorder, childhood disintegrative disorder,* and *pervasive developmental disorder-not otherwise specified* (PDD-NOS), are brain disorders that occur in an estimated 2 to 6 per 1,000 American children. They typically affect the ability to communicate, to form relationships with others, and to respond appropriately to the outside world. The signs of PDDs usually develop by 3 years of age. The symptoms and deficits associated with each PDD may vary among children. For example, while some individuals with autism function at a relatively high level, with speech and intelligence intact, others are developmentally delayed, do not speak, or have serious language difficulty.

Research has made it possible to identify earlier those children who show signs of developing a PDD and thus to initiate early intervention. While there is no single best treatment program for all children with PDDs, both psychosocial and pharmacological interventions can help improve their behavioral and cognitive functioning. NIMH is funding studies of behavioral treatment approaches to determine the best time for treatment to start, the optimum treatment intensity and duration, and the most effective methods to reach both high- and low-functioning children. In addition, research and clinical experience have shown that a range of medications originally developed to treat other disorders with similar symptoms can be effective in treating the symptoms and behaviors that cause impairment for children with PDDs. For many individuals, the use of behavioral or educational support is all that is needed. For others, such interventions, by themselves, may be insufficient. The decision to use medication should be based on the symptoms causing the most impairment and on the potential risks and benefits of using and not using medication.

Schizophrenia

Schizophrenia is a chronic, severe, and disabling brain disorder that affects about 1 percent of the population during their lifetime. Symptoms include hallucinations, false beliefs, disordered thinking, and social withdrawal. Schizophrenia appears to be extremely rare in children; more typically, the illness emerges in late adolescence or early adulthood. However, research studies are revealing that various cognitive and social impairments may be evident early in children who later develop schizophrenia. These and other findings may lead to the development of preventive interventions for children. Only in this decade have researchers begun to make significant headway in understanding the origins of schizophrenia. In the emerging picture, genetic factors, which confer susceptibility to schizophrenia, appear to combine with other factors early in life to interfere with normal brain development. These developmental disturbances eventually appear as symptoms of schizophrenia many years later, typically during adolescence or young adulthood.

Treatments that help manage schizophrenia have improved significantly in recent years. As in adults, antipsychotic medications are especially helpful in reducing hallucinations and delusions in children and adolescents. The newer generation "atypical" antipsychotics, such as olanzapine and clozapine, may also help improve motivation and emotional expressiveness in some patients. Children with schizophrenia and their families can also benefit from supportive counseling, psychotherapies, and social skills training aimed at helping them cope with the illness. Special education and/or other accommodations may be necessary for children with schizophrenia to succeed in the classroom.

Part Three

Education

Chapter 11

Preparing Children for School

Ready to Learn

How well children will learn and develop and how well they will do in school depends on a number of things, including the children's health and physical well-being, their social and emotional preparation and their language skills and general knowledge of the world.

Good Health and Physical Well-Being

Seeing to it that your preschool child has nutritious food, enough exercise, and regular medical care gives him a good start in life and lessens the chances that he will have serious health problems or trouble learning later on.

Food

Preschoolers require a healthy diet. After your child is born, she requires nutritious food to keep her healthy. School-aged children can concentrate better in class if they eat balanced meals that include

Excerpted from "Helping Your Preschool Child," U.S. Department of Education, Office of Intergovernmental and Interagency Affairs, Washington, D.C., 20202, revised 2002. To order copies of this publication in English or Spanish write to: ED Pubs, Education Publications Center, U.S. Department of Education, P.O. Box 1398, Jessup, MD 20794-1398: or call in your request toll-free: 877-433-7827; or order on-line at: www.ed.gov/pubs/edpubs.html. This publication is also available on the Department's website at: www.ed.gov/pubs.

servings of breads and cereals; fruits and vegetables; meat, poultry and fish and meat alternatives (such as eggs and dried beans and peas); and milk, cheese and yogurt. You should see to it that your child does not eat too many fatty foods and sweets.

Children aged 2–5 generally can eat the same foods as adults but in smaller portions. Your child's doctor or medical clinic adviser can provide you with advice on what to feed a baby or a toddler who under the age of 2.

If you need food for your child, federal, state, and local programs can help. For example, the federal nutrition program, called the Special Supplemental Food Program for Women, Infants, and Children (WIC), distributes food to low-income women and their children across the country. Food stamp programs also are available. If you want more information or want to find out if you are eligible for food stamps, call or visit your local or state health department. Your local librarian can help you find names, addresses and phone numbers.

Exercise

Preschoolers need opportunities to exercise. To learn to control and coordinate the large muscles in his arms and legs, your child needs to throw and catch balls, run, jump, climb, and dance to music. To learn to control and coordinate the small muscles in his hands and fingers, he needs to color with crayons, put together puzzles, use blunt-tipped safety scissors, zip his jacket, and grasp small objects such as coins.

If you suspect that your child has a disability, see a doctor as soon as possible. Early intervention can help your child to develop to his full potential.

Medical Care

Preschoolers require regular medical checkups, immunizations, and dental care. It's important for you to find a doctor or a clinic where your child can receive routine health care as well as special treatment if she becomes sick or injured.

Early immunizations can help prevent a number of diseases including measles, mumps, German measles (rubella), diphtheria, tetanus, whooping cough, hib (*Haemophilus influenzae* type b), polio, and tuberculosis. These diseases can have serious effects on your child's physical and mental development. Talk to your doctor about the benefits and risks of immunization.

Beginning by the age of 3 at the latest, your child also should have regular dental checkups.

Social and Emotional Preparation

Children start school with different degrees of social and emotional maturity. These qualities take time and practice to learn. Give your child opportunities at home to begin to develop the following positive qualities.

- **Confidence:** Children must feel good about themselves and believe they can succeed. Confident children are more willing to attempt new tasks—and try again if they don't succeed the first time.

- **Independence:** Children must learn to do things for themselves.

- **Motivation:** Children must want to learn.

- **Curiosity:** Children are naturally curious and must remain so to get the most out of learning opportunities.

- **Persistence:** Children must learn to finish what they start.

- **Cooperation:** Children must be able to get along with others and learn to share and take turns.

- **Self-control:** Children must learn that there are good and bad ways to express anger. They must understand that some behaviors, such as hitting and biting, are not acceptable.

- **Empathy:** Children must have an interest in others and understand how others feel.

Here are some things that you can do to help your child develop these qualities.

- Show your child that you care about him and that you are dependable. Children who feel loved are more likely to be confident. Your child must believe that no matter what, someone will look out for him. Give your baby or toddler plenty of attention, encouragement, hugs, and lap time.

- Set a good example. Children imitate what they see others do and what they hear others say. When you exercise and eat nourishing food, your child is more likely to do so as well. When you treat others with respect, your child probably will, too. If you share things with others, your child also will learn to be thoughtful of others' feelings.

- Provide opportunities for repetition. It takes practice for a child to crawl, pronounce new words, or drink from a cup. Your child doesn't get bored when she repeats things. Instead, by repeating things until she learns them, your child builds the confidence she needs to try new things.

- Use appropriate discipline. All children need to have limits set for them. Children whose parents give them firm but loving discipline generally develop better social skills and do better in school than do children whose parents set too few or too many limits. Here are some ideas.

  - Direct your child's activities, but don't be too bossy.

  - Give reasons when you ask your child to do something. Say, for example, "Please move your truck from the stairs so no one falls over it"; not, "Move it because I said so."

  - Listen to your child to find out how he feels and whether he needs special support.

  - Show love and respect when you are angry with your child. Criticize your child's behavior but not the child. Say, for example, "I love you, but it's not okay for you to draw pictures on the walls. I get angry when you do that."

  - Help your child make choices and work out problems. You might ask your 4-year-old, for example, "What can we do to keep your brother from knocking over your blocks?"

  - Be positive and encouraging. Praise your child for a job well done. Smiles and encouragement go much further to shape good behavior than harsh punishment.

- Let your child do many things by herself. Young children need to be watched closely. However, they learn to be independent and to develop confidence by doing tasks such as dressing themselves and putting their toys away. It's important to let your child make choices, rather than deciding everything for her.

- Encourage your child to play with other children and to be with adults who are not family members. Preschoolers need social opportunities to learn to see the point of view of others. Young children are more likely to get along with teachers and classmates if they have had experiences with different adults and children.

- Show a positive attitude toward learning and toward school. Children come into this world with a powerful need to discover and to explore. If your child is to keep her curiosity, you need to encourage it. Showing enthusiasm for what your child does ("You've drawn a great picture!") helps to make her proud of her achievements.

Children also become excited about starting school when their parents show excitement about this big step. As your child gets ready to enter kindergarten, talk to him about school. Talk about the exciting things that he will do in kindergarten, such as making art projects, singing, and playing games. Be enthusiastic as you describe all the important things that he will learn from his teacher—how to read, how to how to count, and how to measure and weigh things.

Language and General Knowledge

Children can develop language skills only if they have many op-portunities to talk, listen, and use language to solve problems and learn about the world.

Long before your child enters school, you can do many things to help her develop language. You can:

- Give your child opportunities to play. Play is how children learn. It is the natural way for them to explore, to become creative, to learn to make up and tell stories and to develop social skills. Play also helps children learn to solve problems—for example, if her wagon tips over, a child must figure out how to get it up-right again. When they stack up blocks, children learn about colors, numbers, geometry, shapes, and balance. Playing with others helps children learn how to negotiate.

- Support and guide your child as she learns a new activity. Par-ents can help children learn how to do new things by "scaffold-ing," or guiding their efforts. For example, you as you and your toddler put together a puzzle, you might point to a piece and say, "I think that this is the piece we need for this space. Why don't you try it?" Then have the child piece up the piece and place it correctly. As the child becomes more aware of how the pieces fit into the puzzle, you can gradually withdraw your sup-port.

- Talk to your child, beginning at birth. Your baby needs to hear your voice. Voices from a television or radio can't take the place of your voice because they don't respond to your baby's coos and babbles. Your child needs to know that when he makes a certain sound, for example, "mamamamamama," that his mother will respond—she will smile and talk back to him. The more you talk to your baby, the more he will learn and the more he will have to talk about as he gets older. Everyday activities provide opportunities to talk, sometimes in detail, about what's happening around him. As you give your child a bath, for example, you might say, "First let's stick the plug in the drain. Now let's turn on the water. Do you want your rubber duck? That's a good idea. Look, the duck is yellow, just like the rubber duck we saw on 'Sesame Street.'"

- Listen to your child. Children have their own special thoughts and feelings, joys and sorrows, hopes and fears. As your child's language skills develop, encourage her to talk about her thoughts and feelings. Listening is the best way to learn what's on her mind and to discover what she knows and doesn't know and how she thinks and learns. It also shows your child that her feelings and thoughts are valuable.

- Ask your child questions, particularly questions that require him to give more than a "yes" or "no" response. If, as you walk with your toddler in a park, he stops to pick up leaves, you might point out how the leaves are the same and how they are different. With an older child, you might ask, "What else grows on trees?"

- Answer your child's questions. Asking questions is a good way for your child to learn to compare and to classify things—different kinds of dogs, different foods, and so forth. Answer your child's questions thoughtfully and, whenever possible, encourage her to answer her own questions. If you don't know the answer to a question, say so. Together with your child, try to find the answer.

- Read aloud to your child every day. Children of all ages love to be read to—even babies as young as six weeks. Although your child doesn't understand the story or poem that you read, reading together gives her a chance to learn about language and enjoy the sound of your voice. You don't have to be an excellent reader for your child to enjoy reading aloud together. Just by allowing her to connect reading with the warm experiences of being with you, you can create in her a lifelong love of reading. Be aware of your child's television viewing. Good television programs can introduce children to new worlds and promote learning, but poor programs or too much TV watching can be harmful. It's up to you to decide how much TV and what kinds of shows your child should watch.

- Be realistic about your child's abilities and interests. Set high standards and encourage your child to try new things. Children who aren't challenged become bored. But children who are pushed along too quickly or who are asked to do things that don't interest them can become frustrated and unhappy.

- Provide opportunities for your child to do and see new things. The more varied the experiences that she has, the more she will learn about the world. No matter where you live, your community can provide new experiences. Go for walks in your neighborhood or go places on the bus. Visit museums, libraries, zoos, and other places of interest. If you live in the city, spend a day in the country. If you live in the country, spend a day in the city. Let your child hear and make music, dance, and paint. Let her participate in activities that help to develop her imaginations and let her express her ideas and feelings.

Activities for Preschoolers: Children 3 to 5 Years Old

What to Expect

Between their third and fourth birthdays, children:

- Start to play with other children, instead of next to them;
- Are more likely to take turns and share and begin to understand that other people have feelings and rights;
- Are increasingly self-reliant and probably can dress with little help;
- May develop fears ("Mommy, there's a monster under my bed.") and have imaginary companions;
- Have greater large-muscle control than toddlers and love to run, skip, jump with both feet, catch a ball, climb downstairs, and dance to music;
- Have greater small-muscle control than toddlers, which is reflected in their drawings and scribbles;
- Match and sort things that are alike and unlike;
- Recognize numerals;
- Like silly humor, riddles, and practical jokes;

- Understand and follow spoken directions;
- Use new words and longer sentences;
- Are aware of rhyming sounds in words;
- May attempt to read, calling attention to themselves and showing pride in their accomplishment;
- Recognize print around them on signs or in logos;
- Know that each alphabet letter has a name and identify at least 10 alphabet letters, especially those in their own names; and
- "Write," or scribble messages.

Between their fourth and fifth birthdays, children:

- Are active and have lots of energy and may be aggressive in their play;
- Enjoy more group activities, because they have longer attention spans;
- Like making faces and being silly;
- May form cliques with friends and may change friendships quickly;
- Have better muscle control in running, jumping, and hopping;
- Recognize and write the numerals 1–10;
- Recognize shapes such as circles, squares, rectangles, and triangles;
- Love to make rhymes, say nonsense words, and tell jokes;
- Know and use words that are important to school work, such as the names for colors, shapes, and numbers; know and use words that are important to daily life, such as street names and addresses;
- Know how books are held and read and follow print from left to right and from top to bottom of a page when listening to stories read aloud;
- Recognize the shapes and names of all letters of the alphabet and know the sounds of some letters; and
- Write some letters, particularly those in his own name.

What Preschoolers Need

3- to 4-year-old children require opportunities to:

- Play with other children so they can learn to listen, take turns, and share;

- Develop more physical coordination—for example, by hopping on both feet;

- Develop their growing language abilities through books, games, songs, science, math, and art activities;

- Develop more self-reliance skills—for example, learning to dress and undress themselves;

- Count and measure;

- Participate actively with adults in reading-aloud activities;

- Explore the alphabet and print; and

- Attempt to write messages.

4- to 5-year-old children need opportunities to:

- Experiment and discover, within limits;

- Develop their growing interest in school subjects, such as science, music, art, and math;

- Enjoy activities that involve exploring and investigating;

- Group items that are similar (for example, by size, color, or shape);

- Use their imaginations and curiosity;

- Develop their language skills by speaking and listening; and

- See how reading and writing are both enjoyable and useful (for example, by listening to stories and poems, seeing adults use books to find information, and dictating stories to adults).

What about Kindergarten?

As the first day of school approaches, you may want to do a few things to set your child on the path to school success.

1. Find out if the school that your child will attend has a registration deadline. Some schools have a limited number of slots

for children. Start early to find out your school's policy and the procedures.

2. Learn as much as you can about the school your child will attend before the school year begins. Schools—even schools in the same district—can differ greatly. Don't rely only on information about kindergarten that you have received from other parents—their schools might have different requirements and expectations. You will want to find out the following:

    - The principal's name;
    - The name of your child's teacher;
    - What forms you need to fill out;
    - What immunizations are required before your child enters school;
    - A description of the kindergarten program;
    - The yearly calendar and daily schedule for kindergarten children;
    - Procedures for transportation to and from school;
    - Available food services; and
    - How you can become involved in your child's education and in the school.

    Some schools will send you this information. In addition, some schools will hold orientation meetings in the spring for parents who expect to enroll their children in kindergarten the following fall. If your school doesn't plan such a meeting, call the principal's office to ask for information and to arrange a visit.

3. Find out in advance what the school expects from new kindergarten students. If you know the school's expectations a year or two ahead of time, you will be in a better position to prepare your child. Sometimes parents and caregivers don't think the school's expectations are right for their children. For example, they may think that the school doesn't adequately provide for differences in children's learning and development, or that its academic program is not strong enough. If you don't agree with your school's expectations for your child, you may want to meet with the principal or kindergarten teacher to talk about the expectations.

4. Visit the school with your child. Walk up and down the hallways to help her learn where different rooms—her classroom, the library, the gym, the cafeteria—are. Let your child observe other children and their classrooms.

5. Talk with your child about school. During your visit, make positive comments about the school—your good attitude will rub off! ("Look at all the boys and girls painting in this classroom. Doesn't that look like fun!") At home, show excitement about the big step in your child's life. Let him know that starting school is a very special event.

   Talk with your child about the teachers she will have and how they will help her learn new things. Encourage your child to consider teachers to be wise friends to whom she should listen and show respect. Explain to your child how important it is to go to class each day. Explain how important and exciting the things that she will learn in school are—reading, writing, math, science, art, and music.

6. Consider volunteering to help out in the school. Your child's teacher may appreciate having an extra adult to help do everything from passing out paper and pencils to supervising children on the playground. Volunteering is a good way to learn more about the school and to meet its staff and to meet other parents.

When the long-awaited first day of kindergarten arrives, go to school with your child (but don't stay too long). And be patient. Many young children are overwhelmed at first, because they haven't had much experience in dealing with new situations. They may not like school immediately. Your child may cry or cling to you when you say goodbye each morning, but with support from you and his teacher, this can change rapidly.

As your child leaves home for her first day of kindergarten, let her know how proud of her you are.

Chapter 12

Getting Ready for the First Day of School

Kindergarten is now a nearly universal experience for children in the United States. Many children make the transition to school without difficulty. Other children may be wary of their new surroundings, but they adjust over time. Wariness in new situations is not all bad; it indicates an ability to discern who may and who may not be trustworthy.

This chapter discusses some ways parents can help prepare children new to school before the year begins, common problems faced by children just beginning school, and strategies parents can use to help their child adapt to the new environment.

Getting Ready

The details of registration, immunization requirements, and information about arrangements for transportation, snacks, or meals are best attended to by the responsible adults well ahead of September. It is often helpful to find out from the school what school personnel expect of entering kindergartners in terms of self-reliance. Are they

From "Getting Ready for School," by Lilian Katz, Ph.D., in *Parent News*, May-June 2000, National Parent Information Network (NPIN), Educational Resources Information Center (ERIC), Clearinghouse on Elementary and Early Childhood Education (EECE). The full text including references is available online at http://npin.org/pnews/2000/pnew500/feat500.html. Additional information is available from NPIN online at http://npin.org and from ERIC EECE at www.ericeece.org.

expected to know their address and phone number? Do they need to know how to tie their shoes and zip jackets?

Many schools provide introductory packets or booklets for parents of kindergartners or new first-graders, and they distribute this information during registration (and often earlier, upon request). Other ways to find out about the school's expectations include calling and requesting any other introductory material that is available, visiting the school—including the building, playgrounds, lunchroom, restrooms, and classrooms—and asking for a meeting with the most likely teacher of your child.

If your child shows no special apprehension about entering the new school environment, it is best for you to be matter-of-fact about it, too, and to take any opportunities as they arise for informal chats with the child about what is likely to be ahead.

Acknowledge and Accept Uneasiness about the New School

For children who show some concern about what the new experience is likely to include, it is easier to help them through the adjustment period if you are reasonably sure the new environment is a sensitive and responsive one. Your confidence that school will be a good experience will make it possible for you to reassure your child that he or she will be all right and that the adults in the new situation will understand the child's feelings and be ready to help with difficult moments. Many children pick up their parents' uncertainties and anxieties and persist in behavior that will either get them reassurance or, in extreme cases, provoke a change in plans.

A parent's uncertainty about what is in store for his or her child may be caused by concern about the quality of education offered in the school or about the curriculum and teaching practices in classrooms. Many parents find that their concerns stimulate their active participation in school activities, volunteering in class, and taking part in discussions of school plans and new curriculum approaches. If inquiries into the school's curriculum and teaching practices do not reassure you, and other options for schooling are not available to you, then it may be best to focus on simply reassuring your child that you will be glad to help him to do well and are always ready and willing to talk with him about his experiences.

For some parents, their child's entry into school arouses apprehension or unpleasant school memories from their own childhood. Such hesitation may be based on a parent's experience with schools that were insufficiently aware or sensitive to his or her cultural background and needs. In such cases, it may be helpful to contact a neighbor or friend who has already had experience in the school or class that your child will enter and to discuss your concerns and perhaps visit the school with her.

The young child, however, is unlikely to be concerned about such things as curriculum and teaching methods, or to be too concerned about her parents' experiences in school. She is more apt to wonder what it might be like on the school bus with many other children of different ages and sizes, what she will do when she has to go to the bathroom and where it is, how meals will be managed, where she will put her coat, or what the new rules will be like. Some children want to be sure about where they will be dropped off when they arrive at school, who will meet them there, and who will meet them when they return home after school. Relaxed informative discussion of such details, and even rehearsal of some of the procedures, can reduce apprehension.

For children with little or no previous experience in large group settings, a casual visit together with your child to the school grounds, a walk through the hallways, and a visit in the classroom—plus a brief meeting with the teacher—can assure both of you that the new experience will be manageable.

Inviting to your home a neighborhood friend who is also going to start school with your child, or an "experienced" first-grader, can often provide a relaxed setting to discuss going to school and provide a "buddy" who can help reduce the strangeness of the new experience. Also, if kindergarten is to be the child's first experience in a large group setting, giving the child some advance experience of being apart from you and from home for brief periods before school begins, perhaps visiting a friend at her house for a few afternoons before school starts, can help build confidence in her capacity to cope with the new phase in her life. Most likely, however, your child has already been away from home for a good part of the day in a preschool program of some kind, and she has probably already developed useful coping skills for entering a group.

Be Matter-of-Fact about What's ahead

Instead of asking your child at the moment she leaves for school "Are you okay?" indicate that you believe he or she will do fine, that there will be people in school ready to be helpful when necessary, and say something like "I know you'll get used to it all in no time!"

Be careful, however, not to promise that it will be exciting and fun from the word "go." For some children, that may be so. But for most, some upset at entering a new environment that is large and swarming with strange children and adults should be expected. Accept the child's feelings without dwelling on them, and let her know that you understand it takes time to get used to the new people, places, routines, and rules.

When a child talks very excitedly about what she or he expects, tone it down a bit so as not to add to excessively high expectations. In fact, it is a good idea to say to the child, in an informal context, something like "You'll make some new friends and have lots of good experiences in kindergarten. But most likely there will be moments when you wish you were at home (or back in your old preschool)." Such statements prepare the child in a way that when these inevitable moments arise they are not unstrung by them. As the saying goes, to be forewarned is to be forearmed.

Some young children are very eager to get to the big school and are unprepared for differences from their earlier group experiences in a preschool or child care setting. In kindergarten or first grade, it is harder to get the teacher's attention than in a preschool group. In kindergarten, they will have to work in larger groups and observe some rules about getting along with new adults and children. Furthermore, in school, children are expected to be slightly more self-reliant and to be able to do many more things for themselves than was expected in preschool. Parents can often help by providing practice with dressing, buttoning and unbuttoning, zippers, and the like. For many children, confidence in their ability to handle these details frees them to attend to the more important aspects of this important new phase in their lives.

Resistance to Going to School: School Phobia and School Refusal

If your child has had few previous group experiences, then some degree of anxiety on separation—for both child and parents—is to be expected and is not a cause for alarm. If your child is reluctant to go to school, try to resist offering a reward or a bribe, such as promising a special treat for quiet separation; by doing so, you may signal that she or he has cause to be upset. Instead, it is best to express your confidence in the child's ability to gradually get used to the new situation and to do well in it.

School phobia, currently referred to by psychologists as school refusal in its mild form, occurs in only about 5% to 10% of children. Full-blown school phobia is very rare, occurring in only 1% as a form of severe phobia (Murray, 1997). At some time during their school experience, however, many children occasionally suffer from some of the symptoms generally associated with school phobia.

School refusal takes many forms such as crying, shyness, tantrums, petulance, persistent clinging, and, in many cases, illnesses such as sore throats, stomachaches, headaches, and the like. These illnesses often occur shortly before it is time to leave for school, tend to subside when the child stays home, and often reappear the next morning.

Occasionally, school refusal occurs after a long break from school such as the summer holidays. In such cases, children anticipate problems on their return to school. For example, they may be responding to underlying worry about their abilities to do well enough in class or about relationships with peers. Parents can usually help the child talk through such fears. Persistent cases of such school refusal usually require professional assistance to prevent them from becoming a serious pattern of behavior.

Conclusion

Many parents worry about preparing their children for the transition to the "big school." Even if your child has had a year or two of preschool or child care, the transition to school can be eased by good preparation at home, working with the school, and maintaining an open, matter-of-fact communication strategy with children.

Chapter 13

Helping Your Child Become a Reader

Talking and Listening

Scientists who study the brain have found out a great deal about how we learn. They have discovered that babies learn much more from the sights and sounds around them than we thought previously. You can help your baby by taking advantage of her hunger to learn.

From the very beginning, babies try to imitate the sounds that they hear us make. They "read" the looks on our faces and our movements. That's why it is so important to talk, sing, smile, and gesture to your child. Hearing you talk is your baby's very first step toward becoming a reader, because it helps her to love language and to learn words.

As your child grows older, continue talking with her. Ask her about the things she does. Ask her about the events and people in the stories you read together. Let her know you are listening carefully to what she says. By engaging her in talking and listening, you are also encouraging your child to think as she speaks. In addition, you are showing that you respect her knowledge and her ability to keep learning.

Excerpted from "Helping Your Child Become a Reader," U.S. Department of Education, Office of Intergovernmental and Interagency Affairs, Washington, D.C., 20202, revised 2002. To order copies of this publication in English or Spanish write to: ED Pubs, Education Publications Center, U.S. Department of Education, P.O. Box 1398, Jessup, MD 20794-1398: or call in your request toll-free: 877-433-7827; or order on-line at: www.ed.gov/pubs/edpubs.html. This publication is also available on the Department's website at: www.ed.gov/pubs.

Reading Together

Reading books with their children is one of the most important things that parents can do to help their children become readers.

What Does It Mean?

From the earliest days, talk with your child about what you are reading. You might point to pictures and name what is in them. When he is ready, have him do the same. Ask him, for example, if he can find the little mouse in the picture, or do whatever is fun and right for the book. Later on, as you read stories, read slowly and stop now and then to think aloud about what you've read. From the time your child is able to talk, ask him such questions about the story as, "What do you think will happen next?" or "Do you know what a palace is?" Answer his questions and, if you think he doesn't understand something, stop and talk more about what he asked. Don't worry if you occasionally break the flow of a story to make clear something that is important. However, don't stop so often that the child loses track of what is happening in the story.

Look for Books

The books that you pick to read with your child are very important. If you aren't sure of what books are right for your child, ask a librarian to help you choose titles.

Introduce your child to books when she is a baby. Let her hold and play with books made just for babies: board books with study cardboard covers and thick pages, cloth books that are soft and washable, touch-and-feel books, or lift-the-flap books that contain surprises for your baby to discover.

As your child grows into a preschooler and kindergartner, the two of you can look for books that have longer stories and more words on the pages. Also look for books that have repeating words and phrases that she can begin to read or recognize when she sees them. By early first grade, add to this mix some books designed for beginning readers, including some books that have chapters and some books that show photographs and provide true information rather than make-believe stories.

Keep in mind that young children most often enjoy books about people, places, and things that are like those they know. The books can be about where you live or about parts of your culture, such as your religion, your holidays, or the way that you dress. If your child has special interests, such as dinosaurs or ballerinas, look for books about those interests.

From your child's toddler years through early first grade, you also should look for books of poems and rhymes. Remember when your baby heard your talking sounds and tried to imitate them? Rhymes are an extension of that language skill. By hearing and saying rhymes, along with repeated words and phrases, your child learns about spoken sounds and about words. Rhymes also spark a child's excitement about what comes next, which adds fun and adventure to reading.

Show Your Child That You Read

When you take your child to the library, check out a book for yourself. Then set a good example by letting your child see you reading for yourself. Ask your child to get one of her books and sit with you as you read your book, magazine, or newspaper. Don't worry if you feel uncomfortable with your own reading ability. It's the reading that counts. When your child sees that reading is important to you, she may decide that it is important to her, too.

Learning about Print and Books

Reading together is a perfect time to help a late toddler or early preschooler learn what print is. As you read aloud, stop now and then and point to letters and words, then point to the pictures they stand for. Your child will begin to understand that the letters form words and that words name pictures. He will also start to learn that each letter has its own sound—one of the most important things your child can know when learning to read.

By the time children are 4, most have begun to understand that printed words have meaning. By age 5, most will begin to know that not just the story but the printed words themselves go from left to right. Many children will even start to identify some capital and small letters and simple words.

In late kindergarten or early first grade, your child may want to read on his own. Let him! But be sure that he wants to do it. Reading should be some thing he is proud of and eager to do and not a lesson.

How Does a Book Work?

Children are fascinated by how books look and feel. They see how easily you handle and read books, and they want to do the same. When your toddler watches you handle books, she begins to learn that a book is for reading, not tearing or tossing around. Before she is 3, she may even pick one up and pretend to read, an important sign that she is beginning to know what a book is for. As your child becomes a preschooler, she is learning that:

- A book has a front cover.
- A book has a beginning and an end.
- A book has pages.
- A page in a book has a top and a bottom.
- You turn pages one at a time to follow the story.
- You read a story from left to right of a page.

As you read with your 4- or 5-year-old, begin to remind her about these things. Read the title on the cover. Talk about the picture on the cover. Point to the place where the story starts and, later, where it ends. Let your child help turn the pages. When you start a new page, point to where the words of the story continue and keep following the words by moving your finger beneath them. It takes time for a child to learn these things, but when your child does learn them, she has solved some of reading's mysteries.

Early Efforts to Write

Writing and reading go hand in hand. As your child is learning one, he is learning the other. You can do certain things to make sure that he gets every opportunity to practice both. When he is about 2 years old, for example, give your child crayons and paper and encourage him to draw and scribble. He will have fun choosing which colors to use and which shapes to make. As he holds and moves the crayons, he will also develop muscle control. When he is a late toddler or early pre-schooler, he will become as eager to write as he is to read.

Your preschool child's scribbles or drawings are his first writing. He will soon begin to write the alphabet letters. Writing the letters helps your child learn about their different sounds. His very early learning about letters and sounds gives him ideas about how to begin spelling words. When he begins writing words, don't worry that he doesn't spell them correctly. Instead, praise him for his efforts! In fact, if you look closely, you'll see that he's made a pretty good try at spelling a word for the first time. Later on, with help from teachers (and from you), he will learn the right way to spell words. For the moment, however, he has taken a great step toward being a writer.

Reading in Another Language

If your child's first language is not English, she can still become an excellent English reader and writer. She is on her way to successful English reading if she is beginning to learn many words and is interested in learning to read in her first language. You can help by supporting her in her first language as she learns English. Talk with her, read with her, encourage her to draw and write. In other words, do the same kinds of activities just discussed, but do them in your child's first language.

If You Think There's a Problem

Your child may resist being read to or joining with you in the activities in this chapter. If so, keep trying the activities, but keep them playful. Remember that children vary a great deal in the ways that they learn. Don't be concerned if your child doesn't enjoy a certain activity that her friend of the same age loves. It is important, though, to keep an eye on how your child is progressing.

When a child is having a language or reading problem, the reason might be simple to understand and deal with, or it might be complicated and require expert help. Often, children may just need more time to develop their language skills. On the other hand, some children might have trouble seeing, hearing, or speaking. Others may have a learning disability. If you think your child may have some kind of physical or learning problem, it is important to get expert help quickly.

If your child is in school and you think that she should have stronger language skills, ask for a private meeting with her teacher. (You may feel more comfortable taking a friend, relative, or someone else in your community with you.) In most cases, the teacher, or perhaps the principal, will be able to help you to understand how your child is doing and what you might do to help her.

There is a law—the Individuals with Disabilities Education Act (IDEA)—that may allow you to get certain services for your child from your school district. Your child might qualify to receive help from a speech and language therapist or other specialist, or she might qualify to receive materials designed to match her needs. You can learn about your special education rights and responsibilities by requesting that the school give you, in your first language, a summary of legal rights.

The good news is that no matter how long it takes, most children can learn to read. Parents, teachers, and other professionals can work together to determine if a child has a learning disability or other problem, and then provide the right help as soon as possible. When a child gets such help, chances are very good that she will develop the skills she needs to succeed in school and in life. Nothing is more important than your support for your child as she goes through school. Make sure she gets any extra help she needs as soon as possible, and always encourage her and praise her efforts.

A Reading Checklist

There are many ways that you can encourage your child to become a reader. Here are some questions that you can ask yourself to make sure that you are keeping on track:

For Babies (6 weeks to 1 year)

- Do I provide a comfortable place for our story time? Is my child happy to be in this place?

- Am I showing my child the pictures in the book? Am I changing the tone of my voice as I read to show emotion and excitement?

- Am I paying attention to how my child responds? What does she especially like? Is she tired and ready to stop?

For Toddlers (1 to 3 years)

All of the questions above, plus:

- Does my child enjoy the book we are reading?

- Do I encourage my child to "pretend read," joining in where he has memorized a word or phrase?

- When I ask questions, am I giving my child enough time to think and answer?

- Do I tie ideas in the book to things that are familiar to my child? Do I notice if he does this on his own?

- Do I let my child know how much I like his ideas and encourage him to tell me more?

- Do I point out letters, such as the first letter of his name?

For Preschoolers (3 and 4 years)

All of the questions above, plus:

- Do I find ways to help my child begin to identify sounds and letters and to make letter-sound matches?

For Kindergartners (5 years)

All of the questions above, plus:

- Do I find ways to help my child begin to identify some printed words?

- Do I let my child retell favorite stories to show that she knows how the story develops and what's in it?

For Beginning First-Graders (6 years)

All of the questions above, plus:

- Do I give my child the chance to read a story to me using the print, picture clues, his memory—or any combination of these ways that help him make sense of the story?

Remember: Children learn step by step in a process that takes time and patience. They vary a great deal in what holds their interest and in the rate at which they make progress.

Typical Language Accomplishments: Children, Birth to Age 6

Learning to read is built on a foundation of language skills that children start to learn at birth—a process that is both complicated and amazing. Most children develop certain skills as they move through the early stages of learning language. By age 7, most children are reading.

The following list of accomplishments is based on current scientific research in the fields of reading, early childhood education, and child development. Studies continue in their fields, and there is still much still to learn. As you look over the accomplishments, keep in mind that children vary a great deal in how they develop and learn. If you have questions or concerns about your child's progress, talk with the child's doctor, teacher, or a speech and language therapist. For children with any kind of disability or learning problem, the sooner they can get the special help they need, the easier it will be for them to learn.

From ages 3–4, most preschoolers become able to:

- Enjoy listening to and talking about storybooks.
- Understand that print carries a message.
- Make attempts to read and write.
- Identify familiar signs and labels.
- Participate in rhyming games.
- Identify some letters and make some letter-sound matches.
- Use known letters (or their best attempt to write the letters) to represent written language, especially for meaningful words like their names or phrases such as "I love you."

At age 5, most kindergartners become able to:

- Sound as if they are reading when they pretend to read.
- Enjoy being read to.
- Retell simple stories.
- Use descriptive language to explain or to ask questions.
- Recognize letters and letter-sound matches.
- Show familiarity with rhyming and beginning sounds.
- Understand that print is read left-to-right and top-to-bottom.
- Begin to match spoken words with written ones.
- Begin to write letters of the alphabet and some words they use and hear often.
- Begin to write stories with some readable parts.

At age 6, most first-graders can:

- Read and retell familiar stories.
- Use a variety of ways to help with reading a story such as re-reading, predicting what will happen, asking questions, or using visual cues or pictures.

- Decide on their own to use reading and writing for different purposes.

- Read some things aloud with ease.

- Identify new words by using letter-sound matches, parts of words, and their understanding of the rest of a story or printed item.

- Identify an increasing number of words by sight.

- Sound out and represent major sounds in a word when trying to spell.

- Write about topics that mean a lot to them.

- Try to use some punctuation marks and capitalization.

Chapter 14

Helping Your Child with Homework

Homework is important because it can improve children's thinking and memory. It can help them to develop positive study skills and habits that will serve them well throughout their lives. It can encourage them to use time well, to learn independently, and to take responsibility for their work.

But helping children with their homework benefits families as well. It can, for example, be a way for families to learn more about what their children are learning in school and an opportunity for them to communicate both with their children and with teachers and principals.

Why Do Teachers Assign Homework?

Teachers assign homework for many reasons. Homework can help their students:

- review and practice what they've covered in class;

Excerpted from "Helping Your Child with Homework," U.S. Department of Education, Office of Intergovernmental and Interagency Affairs, Washington, D.C., 20202, revised 2002. To order copies of this publication in English or Spanish write to: ED Pubs, Education Publications Center, U.S. Department of Education, P.O. Box 1398, Jessup, MD 20794-1398: or call in your request toll-free: 877-433-7827; or order on-line at: www.ed.gov/pubs/edpubs.html. This publication is also available on the Department's website at: www.ed.gov/pubs.

- get ready for the next day's class;

- learn to use resources, such as libraries, reference materials, and computer websites to find information about a subject;

- explore subjects more fully than classroom time permits;

- extend learning by applying skills they already have to new situations; and

- integrate their learning by applying many different skills to a single task, such as book reports or science projects.

Homework also can help students to develop good study habits and positive attitudes. It can:

- teach them to work independently; and

- encourage self-discipline and responsibility (assignments provide some children with their first chance to manage time and to meet deadlines).

In addition, homework can help create greater understanding between families and teachers and provide opportunities for increased communication. Monitoring homework keeps families informed about what their children are learning and about the policies and programs of the teacher and the school.

Does Homework Help Children Learn?

Homework helps your child do better in school when the assignments are meaningful, are completed successfully, and are returned to her with constructive comments from the teacher. An assignment should have a specific purpose, come with clear instructions, be fairly well matched to a child's abilities, and help to develop a child's knowledge and skills.

In the early grades, homework can help children to develop the good study habits and positive attitudes. From third through sixth grades, small amounts of homework, gradually increased each year, may support improved school achievement. In seventh grade and beyond, students who complete more homework score better on standardized tests and earn better grades, on the average, than do students who do less homework. The difference in test scores and grades between students who do more homework and those who do less increases as students move up through the grades.

What's the Right Amount of Homework?

The right amount of homework depends on the age and skills of the child. National organizations of parents and teachers suggest that children in kindergarten through second grade can benefit from 10 to 20 minutes of homework each school day. In third through sixth grades, children can benefit from 30 to 60 minutes a school day. In seventh through ninth grades, students can benefit from spending more time on homework and the amount may vary from night to night.

Amounts that vary from these guidelines are fine for some children and in some situations. For example, because reading at home is especially important for children, reading assignments might push the time on homework a bit beyond the amounts suggested here.

If you are concerned that your child has either too much or too little homework, talk with his teacher and learn about her homework policies.

How to Help: Show That You Think Education and Homework Are Important

Children need to know that their family members think homework is important. If they know their families care, children have a good reason to complete assignments and to turn them in on time. You can do many things to show your child that you value education and homework.

- Set a regular time for homework
- Pick a place
- Remove distractions
- Provide supplies and identify resources
- Set a good example
- Be interested

How to Help: Monitor Assignments

Children are more likely to complete homework successfully when parents monitor their assignments. How closely you need to monitor your child depends upon her age, how independent she is, and how well she does in school. Whatever the age of your child, if she is not getting assignments done satisfactorily, she requires more supervision.

Here are some ways to monitor your child's assignments.

- Ask about the school's homework policy

- Be available
- Look over completed assignments
- Monitor time spent viewing TV and playing video games

How to Help: Provide Guidance

The basic rule is, "Don't do the assignments yourself." It's not your homework—it's your child's. "I've had kids hand in homework that's in their parents' handwriting," one eighth-grade teacher complains. Doing assignments for your child won't help him understand and use information. And it won't help him become confident in his own abilities.

Here are some ways that you can provide guidance without taking over your child's homework.

- Help your child get organized.
- Encourage good study habits.
    - Help your child manage time to complete assignments.
    - Help your child to get started when he has to do research reports or other big assignments.
    - Give practice tests.
    - Help your child avoid last-minute cramming.
    - Talk with your child about how to take a test.
- Talk about the assignments.
- Watch for frustration.
- Give praise.

How to Help: Talk with Teachers to Resolve Problems

Homework problems often can be avoided when families and caregivers value, monitor, and guide their children's work on assignments. Sometimes, however, helping in these ways is not enough. If you have problems, here are some suggestions for how to deal with them.

Tell the Teacher about Your Concerns

You may want to contact the teacher if

- your child refuses to do her assignments, even though you've tried hard to get her to do them;

- the instructions are unclear;

- you can't seem to help your child get organized to finish the assignments;

- you can't provide needed supplies or materials;

- neither you nor your child can understand the purpose of the assignments;

- the assignments are too hard or too easy;

- the homework is assigned in uneven amounts—for instance, no homework is given on Monday, Tuesday, or Wednesday, but on Thursday four assignments are made that are due the next day; or

- your child has missed school and needs to make up assignments.

In some cases, the school guidance counselor or principal also may be helpful in resolving problems.

Work with the Teacher

Continuing communication with teachers is very important in solving homework problems. As you work with your child's teacher, here are some important things to remember:

- Talk with each of your child's teachers early in the school year. Get acquainted before problems arise and let each teacher know that you want to be kept informed.

- Contact the teacher as soon as you suspect your child has a homework problem (as well as when you think he's having any major problems with his schoolwork). By alerting the teacher, you can work together to solve a problem in its early stages.

- Request a meeting with the teacher to discuss homework problems. Tell him briefly why you want to meet. Believe that the teacher wants to help you and your child, even if you disagree about something. Don't go to the principal without giving the teacher a chance to work out the problem with you and your child.

- Let the teacher know whether your child finds the assignments too hard or too easy. (Teachers also like to know when their students are particularly excited about an assignment.)

- During your meeting with the teacher, explain what you think is going on. In addition, tell the teacher if you don't know what the problem is. Sometimes a student's version of what's going on isn't the same as the teacher's version.

- Work out a way to solve or lessen the problem. The strategy will depend on what the problem is, how severe it is, and what the needs of your child are. For instance:

  - Is the homework often too hard? Maybe your child has fallen behind and will need extra help from the teacher or a tutor to catch up.

  - Does your child need to make up a lot of work because of absences? The first step might be working out a schedule with the teacher.

  - Does your child need extra support beyond what home and school can give her? Ask the teacher, school guidance counselor, or principal if there are mentor programs in your community. Mentor programs pair a child with an adult volunteer who assists with the child's special needs. Many schools, universities, community organizations, churches, and businesses offer excellent mentoring programs.

- Make sure that communication is clear. Listen to the teacher and don't leave until you're sure that you understand what's being said. Make sure, too, that the teacher understands what you have to say. If, after the meeting, you realize you don't understand something, call the teacher to clarify.

- At the end of the meeting, it may help to summarize what you've agreed to do.

- Follow up to make sure that the approach you agreed to is working.

Homework can bring together children, families, and teachers in a common effort to improve children's learning.

Helping your child with homework is an opportunity to improve your child's chances of doing well in school and life. By helping your child with homework, you can help him learn important lessons about discipline and responsibility. You can open up lines of communication—between you and your child and you and the school. You are in a unique position to help your child make connections between school work and the "real world," and thereby bring meaning (and some enjoyment) to your child's homework experience.

Chapter 15

Recognizing and Developing Your Child's Special Talents

All children have special talents that need to be noticed and nurtured so they will do well in school and in their later lives. In the past, poor students, students with limited English language skills, and students from diverse cultures have been overlooked by schools when they selected children for programs for the gifted. Schools used a very narrow definition of intelligence that did not account for the different ways that children show their abilities, or for the fact that some children have difficulty in showing their talents at all. Now, though, schools are using broader and fairer methods to identify children with special talents, and the students in gifted programs represent much more varied backgrounds.

Parents can be very important in helping their children develop their talents by working with them at home. Parents can also make schools aware of their children's talents, and work with them to make sure that their children are in a program that challenges them intellectually and responds to their educational and emotional needs.

What Families Can Do at Home

Children's talents should be developed as early as possible so they can achieve their full potential. Parents don't need to be very educated

"How to Recognize and Develop Your Children's Special Talents," by Wendy Schwarz, 1997, National Parent Information Network (NPIN), Educational Resources Information Center (ERIC). This article is provided courtesy of the ERIC Clearinghouse on Urban Education. Despite the older date of this article, the suggested guidelines are still appropriate. Additional information is available from NPIN online at http://npin.org.

themselves—or have a great deal of money, or even time—to help their children learn and improve their ability to think and communicate. Here are some things to do at home:

- Set high academic goals for your children. Tell them that success is possible, that they will benefit later in life from doing well in school, and that families and their teachers expect them to do well. Help them develop a sense of pride in their identity, both personal and cultural.

- Talk to and play with your children. Have conversations about current events, what's happening in the neighborhood, and what you all did during the day. As you go through your daily routine, explain what you are doing and why. Encourage your children to ask questions that you can answer or help them answer. Make up stories together. Read to them, play games, and do puzzles together.

- Ask your children to pay attention to the way people speak on the radio and TV. Talk about why learning to use good English speech patterns will help them in school and later in life.

- Pay attention to what your children like to do, such as a hobby, drawing, or working with numbers. Help them develop those skills or find out where in the community they can participate in learning enrichment activities. Start early, Head Start, and other preschool programs can give your children many advantages.

- Take your children to places where they can learn. Find out about story times at the library and bookstores, and about children's events at museums and community centers. Check out free books and games at the library.

- Take a parenting course in the community or at school that teaches how to develop children's talents.

- Find a mentor in your family or community who can help your children develop their talents and serve as a role model for academic achievement.

- Find out about early talent identification programs so that when your children begin preschool or school they will receive an education that challenges them. Also find out about local community or religious preschools and after-school enrichment programs.

- Set up a quiet study space for your children and help them with their homework, or find them an after-school program that provides a place for studying without distractions.

How Families Can Work with Schools

All parents are partners in their children's education, and all parents have a place in their children's school, regardless of their own education or economic status. Parents should also know that their children can get a good education in public schools, but they may need to help school people understand how their children's talents can best be developed. Here are some ways for parents to work with schools:

- Ask the school to provide training in recognizing signs of talent and intelligence in children. Some schools give out a "parent nomination form" so parents can check off ways that their children are gifted.

- Find out about enrichment programs for gifted students and tell the school about all your children's talents and why you think your children should be placed in such a program.

- Lobby the school for early and bias-free assessment of children's talent and intelligence. All the abilities of all children should be considered.

- Pay attention to the curriculum and instruction in your children's gifted program to be sure it is successful with their learning style. Some schools distribute a newsletter about their special programs to keep parents informed; ask your school to do this, or even volunteer to help produce it.

- Be sure that your children are given the support they need to be retained in the program. Ask for enrichment or tutoring if your children aren't doing well in a gifted program.

- Ask for—or help create—a support system for parents. It can include workshops and dissemination of information about ways to help develop children's talent at home, and about enrichment materials for use at home and ways to get them at minimum cost.

What Programs Are Most Successful with Gifted Multicultural Students

Children with many different learning styles, educational backgrounds, and academic and social skills participate in programs for specially talented students. The following curriculum and teaching strategies are especially effective in multicultural gifted programs.

Parents can work with schools to make sure that their children's education includes:

- An orientation toward achievement and success, and high expectations.
- One-to-one teaching and small learning groups of students.
- Mentoring by adults or older gifted students.
- Special attention to development of communication skills, particularly for bilingual students and those who speak non-standard English.
- A multicultural focus and instruction based on the children's experience.
- Use of community resources.

Chapter 16

Perfectionist Students

Perfectionist students are not satisfied with merely doing well or even with doing better than their peers. They are satisfied only if they have done a job perfectly, so that the result reveals no blemishes or weaknesses. To the extent that perfectionism involves striving for difficult but reachable goals, it involves the success-seeking aspects of healthy achievement motivation and functions as an asset to the student and as an ally to the teacher.

Even a success-seeking version of perfectionism, however, can become a problem to the extent that the student begins to focus not so much on meeting personal goals as on winning competitions against classmates.

Problems associated with forms of perfectionism that focus on seeking success are relatively minor, however, compared to the problems associated with forms of perfectionism that focus on avoiding failure. Fear of failure (or of blame, rejection, or other anticipated social consequences of failure) can be destructive to achievement motivation, especially if it is powerful and persistent. Victims of such fear typically try to avoid or escape as quickly as possible from achievement situations in which their performance will be judged according to standards of excellence.

Reprinted with permission from "The Perfectionist Student," Pediatric Development and Behavior, adapted from *Teaching Problem Students*, by Jere Brophy (New York: Guliford, 1996), revised June 1997 and July 2000; the text and additional are information available online from Pediatric Development and Behavior at www.dbpeds.org.

When escape is not possible, they try to protect their self-esteem either by expressing very low aspirations that will be easy to fulfill or by expressing impossibly high aspirations that they have no serious intention of striving to fulfill. In the school setting, many such students become alienated underachievers.

Characteristics of Perfectionist Students

The following are symptoms of student perfectionism:

- performance standards that are impossibly high and unnecessarily rigid
- motivation more from fear of failure than from pursuit of success
- measurement of one's own worth entirely in terms of productivity and accomplishment
- all-or-nothing evaluations that label anything other than perfection as failure
- difficulty in taking credit or pleasure, even when success is achieved, because such achievement is merely what is expected
- procrastination in getting started on work that will be judged
- long delays in completing assignments, or repeatedly starting over on assignments, because the work must be perfect from the beginning and continue to be perfect as one goes along

Other symptoms commonly observed in perfectionist students include unwillingness to volunteer to respond to questions unless certain of the correct answer, overly emotional and "catastrophic" reactions to minor failures, and low productivity due to procrastination or excessive "start overs."

Coping with Perfectionist Students

Perfectionist students need to relearn performance norms and work expectations. They need to learn that:

1. Schools are places to learn knowledge and skills, not merely to demonstrate them.

2. Errors are normal, expected, and often necessary aspects of the learning process.

3. Everyone makes mistakes, including the teacher.

4. There is no reason to devalue oneself or fear rejection or punishment just because one has made a mistake.

5. It is usually more helpful to measure progress by comparing where one is now with where one was, rather than by comparing oneself with peers or with ideals of perfection.

Swift and Spivack emphasized that helping perfectionists develop more realistic expectations is a process that needs to be couched within a context of acceptance of their motivation to achieve and their need to feel satisfied with their accomplishments. Thus, instead of dismissing their concerns as unfounded (and expecting them to accept this view), teachers can use active listening methods to encourage these students to express their concerns, make it clear that they take those concerns seriously, and engage in collaborative planning with the students concerning steps that might alleviate the problem. The goal is to help perfectionist students achieve a 20- or 30-degree change rather than a 180-degree turnaround.

Teachers want students to retain their desire to aim high and put forth their best efforts, but to learn to do so in ways that are realistic and productive rather than rigid and compulsive.

Intervention efforts are likely to feature some form of cognitive restructuring. The following teacher strategies for working with perfectionists are suggested:

- Give permission to make mistakes, or divide assignments into outline, rough draft, and final draft stages, with perfection promoted only for the final draft.
- Discuss appropriate reactions to making mistakes.
- Frequently use ungraded assignments or assignments that call for creative, individual responses rather than correct answers.

If necessary, place limits on perfectionist procrastination by limiting the time that can be spent on an assignment or by limiting the amount of correcting allowed.

Teachers must be careful to be sure that the assistance they provide does not make these students too dependent on them, to the point that they seek teacher clarification and approval of every step of their work. The goal is to gradually guide the student toward an independent work posture.

Strategies of Effective Teachers

Studies have shown that effective teachers make an attempt to appeal to, persuade, or change the attitudes of perfectionist students, and to support their efforts to change, by doing the following:

- building a friendly, supportive learning environment
- establishing the expectation that mistakes are a normal part of the learning process
- presenting themselves as helpful instructors concerned primarily with promoting student learning, rather than as authority figures concerned primarily with evaluating student performance
- articulating expectations that stress learning and improvement over perfect performance on assignments
- explaining how perfectionism is counterproductive
- reassuring perfectionist students that they will get the help they need to achieve success, following through with help, and communicating teacher approval of students' progress and accomplishments.

Effective teachers identified the most ineffective strategies for dealing with perfectionist students as criticizing or nagging, threatening punishment for failure to change, controlling or suppressing perfectionist tendencies, and ignoring or denying the problem rather than dealing with it.

Conclusion

Perfectionists often show unsatisfactory achievement progress because they are more concerned about avoiding mistakes than with learning. They are inhibited about classroom participation and counterproductively compulsive in their work habits. Identifying perfectionist students is possible by observing their behaviors and talking with them about habits and practices that interfere with class participation and performance on assignments.

Effective teachers take perfectionist students seriously, communicating understanding and approval of their desire to do well and sympathizing with the students' feelings of embarrassment and frustration. Teachers can learn to support and reinforce the success-seeking aspects of achievement motivation while working to reduce unrealistic goal setting.

Chapter 17

Learning Disabilities

Chapter Contents

Section 17.1

What Are Learning Disabilities?

Excerpted from "Learning Disabilities," Fact Sheet 7 (FS7), National Information Center for Children and Youth with Disabilities (NICHCY), January 2003. The full text of this document including references is available online at http://www.nichcy.org/pubs/factshe/fs7txt.htm. Information about educational resources is included in Chapter 57.

What Are Learning Disabilities?

Learning disability is a general term that describes specific kinds of learning problems. A learning disability can cause a person to have trouble learning and using certain skills. The skills most often affected are reading, writing, listening, speaking, reasoning, and doing math.

Learning disabilities (LD) vary from person to person. One person with LD may not have the same kind of learning problems as another person with LD. One may have trouble with reading and writing. Another person with LD may have problems with understanding math. Still another person may have trouble in each of these areas, as well as with understanding what people are saying.

Researchers think that learning disabilities are caused by differences in how a person's brain works and how it processes information. Children with learning disabilities are not "dumb" or "lazy." In fact, they usually have average or above average intelligence. Their brains just process information differently.

The definition of "learning disability" comes from the Individuals with Disabilities Education Act (IDEA). The IDEA is the federal law that guides how schools provide special education and related services to children with disabilities.

There is no "cure" for learning disabilities. They are life-long. However, children with LD can be high achievers and can be taught ways to get around the learning disability. With the right help, children with LD can and do learn successfully.

IDEA's Definition of "Learning Disability"

Our nation's special education law, the Individuals with Disabilities Education Act, defines a specific learning disability as: ". . . a disorder in one or more of the basic psychological processes involved in understanding or in using language, spoken or written, that may manifest itself in an imperfect ability to listen, think, speak, read, write, spell, or do mathematical calculations, including conditions such as perceptual disabilities, brain injury, minimal brain dysfunction, dyslexia, and developmental aphasia."

However, learning disabilities do not include, "...learning problems that are primarily the result of visual, hearing, or motor disabilities, of mental retardation, of emotional disturbance, or of environmental, cultural, or economic disadvantage." 34 Code of Federal Regulations §300.7(c)(10)

How Common Are Learning Disabilities?

As many as one out of every five people in the United States has a learning disability. Almost three million children (ages 6 through 21) have some form of a learning disability and receive special education in school. In fact, over half of all children who receive special education have a learning disability (*Twenty-third Annual Report to Congress*, U.S. Department of Education, 2001).

What Are the Signs of a Learning Disability?

There is no one sign that shows a person has a learning disability. Experts look for a noticeable difference between how well a child does in school and how well he or she could do, given his or her intelligence or ability. There are also certain clues that may mean a child has a learning disability. We've listed a few below. Most relate to elementary school tasks, because learning disabilities tend to be identified in elementary school. A child probably won't show all of these signs, or even most of them. However, if a child shows a number of these problems, then parents and the teacher should consider the possibility that the child has a learning disability.

When a child has a learning disability, he or she:

- may have trouble learning the alphabet, rhyming words, or connecting letters to their sounds;

- may make many mistakes when reading aloud, and repeat and pause often;

- may not understand what he or she reads;

- may have real trouble with spelling;

- may have very messy handwriting or hold a pencil awkwardly;

- may struggle to express ideas in writing;

- may learn language late and have a limited vocabulary;

- may have trouble remembering the sounds that letters make or hearing slight differences between words;

- may have trouble understanding jokes, comic strips, and sarcasm;

- may have trouble following directions;

- may mispronounce words or use a wrong word that sounds similar;

- may have trouble organizing what he or she wants to say or not be able to think of the word he or she needs for writing or conversation;

- may not follow the social rules of conversation, such as taking turns, and may stand too close to the listener;

- may confuse math symbols and misread numbers;

- may not be able to retell a story in order (what happened first, second, third); or

- may not know where to begin a task or how to go on from there.

If a child has unexpected problems learning to read, write, listen, speak, or do math, then teachers and parents may want to investigate more. The same is true if the child is struggling to do any one of these skills. The child may need to be evaluated to see if he or she has a learning disability.

What about School?

Learning disabilities tend to be diagnosed when children reach school age. This is because school focuses on the very things that may be difficult for the child—reading, writing, math, listening, speaking, and reasoning. Teachers and parents notice that the child is not learning as expected. The school may ask to evaluate the child to see what is causing the problem. Parents can also ask for their child to be evaluated.

With hard work and the proper help, children with LD can learn more easily and successfully. For school-aged children (including preschoolers), special education and related services are important sources of help. School staff work with the child's parents to develop an Individualized Education Program, or IEP. This document describes the child's unique needs. It also describes the special education services that will be provided to meet those needs. These services are provided at no cost to the child or family.

Supports or changes in the classroom (sometimes called "accommodations") help most students with LD. Some common accommodations are listed below in "Tips for Teachers." Assistive technology can also help many students work around their learning disabilities. Assistive technology can range from "low-tech" equipment such as tape recorders to "high-tech" tools such as reading machines (which read books aloud) and voice recognition systems (which allow the student to "write" by talking to the computer).

It's important to remember that a child may need help at home as well as in school. The resources listed below will help families and teachers learn more about the many ways to help children with learning disabilities.

Tips for Parents

- *Learn about LD.* The more you know, the more you can help yourself and your child.

- *Praise your child when he or she does well.* Children with LD are often very good at a variety of things. Find out what your child really enjoys doing, such as dancing, playing soccer, or working with computers. Give your child plenty of opportunities to pursue his or her strengths and talents.

- *Find out the ways your child learns best.* Does he or she learn by hands-on practice, looking, or listening? Help your child learn through his or her areas of strength.

- *Let your child help with household chores.* These can build self-confidence and concrete skills. Keep instructions simple, break down tasks into smaller steps, and reward your child's efforts with praise.

- *Make homework a priority.* Read more about how to help your child be a success at homework. (See Chapter 14.)

183

- *Pay attention to your child's mental health* (and your own). Be open to counseling, which can help your child deal with frustration, feel better about himself or herself, and learn more about social skills.

- *Talk to other parents whose children have learning disabilities.* Parents can share practical advice and emotional support. Call NICHCY (800-695-0285) and ask how to find parent groups near you. Also let us put you in touch with the parent training and information (PTI) center in your state.

- *Meet with school personnel and help develop an educational plan to address your child's needs.* Plan what accommodations your child needs, and don't forget to talk about assistive technology.

- *Establish a positive working relationship with your child's teacher.* Through regular communication, exchange information about your child's progress at home and at school.

Tips for Teachers

- *Learn as much as you can about the different types of LD.* The resources and organizations at the end of this document can help you identify specific techniques and strategies to support the student educationally.

- *Seize the opportunity to make an enormous difference in this student's life.* Find out and emphasize what the student's strengths and interests are. Give the student positive feedback and lots of opportunities for practice.

- *Review the student's evaluation records to identify where specifically the student has trouble.* Talk to specialists in your school (for example, special education teacher) about methods for teaching this student.

- *Provide instruction and accommodations to address the student's special needs.* Examples include:
  - breaking tasks into smaller steps, and giving directions verbally and in writing;
  - giving the student more time to finish schoolwork or take tests;
  - letting the student with reading problems use textbooks-on-tape;

- letting the student with listening difficulties borrow notes from a classmate or use a tape recorder; and

- letting the student with writing difficulties use a computer with specialized software that spell checks, grammar checks, or recognizes speech.

- *Learn about the different testing modifications* that can really help a student with LD show what he or she has learned.

- *Teach organizational skills, study skills, and learning strategies.* These help all students but are particularly helpful to those with LD.

- *Work with the student's parents to create an educational plan tailored to meet the student's needs.*

- *Establish a positive working relationship with the student's parents.* Through regular communication, exchange information about the student's progress at school.

Section 17.2

Frequently Asked Questions about Dyslexia and Other Specific Learning Disabilities

"Frequently Asked Questions (FAQs)," © 2002 The International Dyslexia Association®; reprinted with permission. Visit the International Dyslexia Association website online at http://interdys.org.

What is dyslexia?

- Dyslexia is one of several distinct learning disabilities. It is a specific language-based disorder of constitutional origin characterized by difficulties in single word decoding, usually reflecting insufficient phonological processing abilities. These difficulties in single word decoding are often unexpected in relation to age and other cognitive and academic abilities; they are not the result

185

of generalized developmental disability or sensory impairment. Dyslexia is manifest by variable difficulty with different forms of language, often including, in addition to problems reading, a conspicuous problem with acquiring proficiency in writing and spelling. The Definition of Dyslexia as adopted by the Research Committee of International Dyslexia Association, May 11, 1994 and by the National Institutes of Health, 1994.

- Studies show that individuals with dyslexia process information in a different area of the brain than do non-dyslexics.

- Many people who are dyslexic are of average to above average intelligence.

Are there other learning disabilities besides dyslexia?

Dyslexia is one type of learning disability. Others include:

- **Dyscalculia:** A mathematical disability in which a person has unusual difficulty solving arithmetic problems and grasping math concepts.

- **Dysgraphia:** A neurological-based writing disability in which a person finds it hard to form letters or write within a defined space.

Are attention deficit disorder (ADD) and attention deficit hyperactive disorder (ADHD) learning disabilities?

- No, they are behavioral disorders.

- An individual can have more than one learning or behavioral disability. In various studies as many as 50% of those diagnosed with a learning or reading difference have also been diagnosed with ADHD.

- Although disabilities may co-occur, one is not the cause of the other.

How common are language-based learning disabilities?

- 15–20% of the population have a language-based learning disability.

- Of the students with specific learning disabilities receiving special education services, 70–80% have deficits in reading.

- Dyslexia is the most common cause of reading, writing, and spelling difficulties.

- Dyslexia affects males and females nearly equally, and people from different ethnic and socio-economic backgrounds as well.

Can individuals who are dyslexic learn to read?

- Yes, it is never too late to learn to read, process, and express information more efficiently.

- Research shows that programs utilizing multisensory structured language techniques can help adults and children learn to read.

How do people get dyslexia?

The causes for dyslexia are neurobiological and genetic. Research shows that individuals inherit the genetic links for dyslexia. If one of your grandparents, parents, aunts or uncles is dyslexic, then chances are that one or more of your children will be dyslexic.

Is there a cure for dyslexia?

- No, dyslexia is not a disease. There is no cure.

- With proper diagnosis, appropriate instruction, hard work, and support from family, friends, employers, and others, people who are dyslexic can lead successful and productive lives.

Am I limited to doing specific types of work?

No, individuals can succeed in varied fields despite their dyslexia. Examples include:

- **Ann Bancroft:** First woman in history to cross the ice to both the North and South Poles.

- **David Boies:** Trial lawyer whose high-profile clients have included former U.S. Vice President Al Gore, Jr., Napster, and the U.S. Justice Department in its antitrust suit against Microsoft.

- **Erin Brokovich:** Real-life heroine who exposed a cover-up by a major California utility that was contaminating the local water supply. Their actions had severe, even deadly consequences to the members of the community. With her help, the townspeople were awarded a $333 million settlement, the largest ever in a U.S. direct-action lawsuit. (Julia Roberts played her in the movie with the same name.)

- **Stephen J. Cannell:** Author and Emmy Award-winning TV producer and writer, who has created or co-created more than 38 shows, of which he has scripted more than 350 episodes and produced or executive produced more than 1,500 episodes. His hits include "The Rockford Files," "A-Team," "21 Jump Street," "Wiseguy," "Renegade" and "Silk Stalkings."

- **Whoopi Goldberg:** Actor and comedian, winner of an Academy Award for her supporting role in "Ghost," also an Academy Award nomination for her role in "The Color Purple."

None of these people are letting dyslexia hold them back, so don't let it get you down.

Sources

- *Basic Facts about Dyslexia: What Every Layperson Ought to Know*, Copyright 1993, 2nd ed. 1998. The International Dyslexia Association, Baltimore, MD.

- *Learning Disabilities: Information, Strategies, Resources*, Copyright 2000. Coordinated Campaign for Learning Disabilities, a collaboration of the leading U.S. non-profit learning disabilities organizations. Used with permission.

- Research studies sponsored by the National Institute of Child Health and Human Development, National Institutes of Health, Bethesda, MD.

Section 17.3

Common Warning Signs of Learning Disabilities: A Checklist

"Common Warning Signs of Learning Disabilities: A Brief Checklist," © 2000 National Center for Learning Disabilities (NCLD); reprinted with permission. Additional information is available from NCLD online at www.ld.org.

Although most children experience difficulties with learning and behavior from time to time, a consistent pattern of the behaviors (listed below), over time, should be considered an indication to seek further advice, information, or help when someone is not performing these tasks as people their same age do.

Preschool

Does the child have trouble with or delayed development in:

- Learning the alphabet
- Rhyming words
- Connecting sounds and letters
- Counting and learning numbers
- Being understood when he or she speaks to a stranger
- Using scissors, crayons, and paints
- Reacting too much or too little to touch
- Using words or, later, stringing words together into phrases
- Pronouncing words
- Walking forward or up and down stairs
- Remembering the names of colors
- Dressing self without assistance

Elementary School

Does the child have trouble with:

- Learning new vocabulary
- Speaking in full sentences
- Understanding the rules of conversation
- Retelling stories
- Remembering newly learned information
- Playing with peers
- Moving from one activity to another
- Expressing thoughts orally or in writing
- Holding a pencil
- Handwriting
- Computing math problems at his or her grade level
- Following directions
- Self-esteem
- Remembering routines
- Learning new skills
- Understanding what he or she reads
- Succeeding in one or more subject areas
- Drawing or copying shapes
- Understanding what information presented in class is important
- Modulating voice (may speak to loudly or in a monotone)
- Keeping notebook neat and assignments organized
- Remembering and sticking to deadlines
- Understanding how to play age-appropriate board games

Chapter 18

Attention Deficit Hyperactivity Disorder

Questions and Answers about AD/HD

What is AD/HD?

Attention deficit hyperactivity disorder (AD/HD) is a condition that can make it hard for a person to sit still, control behavior, and pay attention. These difficulties usually begin before the person is 7 years old. However, these behaviors may not be noticed until the child is older.

Doctors do not know just what causes AD/HD. However, researchers who study the brain are coming closer to understanding what may cause AD/HD. They believe that some people with AD/HD do not have enough of certain chemicals (called neurotransmitters) in their brain. These chemicals help the brain control behavior.

Parents and teachers do not cause AD/HD. Still, there are many things that both parents and teachers can do to help a child with AD/HD.

How common is AD/HD?

As many as 5 out of every 100 children in school may have AD/HD. Boys are three times more likely than girls to have AD/HD.

From Fact Sheet 19 (FA19), National Information Center for Children and Youth with Disabilities (NICHCY), September 2002. For more information from NICHCY, visit their website at www.nichcy.org or call 800-695-0285.

What are the signs of AD/HD?

There are three main signs, or symptoms, of AD/HD. These are:

- problems with paying attention,
- being very active (called hyperactivity), and
- acting before thinking (called impulsivity).

More information about these symptoms is listed in a book called the *Diagnostic and Statistical Manual of Mental Disorders* (DSM), which is published by the American Psychiatric Association (2000). Based on these symptoms, three types of AD/HD have been found:

- *inattentive type,* where the person can't seem to get focused or stay focused on a task or activity;
- *hyperactive-impulsive type*, where the person is very active and often acts without thinking; and
- *combined type,* where the person is inattentive, impulsive, and too active.

Inattentive type: Many children with AD/HD have problems paying attention. Children with the inattentive type of AD/HD often:

- do not pay close attention to details;
- can't stay focused on play or school work;
- don't follow through on instructions or finish school work or chores;
- can't seem to organize tasks and activities;
- get distracted easily; and
- lose things such as toys, school work, and books. (APA, 2000, pp. 85–86)

Hyperactive-impulsive type: Being too active is probably the most visible sign of AD/HD. The hyperactive child is "always on the go." (As he or she gets older, the level of activity may go down.) These children also act before thinking (called impulsivity). For example, they may run across the road without looking or climb to the top of very tall trees. They may be surprised to find themselves

192

in a dangerous situation. They may have no idea of how to get out of the situation.

Hyperactivity and impulsivity tend to go together. Children with the hyperactive-impulsive type of AD/HD often may:

- fidget and squirm;

- get out of their chairs when they're not supposed to;

- run around or climb constantly;

- have trouble playing quietly;

- talk too much;

- blurt out answers before questions have been completed;

- have trouble waiting their turn;

- interrupt others when they're talking; and

- butt in on the games others are playing. (APA, 2000, p. 86)

Combined type: Children with the combined type of AD/HD have symptoms of both of the types described above. They have problems with paying attention, with hyperactivity, and with controlling their impulses.

Of course, from time to time, all children are inattentive, impulsive, and too active. With children who have AD/HD, *these behaviors are the rule, not the exception.*

These behaviors can cause a child to have real problems at home, at school, and with friends. As a result, many children with AD/HD will feel anxious, unsure of themselves, and depressed. These feelings are not symptoms of AD/HD. They come from having problems again and again at home and in school.

How do you know if a child has AD/HD?

When a child shows signs of AD/HD, he or she needs to be evaluated by a trained professional. This person may work for the school system or may be a professional in private practice. A complete evaluation is the only way to know for sure if the child has AD/HD. It is also important to:

- rule out other reasons for the child's behavior, and

- find out if the child has other disabilities along with AD/HD.

What about treatment?

There is no quick treatment for AD/HD. However, the symptoms of AD/HD can be managed. It's important that the child's family and teachers:

- find out more about AD/HD;

- learn how to help the child manage his or her behavior;

- create an educational program that fits the child's individual needs; and

- provide medication, if parents and the doctor feel this would help the child.

What about school?

School can be hard for children with AD/HD. Success in school often means being able to pay attention and control behavior and impulse. These are the areas where children with AD/HD have trouble.

There are many ways the school can help students with AD/HD. Some students may be eligible to receive special education services under the Individuals with Disabilities Education Act (IDEA). Under the newest amendments to IDEA, passed in 1997, AD/HD is specifically mentioned under the category of "Other Health Impairment" (OHI). We've included the IDEA's definition of OHI below. Other students will not be eligible for services under IDEA. However, they may be eligible for services under a different law, Section 504 of the Rehabilitation Act of 1973. In both cases, the school and the child's parents need to meet and talk about what special help the student needs.

Most students with AD/HD are helped by supports or changes in the classroom (called adaptations). Some common changes that help students with AD/HD are listed under "Tips for Teachers" below. More information about helpful strategies can be found in the National Information Center for Children and Youth with Disabilities (NICHCY)'s briefing paper called "Attention-Deficit/Hyperactivity Disorder."

IDEA's Definition of "Other Health Impairment"

Many students with ADHD now may qualify for special education services under the "Other Health Impairment" category within the

Individuals with Disabilities Education Act (IDEA). IDEA defines "other health impairment" as:

> ". . . having limited strength, vitality or alertness, including a heightened alertness to environmental stimuli, that results in limited alertness with respect to the educational environment, that is due to chronic or acute health problems such as asthma, attention deficit disorder or attention deficit hyperactivity disorder, diabetes, epilepsy, a heart condition, hemophilia, lead poisoning, leukemia, nephritis, rheumatic fever, and sickle cell anemia; and adversely affects a child's educational performance." 34 Code of Federal Regulations §300.7(c)(9)

Tips for Parents

- Learn about AD/HD. The more you know, the more you can help yourself and your child.

- Praise your child when he or she does well. Build your child's abilities. Talk about and encourage his or her strengths and talents.

- Be clear, be consistent, be positive. Set clear rules for your child. Tell your child what he or she *should* do, not just what he shouldn't do. Be clear about what will happen if your child does not follow the rules. Have a reward program for good behavior. Praise your child when he or she shows the behaviors you like.

- Learn about strategies for managing your child's behavior. These include valuable techniques such as: charting, having a reward program, ignoring behaviors, natural consequences, logical consequences, and time-out. Using these strategies will lead to more positive behaviors and cut down on problem behaviors. You can read about these techniques in many books.

- Talk with your doctor about whether medication will help your child.

- Pay attention to your child's mental health (and your own). Be open to counseling. It can help you deal with the challenges of raising a child with AD/HD. It can help your child deal with frustration, feel better about himself or herself, and learn more about social skills.

- Talk to other parents whose children have AD/HD. Parents can share practical advice and emotional support.

- Meet with the school and develop an educational plan to address your child's needs. Both you and your child's teachers should get a written copy of this plan.

- Keep in touch with your child's teacher. Tell the teacher how your child is doing at home. Ask how your child is doing in school. Offer support.

Tips for Teachers

- Learn more about AD/HD. The resources and organizations listed in Chapter 57 will help you identify behavior support strategies and effective ways to support the student educationally, such as the following.

- Figure out what specific things are hard for the student. For example, one student with AD/HD may have trouble starting a task, while another may have trouble ending one task and starting the next. Each student needs different help.

- Post rules, schedules, and assignments. Clear rules and routines will help a student with AD/HD. Have set times for specific tasks. Call attention to changes in the schedule.

- Show the student how to use an assignment book and a daily schedule. Also teach study skills and learning strategies, and reinforce these regularly.

- Help the student channel his or her physical activity (for example, let the student do some work standing up or at the board). Provide regularly scheduled breaks.

- Make sure directions are given step by step, and that the student is following the directions. Give directions both verbally and in writing. Many students with AD/HD also benefit from doing the steps as separate tasks.

- Let the student do work on a computer.

- Work together with the student's parents to create and implement an educational plan tailored to meet the student's needs. Regularly share information about how the student is doing at home and at school.

- Have high expectations for the student but be willing to try new ways of doing things. Be patient. Maximize the student's chances for success.

References

Barkley, R. (2000). A new look at ADHD: Inhibition, time, and self-control [video]. New York: Guilford. [Telephone: 800-365-7006. Website: http://www.guilford.com]

—. (2000). *Taking charge of AD/HD: The complete authoritative guide for parents (rev. ed.)* New York: Guilford. (See contact information above.)

Dendy, S. A. Z. (2000). *Teaching teens with ADD and ADHD: A quick reference guide for teachers and parents.* Bethesda, MD: Woodbine House. [Telephone: 800-843-7323. Website: http://www.woodbinehouse.com]

Fowler, M. (1999). *Maybe you know my kid: A parent's guide to identifying, understanding, and helping your child with ADHD* (3rd ed.). Kensington, NY: Citadel. [Telephone: 888-345-2665. Website: http://www.kensingtonbooks.com]

—. (2001). Maybe you know my teen: A parent's guide to helping your adolescent with attention deficit hyperactivity disorder. New York: Broadway Books. (Website: http://www.randomhouse.com)

—. (2002). Attention-deficit/hyperactivity disorder. NICHCY Briefing Paper, 1–24. [Telephone: 800-695-0285. Also available on NICHCY's website, www.nichcy.org.]

National Institutes of Health. (1998). Diagnosis and treatment of attention deficit hyperactivity disorder. NIH Consensus Statement, 16(2), 1–37 [On-line]. Available: odp.od.nih.gov/consensus/cons/110/110_statement.htm

Wodrich, D. L. (2000). *Attention deficit hyperactivity disorder: What every parent wants to know* (2nd ed.). Baltimore, MD: Paul H. Brookes. [Telephone: 800-638-3775. Website: http://brookespublishing.com]

Chapter 19

Questions Often Asked by Parents about Special Education Services

What is special education?

Special education is instruction that is specially designed to meet the unique needs of children who have disabilities. This is done at no cost to the parents. Special education can include special instruction in the classroom, at home, in hospitals or institutions, or in other settings.

Over five million children ages 6 through 21 receive special education and related services each year in the United States. Each of these children receives instruction that is specially designed:

- to meet the child's unique needs (that result from having a disability); and

- to help the child learn the information and skills that other children are learning.

This definition of special education comes from the Individuals with Disabilities Education Act (IDEA), Public Law 105-17.

Excerpted from "Questions Often Asked by Parents about Special Education Services," 4th Edition, National Information Center for Children and Youth with Disabilities (NICHCY), 1999, reviewed by the U.S. Office of Special Education Programs for consistency with the Individuals with Disabilities Education Act Amendments of 1997, Public Law 105-17, and the final implementing regulations published March 12, 1999. The full text is available online at www.nichcy.org/pubs/ideapubs/lg1txt.htm.

Who is eligible for special education?

Certain children with disabilities are eligible for special education and related services. The IDEA provides a definition of a "child with a disability." This law lists 13 different disability categories under which a child may be found eligible for special education and related services. These categories are: autism; deafness; deaf-blindness; hearing impairment; mental retardation; multiple disabilities; orthopedic impairment; other health impairment; serious emotional disturbance; specific learning disability; speech or language impairment; traumatic brain injury; visual impairment, including blindness.

According to the IDEA, the disability must affect the child's educational performance. The question of eligibility, then, comes down to a question of whether the child has a disability that fits in one of IDEA's 13 categories and whether that disability affects how the child does in school. That is, the disability must cause the child to need special education and related services.

How do I find out if my child is eligible for special education?

The first step is to find out if your child has a disability. To do this, ask the school to evaluate your child. Call or write the Director of Special Education or the principal of your child's school. Say that you think your child has a disability and needs special education help. Ask the school to evaluate your child as soon as possible.

The school, however, does not have to evaluate your child just because you have asked. The school may not think your child has a disability or needs special education. In this case, the school may refuse to evaluate your child. It must let you know this decision in writing, as well as why it has refused.

If the school refuses to evaluate your child, there are two things you can do immediately:

- Ask the school system for information about its special education policies, as well as parent rights to disagree with decisions made by the school system. These materials should describe the steps parents can take to challenge a school system's decision.

- Get in touch with your state's Parent Training and Information (PTI) center. The PTI can tell you what steps to take next to find help for your child. Call the National Information Center for Children and Youth with Disabilities NICHCY to find out how to get in touch with your PTI (800-695-0285).

What happens during an evaluation?

Evaluating your child means more than the school just giving your child a test or two. The school must evaluate your child in all the areas where your child may be affected by the possible disability. This may include looking at your child's health, vision, hearing, social and emotional well-being, general intelligence, performance in school, and how well your child communicates with others and uses his or her body. The evaluation must be complete enough (full and individual) to identify all of your child's needs for special education and related services.

The evaluation process involves several steps.

Reviewing existing information. A group of people, including you, begins by looking at the information the school already has about your child. You may have information about your child you wish to share as well. The group will look at information such as:

- your child's scores on tests given in the classroom or to all students in your child's grade;

- the opinions and observations of your child's teachers and other school staff who know your child; and

- your feelings, concerns, and ideas about how your child is doing in school.

Deciding if more information is still needed. The information collected above will help the group decide:

- if your son or daughter has a particular type of disability;

- how your child is currently doing in school;

- whether your child needs special education and related services; and

- what your child's educational needs are.

Group members will look at the information they collected above and see if they have enough information to make these decisions. If the group needs more information to make these decisions, the school must collect it.

Collecting more information about your child. If more information about your child is needed, the school will give your child tests or collect the information in other ways. Your informed written permission is required before the school may collect this information. The evaluation group will then have the information it needs to make the types of decisions listed above.

What happens if my child is not eligible for services?

If the group decides that your child is not eligible for special education services, the school system must tell you this in writing and explain why your child has been found "not eligible." Under the IDEA, you must also be given information about what you can do if you disagree with this decision.

Read the information the school system gives you. Make sure it includes information about how to challenge the school system's decision. If that information is not in the materials the school gives you, ask the school for it.

Also get in touch with your state's Parent Training and Information (PTI) center. The PTI can tell you what steps to take next.

So my child has been found eligible for special education. What next?

The next step is to write what is known as an Individualized Education Program—usually called an IEP. After a child is found eligible, a meeting must be held within 30 days to develop to the IEP.

What is an Individualized Education Program?

An Individualized Education Program (IEP) is a written statement of the educational program designed to meet a child's individual needs. Every child who receives special education services must have an IEP.

The IEP has two general purposes: (1) to set reasonable learning goals for your child; and (2) to state the services that the school district will provide for your child.

What type of information is included in an IEP?

According to the IDEA, your child's IEP must include specific statements about your child. These are listed below.

- Present levels of educational performance

- Annual goals
- Special education and related services to be provided
- Participation with nondisabled children
- Participation in state and district-wide assessments
- Dates and location
- Transition service needs
- Transition services
- Measuring progress

It is very important that children with disabilities participate in the general curriculum as much as possible. That is, they should learn the same curriculum as nondisabled children, for example, reading, math, science, social studies, and physical education, just as nondisabled children do. In some cases, this curriculum may need to be adapted for your child to learn, but it should not be omitted altogether. Participation in extracurricular activities and other nonacademic activities is also important. Your child's IEP needs to be written with this in mind.

For example, what special education services will help your child participate in the general curriculum—in other words, to study what other students are studying? What special education services or supports will help your child take part in extracurricular activities such as school clubs or sports? When your child's IEP is developed, an important part of the discussion will be how to help your child take part in regular classes and activities in the school.

Can my child's IEP be changed?

Yes. At least once a year a meeting must be scheduled with you to review your child's progress and develop your child's next IEP. The meeting will be similar to the IEP meeting described above. The team will talk about:

- your child's progress toward the goals in the current IEP,
- what new goals should be added, and
- whether any changes need to be made to the special education and related services your child receives.

This annual IEP meeting allows you and the school to review your child's educational program and change it as necessary. But you don't have to wait for this annual review. You (or any other team member) may ask to have your child's IEP reviewed or revised at any time.

For example, you may feel that your child is not making good progress toward his or her annual goals. Or you may want to write new goals, because your son or daughter has made such great progress. Call the principal of the school, or the special education director or your child's teacher, and express your concerns. If necessary, they will call the IEP team together to talk about changing your child's IEP.

Will my child be re-evaluated?

Yes. Under the IDEA, your child must be re-evaluated at least every three years. The purpose of this re-evaluation is to find out:

- if your child continues to be a "child with a disability," as defined within the law, and

- your child's educational needs.

Although the law requires that children with disabilities be re-evaluated at least every three years, your child may be re-evaluated more often if you or your child's teacher(s) request it.

What if I disagree with the school about what is right for my child?

You have the right to disagree with the school's decisions concerning your child. This includes decisions about:

- your child's identification as a "child with a disability,"

- his or her evaluation,

- his or her educational placement, and

- the special education and related services that the school provides to your child.

In all cases where the family and school disagree, it is important for both sides to first discuss their concerns and try to compromise. The compromise can be temporary. For example, you might agree to try out a particular plan of instruction or classroom placement for a certain period of time. At the end of that period, the school can check your child's progress. You and other members of your child's IEP team can then meet again, talk about how your child is doing, and decide what to do next. The trial period may help you and the school come to a comfortable agreement on how to help your child.

If you still cannot agree with the school, it's useful to know more about the IDEA's protections for parents and children. The law and regulations include ways for parents and schools to resolve disagreements. These include:

- mediation, where you and school personnel sit down with an impartial third person (called a mediator), talk openly about the areas where you disagree, and try to reach agreement;

- due process, where you and the school present evidence before an impartial third person (called a hearing officer), and he or she decides how to resolve the problem; and

- filing a complaint with the State Education Agency (SEA), where you write directly to the SEA and describe what requirement of IDEA the school has violated. The SEA must either resolve your complaint itself, or it can have a system where complaints are filed with the school district and parents can have the district's decision reviewed by the SEA. In most cases, the SEA must resolve your complaint within 60 calendar days.

Your state will have specific ways for parents and schools to resolve their differences. You will need to find out what your state's policies are. Your local department of special education will probably have these guidelines. If not, contact the state department of education and ask for a copy of their special education policies.

You may also wish to call the Parent Training and Information (PTI) center in your state. They are an excellent resource for parents to learn more about special education.

What if I still have questions and need more information?

You can contact your state's Parent Training and Information (PTI) center. Your PTI will have a lot of information to share about the special education process in your state.

You can also contact NICHCY. We have information on all aspects of the IEP process. We also have information on other issues that are important to families who have a child with a disability. NICHCY staff can send you more publications (see NICHCY's catalog or visit our website at: www.nichcy.org), answer questions, and put you in touch with other organizations who can work with you and your family.

National Information Center for Children and Youth with Disabilities (NICHCY)
P.O. Box 1492
Washington, DC 20013
Toll-Free: 800-695-0285
Fax: 202-884-8441
Website: http://www.nichcy.org
E-mail: nichcy@aed.org

Part Four

Childhood Emergencies: Prevention and First Aid

Chapter 20

Ten Things that Could Save Your Child's Life in an Emergency

Every year in this country nearly 6,700 children under the age of fourteen die and another 50,000 are permanently disabled from preventable injuries. Knowing these ten things could save your child's life.

1. Know How to Spot an Emergency Situation

- An emergency situation exists if you think your child could die or suffer permanent harm unless prompt care is received. If you are not sure, make the call.

2. Know How to Contact Your Local Emergency Service

- In communities that have a 9-1-1 system, simply dialing 9-1-1 in an emergency connects you to Emergency Medical Services (EMS), the police, and fire department.

- Important—Some areas of the country do not have 9-1-1. In these areas, there are different numbers to call for a medical, police, or fire emergency. Find out what they are and

"Emergency! 10 Steps" © 1995 Emergency Medical Services for Children, reviewed and considered current as of May 2003; reprinted with permission. This fact sheet was produced by Emergency Medical Services for Children (EMSC), a federally funded program of the Health Resources and Services Administration's Maternal and Child Health Bureau. For more information, access the EMSC website at www.ems-c.org.

P.L.A.N. — **P**ost **L**ists of **A**ll Emergency **N**umbers on or by every telephone in your home. Seconds count when calling your local ambulance/emergency service, poison control center, and police and fire departments—P.L.A.N. now.

3. Learn CPR and Choking Rescue Procedures for Infants and Children

- Knowing how to perform CPR procedures on a child who has stopped breathing could provide your child with the life-saving support that he or she needs before the professionals arrive.

- Understanding basic choking rescue procedures is essential to saving the life of any child whose airway is blocked by objects lodged in the throat.

- Your local American Red Cross or American Heart Association chapter has information on CPR courses offered in your area. Also check with your local hospital for CPR training, first aid, and child safety courses.

4. Learn the Basics of First Aid

- Knowing how to stop serious bleeding from an open wound, manage shock, handle fractures, and control a fever could provide your child with the right amount of help during an emergency.

- Learning first aid will help you recognize an emergency.

5. Immunize, Immunize, Immunize

- Get all your child's immunizations on time. Failure to do so places your child at serious risk of permanent disability and even death from a preventable illness.

6. Remember What to Do If Your Child Is Involved in a Car Crash

- DO NOT MOVE your child unless in further danger. Moving the child unnecessarily could result in permanent injury.

- Keep the child warm and, if conscious, keep him or her still.

7. Understand What to Do If Your Child Is Poisoned

- If your child has been poisoned, bring the poison (and child, if possible) with you to the phone when calling the poison control center.

- Memorize your local poison control center's number and post it by the phone—P.L.A.N.

- Have Syrup of Ipecac on hand—BUT use only if directed to do so.

8. Learn What to Do in Case Your Child Has a Serious Fall

- DO NOT move any child who is unconscious or has struck his or her head. Doing so may result in a more serious injury or permanent disability.

- Call 9-1-1 or your local emergency number in cases involving any loss of consciousness, blood, or watery fluid coming from the ear or nose, and/or a convulsion/seizure.

- Cover your child with blankets and, if conscious, keep him or her still.

9. Know How to Treat Your Child in Case of a Burn—Stop the Process

- For minor burns without blisters, place the burned area into cold water until pain is gone (about 15 min.). DO NOT use ice.

- For burns with blisters, call your doctor immediately. DO NOT use butter or petroleum jelly.

- Large and/or deep burns require an immediate call to 9-1-1 or your local emergency number. Keep your child warm with a clean sheet and then a blanket until help arrives.

10. Be Prepared to Act in Case Your Child Has a Seizure

- Perform rescue breathing if your child is not breathing. If breathing, lay your child on his or her side.

- Protect your child from other injuries by moving him or her away from dangerous objects.

211

To Learn More

For more information on these safety hints and the Emergency Medical Services for Children Program please contact:

Emergency Medical Services for Children
National Resource Center
111 Michigan Avenue, NW
Washington, DC 20010-2970
Phone: 202-884-4927
Fax: 202-884-6845
Website: http://www.ems-c.org
E-mail: information@emscnrc.com

Chapter 21

First Aid for Common Childhood Injuries

Chapter Contents

Section 21.1

Home First Aid Kit

© 1999 American College of Emergency Physicians® (ACEP), reviewed
and considered current in April 2003; reprinted with permission. For
more health and safety tips, visit ACEP's website at www.acep.org.

The American College of Emergency Physicians (ACEP) recommends that every home be prepared to respond to common medical emergencies by having a Home First Aid Kit. Preventing emergencies is the best way to keep your family healthy and safe. However, you can protect your family and reduce your risk of injury and serious illness by preparing to respond in case one occurs.

Emergency physicians suggest including the items listed below in your Home First Aid Kit. All the items are available from your local pharmacy. For the kit itself, ACEP recommends using a tote bag, because it can hold all the items you need, as well as be visible where it is kept. It also can be easily transported, such as when you go on vacation. Appropriate members of the household should know where it is and how to use each item.

Suggested Contents

First Aid Manual: A valuable resource about health and safety and how to respond to many medical emergencies at home. ACEP also recommends taking a first-aid class, learning CPR, and always seeking immediate medical attention when you need it.

Information

- *Emergency Phone Numbers:* family physician and pediatrician, regional Poison Control Center, and if 911 is not in your area, emergency services for local police, fire department, and ambulance service.

- *List of Allergies:* a separate list for each household member.

- *List of Medications:* a separate list for each household member.

Medicines and Supplies

- *Acetaminophen, Ibuprofen, and Aspirin Tablets:* To relieve headaches, pain, fever, and simple sprains or strains of the body. Have at least two aspirin tablets available at all times in case of heart attack, although use as recommended by your physician. Use appropriate dosages and make sure the medicine is age appropriate. (Aspirin should not be used to relieve flu symptoms or be given to children.)

- *Cough Suppressant:* To relieve coughing. Use appropriate dosages and make sure the medicine is age appropriate.

- *Antihistamine:* To relieve allergies and inflammation. Use appropriate dosages and make sure the medicine is age appropriate.

- *Decongestant Tablets:* To relieve nasal congestion from colds or allergies. Use appropriate dosages and make sure the medicine is age appropriate.

- *Oral Medicine Syringe:* To administer medicine to children.

- *Activated Charcoal and Syrup of Ipecac:* To treat ingestion of certain poisons. Use only on the advice of a Poison Control Center, physician, or emergency department.

- *Fluids* to use for oral re-hydration when treating infant diarrhea.

Bandages and Other Injury/Wound Care Supplies

- *Bandages of Assorted Sizes:* To cover minor cuts and scrapes.

- *Bandage Closures/"Butterfly Bandages"* (one-fourth and one-inch sizes): To tape edges of minor cuts together.

- *Triangular Bandage:* To wrap injuries and make an arm sling.

- *Elastic Wraps:* To wrap wrist, ankle, knee, and elbow injuries.

- *Gauze in Rolls and Two-Inch and Four-Inch Pads:* To dress larger cuts and scrapes.

- *Adhesive Tape:* To keep gauze in place.

- *Sharp Scissors with Rounded Tips:* To cut tape, gauze, or clothes.

- *Safety Pins:* To fasten splints and bandages.

- *Antiseptic Wipes:* To disinfect wounds or clean hands.

- *Disposable, Instant-Activating Cold Packs:* For icing injuries and burns.

- *Tweezers:* For removing small splinters, foreign objects, bee stingers, and ticks from the skin (see first aid manual for proper removal of ticks).

- *Hydrogen Peroxide:* To disinfect and clean wounds.

- *Rubber Gloves:* To protect hands and reduce risk of infection when treating open wounds.

Other Supplies

- *Thermometer:* To take temperatures. For babies under age 1, use a rectal thermometer.

- *Petroleum Jelly:* To lubricate a rectal thermometer.

- *Calamine Lotion:* To relieve itching and irritation from insect bites and stings and poison ivy.

- *Hydrocortisone Cream:* To relieve irritation from rashes.

- *Complete Medical Consent Forms* for your family, which will allow someone to authorize medical treatment in an emergency situation when you're unable to give consent. If you have children, complete a medical consent form for each child and provide them to all caregivers.

Remember to follow the same precautions for medicines in your Home First Aid Kit as with any other medication. Use as recommended by your physician, store out of reach of children, and use products with child safety caps. Check expiration dates, and include other items as recommended by your physician. If someone in your household has a life-threatening allergy, carry appropriate medication with you at all times, such as auto injectable epinephrine.

Section 21.2

How to Care for Cuts, Scrapes, and Abrasions

What is a minor wound?

• Minor wounds are common and are not usually serious.

• Minor wounds usually do not require a doctor's care. Most can be treated at home with first aid.

• A minor wound is a small wound or a wound on just the surface of the skin.

• A minor wound might be a cut, scrape, or abrasion (like a child's skinned knee).

Can I treat it at home or should I seek medical care?

• A cut that goes beyond the top layer of skin may need stitches. Call the doctor.

• Wounds that will not stop bleeding may need stitches. Call the doctor.

• Most other minor wounds can be treated at home with first aid.

How do I care for cuts, scrapes, and abrasions?

• The most important step is to wash the wound with soap and warm water to keep it clean. Pat dry.

• Avoid putting alcohol, hydrogen peroxide, and iodine on the wound. This may actually cause more damage.

- Putting a first-aid ointment, such as Bacitracin, may help prevent infection.

- Cover the wound with a bandage (such as a Band-Aid) to keep out dirt and to prevent infection.

- To help stop bleeding, raise the wounded area. For example, rest a leg on a pillow if a cut to the shin won't stop bleeding.

- Wash the wound with soap and water each day.

- Replace the bandage each day.

What are signs of infection?

- Signs of infection can include redness and swelling.

- Other signs are pain or tenderness.

- Any pus (cream or greenish fluid) draining from the wound could indicate infection.

- Red streaks on the skin near the wound could be a sign of infection. This type of infection is more serious, especially if the child also has a fever. See the doctor right away.

When should I call the doctor?

- People who have illnesses that weaken the immune system, such as diabetes or cancer, should see a doctor if they are wounded. They are more likely to get an infection.

- If you think your child needs stitches, call the doctor right away.

- Call the doctor immediately if your child has red streaks on his skin around the wound, especially if he also has a fever.

- Call the doctor if you think your child's wound is infected.

- If there is risk of infection, call the doctor to see if your child has had a tetanus shot within the last 5 years.

- Call the doctor if you have questions or concerns.

Section 21.3

When to Seek Medical Care for Serious Cuts

From "Emergency Physicians Want Americans to Know When to Seek Medical Care for Serious Cuts," © 1999 American College of Emergency Physicians® (ACEP); reprinted with permission. For more health and safety tips, visit ACEP's website at www.acep.org.

A slip with a kitchen knife, a fall from a bicycle, or an accident on the playground may all cause serious lacerations that require an emergency physician's care. In fact, each year nearly 37 million people visit the emergency department due to an injury, including 11.5 million people who come to be treated for a serious laceration, according to the National Center for Health Statistics. Summer months bring on the year's peak of these injuries as people become more involved in outdoor activities. Yet physicians say that some people who sustain this type of injury wait too long to seek care, making it more difficult for doctors to close the wound, increasing the risk of infection and serious scarring. That is why the American College of Emergency Physicians (ACEP) is urging Americans to practice "Fast Aid First," and learn the basics of emergency wound care.

"I see many patients come into our emergency department with serious open wounds who have waited hours before coming to see us," says Dr. John Moorhead, president of ACEP. "Whether they delayed due to reluctance to appear foolish or simply not understanding how seriously they were injured, blood loss, increased risk of infection, and serious scarring may be the result."

Many lacerations, after only a few hours of delay, will contain enough bacteria that serious infections can occur if the wound is closed. Early treatment improves the chances of successful treatment in all lacerations.

How should you evaluate a wound to determine whether you need to seek immediate medical care? The following guidelines highlight the types of wounds that should prompt immediate treatment:

Wound Warning Signs

- Wounds still bleeding after 5 minutes of steady, firm pressure

- Wounds that appear particularly deep or "gaping" open

- Deep puncture wounds, such as those caused by stepping on a nail

- Wounds that have foreign materials, such as dirt, glass, or metal, embedded in them

- Any cut from animal bites and all human bites

- Any wound that shows signs of infection (for example, fever, swelling, pain, bad smell, fluid draining from area, or increasing pain)

- Problems with movement or sensation after a laceration

Treatments Available

Emergency physicians now have a variety of effective treatments available to close serious wounds and get patients quickly on the road to recovery.

- Topical skin adhesive is one of the newest innovations in skin closure. The physician applies the adhesive on top of the skin while holding the edges of the wound together. For some wounds, the adhesive takes less time to apply than stitches and forms a strong, flexible bond over the top of the wound and does not require a bandage. In some cases, it also may not require an injection of local anesthetic and can be associated with less patient pain and anxiety than sutures. The topical skin adhesive sloughs off the wound as it heals, usually in five to ten days, and does not require a return visit to the physician for suture removal.

- Traditional stitches (or sutures) are often used to close cuts. This involves "sewing" the skin together with a needle and surgical thread. This procedure usually requires an injection of anesthetic. A bandage is generally applied to the wound. After the wound is sufficiently healed, a physician will remove the stitches from the wound. Sometimes, the sutures are absorbed.

- Staples may also be used to close cuts.

- Skin strips are adhesive bands placed on top of the closed wound to hold skin edges together as it heals. This type of treatment is only used on very minor, superficial cuts.

"There are several new treatments available for treating patients with serious lacerations," says Dr. Moorhead. "People shouldn't delay seeking treatment. We can close their wounds quickly and relatively painlessly. You can never know when an emergency is going to occur. Our goal is to remind people that during the summer, when these types of injuries increase, fast action is important."

Section 21.4

Sprains and Strains

"Questions and Answers About Sprains and Strains,"
National Institute of Arthritis and Musculoskeletal and Skin Diseases
(NIAMS), March 1999.

What Is the Difference between a Sprain and a Strain?

A sprain is an injury to a ligament—a stretching or a tearing. One or more ligaments can be injured during a sprain. The severity of the injury will depend on the extent of injury to a single ligament (whether the tear is partial or complete) and the number of ligaments involved.

A strain is an injury to either a muscle or a tendon. Depending on the severity of the injury, a strain may be a simple overstretch of the muscle or tendon, or it can result in a partial or complete tear.

What Causes a Sprain?

A sprain can result from a fall, a sudden twist, or a blow to the body that forces a joint out of its normal position. This results in an overstretch or tear of the ligament supporting that joint. Typically, sprains occur when people fall and land on an outstretched arm, slide into base, land on the side of their foot, or twist a knee with the foot planted firmly on the ground.

Where Do Sprains Usually Occur?

Although sprains can occur in both the upper and lower parts of the body, the most common site is the ankle. The knee is another common site for a sprain. A blow to the knee or a fall is often the cause; sudden twisting can also result in a sprain. Sprains also frequently occur at the wrist, typically when people fall and land on an outstretched hand.

What Are the Signs and Symptoms of a Sprain?

The usual signs and symptoms include pain, swelling, bruising, and loss of the ability to move and use the joint (called functional ability). However, these signs and symptoms can vary in intensity, depending on the severity of the sprain. Sometimes people feel a pop or tear when the injury happens.

Doctors use many criteria to diagnose the severity of a sprain. In general, a grade I, or mild sprain, causes overstretching or slight tearing of the ligaments with no joint instability. A person with a mild sprain usually experiences minimal pain, swelling, and little or no loss of functional ability. Bruising is absent or slight, and the person is usually able to put weight on the affected joint. People with mild sprains usually do not need an x-ray, but one is sometimes performed if the diagnosis is unclear.

When to See a Doctor for a Sprain

- You have severe pain and cannot put any weight on the injured joint.

- The area over the injured joint or next to it is very tender when you touch it.

- The injured area looks crooked or has lumps and bumps (other than swelling) that you do not see on the uninjured joint.

- You cannot move the injured joint.

- You cannot walk more than four steps without significant pain.

- Your limb buckles or gives way when you try to use the joint.

- You have numbness in any part of the injured area.

- You see redness or red streaks spreading out from the injury.

- You injure an area that has been injured several times before.

- You have pain, swelling, or redness over a bony part of your foot.

- You are in doubt about the seriousness of the injury or how to care for it.

A grade II, or moderate sprain, causes partial tearing of the ligament and is characterized by bruising, moderate pain, and swelling. A person with a moderate sprain usually has some difficulty putting weight on the affected joint and experiences some loss of function. An x-ray may be needed to help the doctor determine if a fracture is causing the pain and swelling. Magnetic resonance imaging is occasionally used to help differentiate between a significant partial injury and a complete tear in a ligament.

People who sustain a grade III, or severe sprain, completely tear or rupture a ligament. Pain, swelling, and bruising are usually severe, and the patient is unable to put weight on the joint. An x-ray is usually taken to rule out a broken bone.

When diagnosing any sprain, the doctor will ask the patient to explain how the injury happened. The doctor will examine the affected joint and check its stability and its ability to move and bear weight.

Strains

What Causes a Strain?

A strain is caused by twisting or pulling a muscle or tendon. Strains can be acute or chronic. An acute strain is caused by trauma or an injury such as a blow to the body; it can also be caused by improperly lifting heavy objects or overstressing the muscles. Chronic strains are usually the result of overuse—prolonged, repetitive movement of the muscles and tendons.

Where Do Strains Usually Occur?

Two common sites for a strain are the back and the hamstring muscle (located in the back of the thigh). Contact sports such as soccer, football, hockey, boxing, and wrestling put people at risk for strains. Gymnastics, tennis, rowing, golf, and other sports that require extensive gripping can increase the risk of hand and forearm strains. Elbow strains sometimes occur in people who participate in racquet sports, throwing, and contact sports.

What Are the Signs and Symptoms of a Strain?

Typically, people with a strain experience pain, muscle spasm, and muscle weakness. They can also have localized swelling, cramping, or inflammation and, with a minor or moderate strain, usually some loss of muscle function. Patients typically have pain in the injured area and general weakness of the muscle when they attempt to move it. Severe strains that partially or completely tear the muscle or tendon are often very painful and disabling.

How Are Sprains and Strains Treated?

Reduce Swelling and Pain

Treatment for sprains and strains is similar and can be thought of as having two stages. The goal during the first stage is to reduce swelling and pain. At this stage, doctors usually advise patients to follow a formula of rest, ice, compression, and elevation (RICE) for the first 24 to 48 hours after the injury. The doctor may also recommend an over-the-counter or prescription nonsteroidal anti-inflammatory drug, such as aspirin or ibuprofen, to help decrease pain and inflammation.

For people with a moderate or severe sprain, particularly of the ankle, a hard cast may be applied. Severe sprains and strains may require surgery to repair the torn ligaments, muscle, or tendons. Surgery is usually performed by an orthopedic surgeon.

It is important that moderate and severe sprains and strains be evaluated by a doctor to allow prompt, appropriate treatment to begin. A person who has any concerns about the seriousness of a sprain or strain should always contact a doctor for advice.

RICE Therapy

Rest: Reduce regular exercise or activities of daily living as needed. Your doctor may advise you to put no weight on an injured area for 48 hours. If you cannot put weight on an ankle or knee, crutches may help. If you use a cane or one crutch for an ankle injury, use it on the uninjured side to help you lean away and relieve weight on the injured ankle.

Ice: Apply an ice pack to the injured area for 20 minutes at a time, 4 to 8 times a day. A cold pack, ice bag, or plastic bag filled with crushed ice and wrapped in a towel can be used. To avoid cold injury and frostbite, do not apply the ice for more than 20 minutes.

Compression: Compression of an injured ankle, knee, or wrist may help reduce swelling. Examples of compression bandages are elastic wraps, special boots, air casts, and splints. Ask your doctor for advice on which one to use.

Elevation: If possible, keep the injured ankle, knee, elbow, or wrist elevated on a pillow, above the level of the heart, to help decrease swelling.

Begin Rehabilitation

The second stage of treating a sprain or strain is rehabilitation, the overall goal of which is to improve the condition of the injured part and restore its function. The health care provider will prescribe an exercise program designed to prevent stiffness, improve range of motion, and restore the joint's normal flexibility and strength. Some patients may need physical therapy during this stage.

Section 21.5

Burns

This information was provided by KidsHealth, one of the largest resources online for medically reviewed health information written for parents, kids, and teens. For more articles like this one, visit www.KidsHealth.org or www.TeensHealth.org. © 2001 The Nemours Center for Children's Health Media, a division of The Nemours Foundation.

Burns are one of the leading causes of accidental death in childhood, second only to motor vehicle accidents. Burns are often categorized as first, second, or third degree, based on the severity of damage to the skin.

Types of Burns

- **First-degree burns**, the mildest of the three, are generally caused by brief skin contact with hot water, steam, or hot objects or by overexposure to the sun. First-degree burns cause some blistering, swelling, redness, and pain.

- **Second-degree** (or partial thickness) burns result from contact with chemicals, hot liquids or solids, or from clothing catching on fire. The skin can appear mottled white to cherry red, and the burn is quite painful. Blisters are common.

- **Third-degree** (or full thickness) burns can result from prolonged contact with hot liquids or solids, chemicals, or electricity. Skin can be charred, leathery, or have a very pale appearance. There may be little or no pain because of nerve damage.

All burns should be treated quickly to reduce the temperature of the burned area or to wash off chemicals, which helps reduce damage to the skin and underlying tissue.

What to Do

For First-Degree Burns

- Remove clothing from burned area immediately.

- Run cool water over the burned area or hold a clean, cold compress on the burn until pain subsides. (If water is not available, any cold, drinkable fluid can be used.) Do not use ice. Call your child's doctor for burns to the eyes, mouth, hands, and genital areas, even if they seem mild.

- Do not apply butter, grease, powder, or any other remedies to the burn.

- If the burned area is small, loosely cover it with a sterile gauze pad or bandage.

For Second- and Third-Degree Burns

- Follow the instructions for first-degree burns. Remove all clothing from the burn, except for clothing that is stuck to the skin. Do not break blisters.

- Phone your child's doctor. Keep your child lying down with the burned area elevated.

For Chemical Burns

- Flush the burned area with lots of running water for 5 minutes or more. If the burned area is large, use a tub, shower, buckets of water, or a garden hose.

- Do not remove any of your child's clothing before you've begun flushing the burn with water. As you continue flushing the burn, you can then remove clothing from the burned area.

- If the burned area is large, phone for emergency medical help. Continue to flush the burned area.

- If the burned area is small, flush for another 10 to 20 minutes, apply a sterile gauze pad or bandage, and phone your child's doctor.

- Chemical burns to the mouth or eyes require immediate medical evaluation after thorough flushing with water.

Section 21.6

Eye Injuries

This information was provided by KidsHealth, one of the largest resources online for medically reviewed health information written for parents, kids, and teens. For more articles like this one, visit www.KidsHealth.org or www.TeensHealth.org. © 2001 The Nemours Center for Children's Health Media, a division of The Nemours Foundation.

You can treat many minor eye irritations by flushing the eye, but more serious injuries require medical attention. Injuries to the eye are the most common preventable cause of blindness; so when in doubt, err on the side of caution and call your child's doctor for help.

What to Do:

Routine Irritations
(sand, dirt, and other "foreign bodies" on the eye surface)

- Do not try to remove any "foreign body" except by flushing, because of the risk of scratching the surface of the eye, especially the cornea.

- Wash your hands thoroughly before touching the eyelids to examine or flush the eye.

- Do not touch, press, or rub the eye, and do whatever you can to keep the child from touching it (a baby can be swaddled as a preventive measure).

- Tilt the child's head over a basin with the affected eye down and gently pull down the lower lid, encouraging the child to open her eyes as wide as possible. For an infant or small child, it is helpful to have a second person hold the child's eyes open while you flush.

- Gently pour a steady stream of lukewarm water from a pitcher (do not heat the water) across the eye. Sterile saline solution can also be used.

- Flush for up to 15 minutes, checking the eye every 5 minutes to see if the foreign body has been flushed out.

- Since a particle can scratch the cornea and cause an infection, the eye should be examined by a doctor if there continues to be any irritation afterward.

- If a foreign body is not dislodged by flushing, it will probably be necessary for a trained medical practitioner to flush the eye.

Embedded Foreign Body
(an object penetrates the globe of the eye)

- Call for emergency medical help.

- Cover the affected eye. If the object is small, use an eye patch or sterile dressing. If the object is large, cover the injured eye with a small cup taped in place. The point is to keep all pressure off the globe of the eye.

- Keep your child (and yourself) as calm and comfortable as possible until help arrives.

Chemical Exposure

- Many chemicals, even those found around the house, can damage an eye. If your child gets a chemical in the eye and you know what it is, look on the product's container for an emergency number to call for instructions.

- Flush the eye (see above) with lukewarm water for 15 to 30 minutes. If both eyes are affected, do it in the shower.

- Call for emergency medical help.

- Call your local poison control center for specific instructions. Be prepared to give the exact name of the chemical, if you have it. However, do not delay flushing the eye first.

Black Eye, Blunt Injury, or Contusion

A black eye is often a minor injury, but it can also appear when there is significant eye injury or head trauma. A visit to your doctor or an eye specialist may be required to rule out serious injury, particularly if you're not certain of the cause of the black eye.

For a "simple" black eye:

- Apply cold compresses intermittently: 5 to 10 minutes on, 10 to 15 minutes off. If you are not at home when the injury occurs and there is no ice available, a cold soda will do to start. If you use ice, make sure it is covered with a towel or sock to protect the delicate skin on the eyelid.

- Use cold compresses for 24 to 48 hours, then switch to applying warm compresses intermittently. This will help the body reabsorb the leakage of blood and may help reduce discoloration.

- If the child is in pain, give acetaminophen (not aspirin or ibuprofen, which can increase bleeding).

- Prop the child's head with an extra pillow at night, and encourage her to sleep on the uninjured side of her face (pressure can increase swelling).

- Call your child's doctor, who may recommend an in-depth evaluation to rule out damage to the eye. Call immediately if any of the following symptoms are noted:

  - increased redness

  - drainage from the eye

  - persistent eye pain

  - any changes in vision

  - any visible abnormality of the eyeball

  - visible bleeding on the white part (sclera) of the eye, especially near the cornea

If the injury occurred during one of your child's routine activities such as a sport, follow up by investing in an ounce of prevention—protective goggles or unbreakable glasses are vitally important.

Section 21.7

Ear Emergencies

Updated by Ashutosh Kacker, M.D., Department of Otolaryngology, New York Presbyterian Hospital, New York, NY, January 23, 2002. Copyright © 2002 A.D.A.M., Inc.; reprinted with permission.

Alternative Names

Foreign body lodged in the ear canal

Definition

An ear emergency is any injury to the outer, middle, or inner ear. It can also be an object in the ear.

Considerations

There are multiple causes of damage to the ear, many of them emergencies:

- **Acoustic trauma:** Loud percussions, such as a gun going off, can cause immediate hearing loss and ringing in the ear. If the percussion is close enough and loud enough, it can actually perforate the eardrum.

- **Barotrauma:** Rapid changes in pressure, especially in the presence of blocked eustachian tubes, can cause pain and occasional perforation of the eardrum. Pressure changes occur when flying, scuba diving, and driving in the mountains. A common cause of sudden pressure change and a frequent cause of perforated eardrums is water skiing. Rapid pressure changes occur when the skier falls and hits the water. Being slapped or hit on the ear can also rupture the eardrum and cause hearing loss. There can also be dizziness and ringing in the ear (tinnitus) associated with hearing loss.

- **Foreign bodies:** Children often stick objects into their nose or ears (for unclear reasons). It is not an uncommon occurrence, with foreign bodies in the nose being more common than foreign bodies in the ear. These foreign bodies can be difficult to remove because the ear canal is basically a tube through solid bone that is lined with thin and very sensitive skin. Anything pressing against the skin, such as forceps attempting to grasp the foreign body, can cause excruciating pain.

- **Infection:** Middle ear infections are common in childhood. It causes pain and ruined nights for the child and the parents. Infections can result in temporary loss of hearing, ringing in the ears (tinnitus), and the persistence of fluid in the middle ear. Multiple repeat infections can result in scarring or thickening of the membranes in the middle ear with gradual loss of hearing.

Any significant trauma to the ear should be evaluated by a physician. In children, the decision is often simple because the problem is usually associated with pain. Adults should seek attention if they have trauma that results in ringing (tinnitus), hearing loss, drainage from the ear, blood from the ear, pain, or other problems that appear to result from trauma or infection in the ear.

Special instruments are needed to examine the ear thoroughly and safely remove the foreign body.

Causes

- The most common cause of a perforated eardrum is trauma, such as the deliberate or accidental insertion of an object like cotton swabs, bobby pins, or toothpicks.

- Sudden, excessive changes in pressure, such as an explosion, a blow to the head (ear), flying, scuba diving, falling while water skiing, etc.

- Earache, middle ear infection (otitis).

- Anything inserted into the ear is considered a foreign body, even when inserted with good intent. Types of objects that get lodged in the ear include inserted objects, insects, or airborne objects.

Symptoms

- Bleeding
- Bruising
- Dizziness

- Loss of hearing
- Nausea and vomiting
- Noises in the ear
- Earache
- Redness
- Swelling
- Foreign object visible in the ear
- Sensations of a foreign object in the ear
- Clear liquid coming out of the ear (CSF [cerebral spinal fluid]-brain fluid)

First Aid

1. If there is bleeding from cuts on the outer ear, apply direct pressure. If part of the ear has been cut off, keep the part and get medical help immediately. Cover the injured ear with a sterile dressing shaped to the contour of the ear, and tape it loosely in place. Apply cold compresses over the dressing to help reduce pain and swelling.

2. If there is drainage from inside the ear, cover the outside of the ear with a sterile dressing that conforms to the contour of the ear, and tape it loosely in place. Have the victim lie down on the side with the affected ear down so that it can drain. However, do not move the victim if a neck or back injury is suspected. Get medical help.

3. If the eardrum has been ruptured (initially, there will be severe pain), place sterile cotton gently in the outer ear canal to keep the inside of the ear clean. Get medical help.

First Aid for Object in the Ear

1. Calm and reassure the victim.

2. Do not attempt to remove the foreign object by probing with a cotton swab or any other tool.

3. If the object is clearly visible at the entrance of the ear canal, and it can be easily grasped with tweezers, gently remove it. Then, get medical help to make sure the entire object was removed.

4. If you think a small object may be lodged within the ear, but you cannot see it, do not reach inside the ear canal with tweezers. You can do more harm than good. Get medical help.

5. Try using gravity to get the object out by tilting the head to the affected side. Do not strike the victim's head, but shake it gently in the direction of the ground to try to dislodge the object.

6. If the object is an insect, don't let the victim put a finger in their ear since this may make the insect sting. First, turn the victim's head so that the affected side is up, and wait to see if the insect crawls out. If this doesn't work, try to float the insect out by pouring mineral oil, olive oil, or baby oil into the ear. It should be warm, but not hot. As you pour the oil, you can ease the entry of the oil by straightening the ear canal: pull the ear lobe gently backward and upward for an adult, or backward and downward for a child. The insect should suffocate and may float out in the oil bath. Avoid using oil to remove any object other than an insect, since oil can cause other kinds of objects to swell.

Do Not

- DO NOT block any drainage coming from the ear.
- DO NOT try to clean drainage or irrigate inside the ear.
- DO NOT attempt to remove the foreign object by probing with a cotton swab, pin, or any other tool. To do so will risk pushing the object farther into the ear and damaging the middle ear.
- DO NOT reach inside the ear canal with tweezers.

Call immediately for emergency medical assistance if:

- You suspect any serious head injury.
- First aid methods are unsuccessful and the victim is experiencing pain, reduced hearing, dizziness, or a sensation of something lodged in the ear.

Prevention

- Never put anything in the ear canal without first consulting a physician.

- Never thump the head to try to correct an ear problem.

- Following an ear injury, avoid nose blowing and getting water in the injured ear.

- Teach children not to put things in their ears.

- Avoid cleaning the inner ear canals altogether.

Section 21.8

Objects in the Nose

"Foreign Body in the Nose," updated by Ashutosh Kacker, M.D., Department of Otolaryngology, New York Presbyterian Hospital, New York, NY, August 21, 2001. Copyright © 2002 A.D.A.M., Inc.; reprinted with permission.

Definition

First aid for a foreign object inserted into the nose.

Considerations

Curious young children may insert small objects into their nose in a developmentally normal attempt to explore their own bodies. Potential objects may include food, seeds, dried beans, small toys, crayon pieces, erasers, paper wads, cotton, and beads.

A foreign body allowed to remain in the nose may lead to irritation, infection, and obstruction to breathing.

Causes

Insertion of an object into the nose.

Symptoms

- foul-smelling or bloody nasal discharge
- difficulty breathing through the affected nostril

- irritation
- sensation of something in the nostril

First Aid

1. Do not probe the nose with cotton swabs or other tools. Doing so may push the object further into the nose.

2. Have the victim breathe through the mouth and avoid breathing in sharply (which may force the object in further).

3. Once it is determined which nostril is affected, gently press the other nostril closed and have the victim blow gently through the affected nostril. Avoid blowing the nose too hard or repeatedly.

4. If this method fails, get medical help.

Do Not

- DO NOT try to remove an object that is not visible and easy to grasp; doing so may push the object farther in or cause damage to tissue.

- DO NOT use tweezers or other instruments to remove an object lodged deeply in the nose.

Call immediately for emergency medical assistance if:

- you cannot easily remove a foreign object from the victim's nose.

- you suspect an infection in the nose after removal of a foreign object from the victim's nose.

Prevention

- Keep small objects out of the reach of infants and toddlers.

- Discourage your child from putting foreign objects into body openings.

Section 21.9

Dental Injuries

Most traumatic dental injuries occur in children, but people of all ages can be affected. Whether the injury is a result of an automobile accident, a sports mishap, an altercation, or a bad fall, the severity and type of injury will determine the treatment necessary.

A number of common injuries can involve teeth. Many of them affect the inner soft tissues of the tooth, known as the dental pulp. When the pulp becomes injured or inflamed, root canal treatment may be needed.

What Is Endodontic (Root Canal) Treatment?

To understand endodontic treatment, it helps to know something about the anatomy of the tooth. A soft tissue called the pulp is inside the tooth, under the white enamel and a hard, thick layer called the dentin. The pulp, which contains blood vessels, creates the surrounding hard tissues of the tooth during development.

The pulp extends from the crown, or chewing portion of the tooth, to the tip of the roots where it connects to the tissues surrounding the root. The pulp is important during a tooth's growth and development. However, once a tooth is fully mature, it can survive without the pulp because the tooth continues to be nourished by the tissues surrounding it.

Root canal treatment is necessary when the pulp becomes inflamed or infected. This may happen as a result of deep decay, repeated dental procedures on the tooth, or a blow to the tooth. During endodontic treatment, the damaged pulp is removed. Then the tooth's canals are cleaned and filled to help preserve the tooth.

Types of Injuries

Chipped teeth account for the majority of all dental trauma. The remaining represent more serious problems, including dislodged and knocked-out teeth. Treatment depends on the type, location, and severity of each injury. When any dental injury occurs, the most important thing is to see your dentist or endodontist immediately. The outcome, or prognosis, for your specific injury often depends on how quickly you see your dentist.

Chipped or Fractured Teeth

Most chipped teeth can be repaired with a simple filling. Sometimes a chip will expose the pulp of the tooth. Some exposures can be treated by placing a filling over the injured area. Other exposures, however, may require root canal treatment.

Injuries in the back teeth often include fractured cusps, cracked teeth, and the more serious split teeth. Cracks may or may not extend into the root. If the crack does not extend into the root, the tooth can usually be restored by your dentist with a full crown. If the crack does extend into the root and affects the pulp, root canal treatment is usually necessary in an attempt to save all or a portion of your tooth.

Dislodged Teeth

During an injury, a tooth may be pushed into its socket. This can be one of the more serious injuries. Your endodontist or general dentist may reposition and stabilize your tooth. Root canal treatment is usually started within a few weeks of the injury, and a medication, such as calcium hydroxide, may be put inside the tooth. A permanent root canal filling will be placed at a later date. You should continue to have the tooth monitored periodically by your dentist to assure proper healing.

Sometimes a tooth is pushed partially out of the socket. Repositioning and stabilizing of the tooth are usually necessary. If the pulp remains healthy, no additional treatment may be needed. If the pulp is injured, your dentist or endodontist may need to start root canal treatment. Medication, such as calcium hydroxide, may be placed inside the tooth and should be followed by a permanent root canal filling at a later date.

Avulsed Teeth

If a tooth is completely knocked out of your mouth, time is of the essence. If this type of injury happens to you, pick up your tooth by the crown, or chewing portion. Try not to touch the root. If the tooth is dirty, gently rinse it in water. Do not use soap or any other cleaning agent. If possible, place the tooth back into its socket. Go to the dentist immediately.

If you cannot put the tooth back in its socket, be sure to keep it moist. The less time the tooth spends drying out, the better the chance for saving the tooth. Solutions to keep your tooth moist are available at local drug stores. You can also put the tooth in milk or a glass of water with only a pinch of salt, or you can simply put it in your mouth between your gum and cheek. Bring your tooth to the dentist immediately.

If the tooth has been put back in its socket, your dentist may stabilize the tooth with a splint and check for any other facial injuries. If the tooth has not been put back into its socket, your dentist will examine the tooth to determine if it is still intact and check for other facial injuries. Your dentist will clean the tooth carefully and place it gently back into the socket. Your tooth may need to be stabilized with a splint for a period of time. Depending on the stage of root development, your dentist or endodontist may start root canal treatment. A medication may be placed in the tooth followed by a permanent root canal filling at a later date. The length of time the tooth was out of the mouth and the way the tooth was stored before reaching the dentist may influence the type of treatment you receive. You should contact your physician to see if a tetanus booster is necessary.

Root Fractures

A traumatic injury to the tooth may also result in a horizontal root fracture. The location of the fracture determines the long-term health of the tooth. If the fracture is close to the root tip, the chances for success are better. If the fracture does not result in the two pieces of the root being separated, there is also a better chance for success. However, the nearer the fracture is to the chewing surface of the tooth, the poorer the long-term success rate, regardless of whether the pieces are separated.

Sometimes stabilization with a splint is required for a period of time. If the tissue inside the tooth is damaged, root canal treatment may be needed. A medication may be placed in the canal to prepare the fracture site for the eventual root canal filling.

Do Traumatic Dental Injuries Differ in Children?

Children's permanent or adult teeth that are not fully developed at the time of the injury may need special attention. In an immature adult tooth, the tip of the root, called the apex, is open, and the root canal walls are thin. As the tooth develops, the apex closes and the canal walls thicken. An injured immature tooth may need one of the following two procedures to improve the chances of saving the tooth:

Apexogenesis

One procedure, called apexogenesis, encourages the root to continue developing as it helps heal the pulp. The injured soft tissue is covered with a medication to encourage further root growth. The apex continues to close, and the walls of the root canal thicken. If the pulp heals, no additional endodontic treatment may be necessary. The more mature the root becomes, the better the chances that the tooth can be saved. However, apexogenesis is not always successful. A different procedure, called apexification, may need to be performed.

Apexification

During apexification, the unhealthy pulp tissue is removed. The endodontist places a medication into the root to help a hard tissue form near the apex, or root tip. This hard tissue provides a barrier for the permanent root canal filling. In spite of appropriate treatment, the root canal walls of a tooth treated by apexification will not continue to develop and thicken, making the tooth susceptible to crown or root fractures. Proper restoration will minimize this possibility and maximize protection of your tooth.

Other Injuries

An immature permanent tooth that has been dislodged may require minimal or no treatment other than follow-up until it has matured. If the tooth is severely dislodged, orthodontic or surgical repositioning and stabilization may be necessary.

If an immature permanent tooth has been out of the mouth for less than one hour, the tooth should be placed back in its socket, stabilized, and watched closely by your dentist or endodontist for three to four weeks. During this time, your dentist will look for changes in tooth color, pain, swelling, or loosening of the tooth. If any of these problems arise, an apexification procedure followed by a permanent root canal filling may be needed.

If the immature permanent tooth has been out of the mouth and dry for more than one hour, the tooth may be put back in the socket, filled with a medication, and re-evaluated in six to eight weeks. The long-term health of this tooth is generally poor, so your dentist or endodontist may discuss other treatment options with you.

Will the Tooth Need Any Special Care or Additional Treatment?

The nature of the injury, the length of time from injury to treatment, how your tooth was cared for after the injury, and your body's response all affect the long-term health of the tooth. Timely treatment is particularly important with the dislodged or avulsed tooth to prevent resorption. Resorption occurs when your body, through its own defense mechanisms, begins to reject your own hard tooth structure in response to the traumatic injury. You should return to your dentist or endodontist to have the tooth examined at regular intervals following the injury to ensure that resorption is not occurring and that surrounding tissues continue to heal.

For More Information

If you would like further information about traumatic dental injuries, your endodontist will be happy to talk with you. You may also contact the AAE at:

American Association of Endodontists
211 E. Chicago Ave., Suite 1100
Chicago, IL 60611-2691
Toll-free: 800-872-3636
Phone: 312-266-7255
Fax: 866-451-9020; 312-266-9867
Website: www.aae.org
E-mail: info@aae.org

Chapter 22

Checklists for Preventing Injuries in the Home

All Living Areas

- To prevent asthma attacks, eliminate sources of mold, dust, and insects, such as cockroaches. If you have a pet, keep it and its bedding clean and keep the pet off the furniture.

- If you must smoke, avoid smoking in the house, and especially around children.

- Make sure furnaces, fireplaces, wood-burning stoves, space heaters, and gas appliances are vented properly and inspected annually.

- Use safety gates to block stairways (and other danger areas), safety plugs to cover electrical outlets, and safety latches for drawers and cabinets.

- Keep children and the furniture they can climb on away from windows.

- Install window guards (on windows that are not fire emergency exits).

- To prevent falls, keep hallways and stairways well-lit and use non-slip backing for area rugs.

The checklists included in this chapter are from the U.S. Department of Housing and Urban Development (HUD) website http://www.hud.gov/healthy/, December 2000.

- Keep cleaning solutions, pesticides, and other potentially dangerous substances in their original, labeled containers, and out of the reach of children.

- Test homes built before 1978 for lead paint. Call 1-888-LEADLIST for certified inspectors. Ask your doctor or health department if your child should be tested for lead.

- If you have guns or rifles in your home, store the firearms and ammunition in separate containers and lock them out of the reach of children.

- Learn First Aid and Cardiopulmonary Resuscitation (CPR).

- Keep an updated list of emergency telephone numbers, including your local poison control center, physician, and hospital emergency room, next to every phone in your home.

- Have your home tested for radon. If levels are above EPA's recommended level, call 1-800-557-2366 to find out about ways to reduce the levels.

- Make sure your family knows what to do during a natural disaster. In an earthquake, drop to the floor and get under something sturdy for cover; during a tornado, take shelter in a basement or an interior room without windows; and during a hurricane stay away from windows. Have handy supplies of food, flashlights, and water.

In the Kitchen

- Keep knives, plastic bags, lighters, and matches locked away from children.

- Avoid fires and burns by never leaving cooking food unattended, turning pot handles to the back of the stove, and keeping hot liquids and foods away from the edges of tables and counters.

- Make sure you and your children know the "stop, drop, and roll" procedure in case their clothes catch on fire.

- Keep appliance cords unplugged and tied up. Replace any frayed cords and wires.

- Securely strap young children in high chairs, swings, and other juvenile products.

- Do not give young children hard, round foods that can get stuck in their throats like hard candies, nuts, grapes, popcorn, carrots, and raisins.

- Avoid scald burns by keeping children away from the hot water taps on drinking water coolers.

In the Bathroom

- To prevent poisonings, lock away all medicines and vitamins, even those with child-resistant packaging.

- Have syrup of ipecac on hand, but use only at the recommendation of a poison control center or physician.

- Never leave a young child alone in the bathroom, especially in a bath.

- Before bathing a child, always test bath water with your wrist or elbow to make sure it's not too hot.

- To prevent scalds, set the water heater thermostat to 120° F (Fahrenheit) and install anti-scald devices.

- Make sure bathtubs and showers have non-slip surfaces and grab bars.

- Keep electrical appliances, like hair dryers and curling irons, out of the reach of children and away from water.

In the Bedroom

- Install smoke alarms outside bedrooms and on every level of the home. For added protection, consider installing smoke alarms in each bedroom. Test them at least once a month and change batteries at least once a year.

- Practice fire escape routes and identify an outside meeting place.

- Place a baby to sleep on his or her back in a crib with no pillows or soft bedding underneath.

- Use a crib that meets national safety standards and has a snug-fitting mattress.

- Never use an electric blanket in the bed or crib of a small child or infant.

- Keep small toys, balloons, and small balls away from young children.

- Check age labels for appropriate toys. Make sure toy storage chests have safety lid supports.

- To prevent strangulation, use safety tassels for miniblinds and avoid strings on children's toys and pacifiers.

- Install carbon monoxide (CO) alarms outside bedrooms to prevent CO poisoning.

Chapter 23

Poisoning Prevention

Millions of poisoning exposures occur each year in the United States, resulting in nearly 900,000 visits to emergency departments. About 90 percent of poisonings happen in the home, and more than half of them involve children under age six. Many poisonings can be prevented if safety precautions are taken around the home. If a poisoning occurs, calling a poison control center can help ensure rapid, appropriate treatment.

Preventing Poisonings in the Home

The simple steps that follow, provided by the American Association of Poison Control Centers, can help you protect children from poisons:

- Post the telephone number for your poison control center near your phone, in a place where all family members would be able to find it quickly in an emergency.

- Remove all nonessential drugs and household products from your home. Discard them according to the manufacturer's instructions.

- If you have small children, avoid keeping highly toxic products, such as drain cleaners, in the home, garage, shed, or other place children can access.

From "Poisoning Prevention," SafeUSA™, Centers for Disease Control and Prevention, 2002. More information from SafeUSA™ is available online at www.safeusa.org.

- Buy medicines and household products in child-resistant packaging and be sure that caps are always on tight. Do not remove child-safety caps. Avoid keeping medicines, vitamins, or household products in anything but their original packaging.

- Store all of your medicines and household products in a locked closet or cabinet—including products and medicines with child-resistant containers.

- Crawl around your house, including inside your closets, to inspect it from a child's point of view. You'll likely find a poisoning hazard you hadn't noticed before.

- Never refer to medicine or vitamins as "candy."

- Make sure visiting grandparents, family friends, or other care givers keep their medications away from children. For example, if Grandma keeps pills in her purse, make sure the purse is out of children's reach.

- Keep a bottle of syrup of ipecac in your home—this can be used to induce vomiting. Use it only when the poison control center tells you to.

- Avoid products such as cough syrup or mouth wash that contain alcohol—these are hazardous for young children. Look for alcohol-free alternatives.

- Keep cosmetics and beauty products out of children's reach. Remember that hair permanents and relaxers are toxins as well.

Carbon Monoxide Poisoning

Carbon monoxide (CO) is an invisible, odorless, poisonous gas that can cause sickness and death. The gas is produced by the incomplete burning of fuels such as natural gas, oil, kerosene, coal, and wood. Fuel-burning appliances that are not working properly or are installed incorrectly can produce fatal concentrations of carbon monoxide in your home. Other hazards include burning charcoal indoors and running a car in the garage, both of which can lead to dangerous levels of CO in your home.

Every year, more than 200 Americans die from CO produced by fuel-burning appliances, and several thousand go to emergency departments for treatment for CO poisoning. You can prevent carbon monoxide poisonings in your home by following a few simple tips.

248

- Install carbon monoxide alarms near bedrooms and on each floor of your home. If your alarm sounds, the U.S. Consumer Product Safety Commission suggests that you press the reset button, call emergency services (911 or your local fire department), and immediately move to fresh air (either outdoors or near an open door or window). If you learn that fuel-burning appliances were the most likely cause of the poisoning, have a serviceperson check them for malfunction before turning them back on. Refer to the instructions on your CO alarm for more specific information about what to do if your alarm goes off.

- Symptoms of CO poisoning are similar to the flu, only without a fever (headache, fatigue, nausea, dizziness, shortness of breath). If you experience any of these symptoms, get fresh air immediately and contact a physician for proper diagnosis. Also, open windows and doors, turn off combustion appliances, contact emergency services, and take the steps listed above to ensure your home's safety.

- To keep carbon monoxide from collecting in your home, make sure that any fuel-burning equipment, such as a furnace, stove, or heater, works properly, and never use charcoal or other grills indoors or in the garage. Do not leave your car's engine running while it's in the garage, and consider putting weather stripping around the door between the garage and the house.

Who Is Affected?

Millions of poisoning exposures occur each year in the United States, resulting in nearly 900,000 visits to the emergency department. About 90 percent of poisonings happen in the home, and common household items are often the cause. The poisons involved most often are cleaning products, pain relievers, cosmetics, personal care products, plants, and cough and cold medicines.

Children—especially those under age 6—are at highest risk for unintentional poisonings. Adolescents are also at risk for poisonings, both intentional and unintentional. About half of all poisonings among teens are classified as suicide attempts.

Poison control centers help millions of people each year, ensuring that poisonings are treated rapidly and correctly. Poison control centers managed more than 2 million cases of poison exposure in 1996. About three-quarters of these cases were managed at home over the telephone with the help of specialists trained in poison information.

Poison control centers are extremely cost effective. For every $1 spent on poison control centers, an estimated $7 is saved in medical care costs. By helping people manage emergencies at home, these centers prevent about 50,000 hospitalizations and 400,000 trips to doctors' offices each year.

References

The data and safety tips in this fact sheet were obtained from the following sources:

American Association of Poison Control Centers. "Prevention Tips." Available at http://www.aapcc.org/preventi.htm. Accessed September 10, 1999.

Burt CW, Fingerhut LA. "Injury visits to hospital emergency departments: United States, 1992–95." *Vital and Health Statistics* 13(131). DHHS publication no. 98–1792. Hyattsville, MD: National Center for Health Statistics, 1998.

Committee on Injury and Poison Control Prevention, American Academy of Pediatrics. *Injury Prevention and Control for Children and Youth.* Elk Grove Village, IL: The Academy, 1997.

Litovitz TL, Smilkstein M, Felberg L, Klein-Schwartz W, Berlin R, Morgan JL. "1996 annual report of the American Association of Poison Control Centers Toxic Exposure Surveillance System." *American Journal of Emergency Medicine* 1997; 15(5):44715–500.

Miller TR, Lestina DC. "Costs of poisoning in the United States and savings from poison control centers: A benefit-cost analysis." *Annals of Emergency Medicine* 1997; 29(2):239–245.

U.S. Consumer Product Safety Commission. "Carbon Monoxide Fact Sheet." Available at www.cpsc.gov/cpscpub/pubs/466.html. Accessed September 23, 1999.

Chapter 24

Using Insect Repellents Safely

Mosquitoes, biting flies, and ticks can be annoying and sometimes pose a serious risk to public health. In certain areas of the U.S., mosquitoes can transmit diseases like equine and St. Louis encephalitis. Biting flies can inflict a painful bite that can persist for days, swell, and become infected. Ticks can transmit serious diseases like Lyme disease and Rocky Mountain spotted fever. When properly used, insect repellents can discourage biting insects from landing on treated skin or clothing.

Choosing Insect Repellents

Insect repellents are available in various forms and concentrations. Aerosol and pump-spray products are intended for skin applications as well as for treating clothing. Liquid, cream, lotion, spray, and stick products enable direct skin application. Products with a low concentration of active ingredient may be appropriate for situations where exposure to insects is minimal. Higher concentration of active ingredient may be useful in highly infested areas, or with insect species which are more difficult to repel. And where appropriate, consider nonchemical ways to deter biting insects—screens, netting, long sleeves, and slacks.

From "How to Use Insect Repellents Safely," U.S. Environmental Protection Agency (EPA), http://www.epa.gov/pesticides/factsheets/insectrp.htm, updated 2002.

Using Insect Repellents Safely

The U.S. Environmental Protection Agency (EPA) recommends the following precautions when using insect repellents:

- Apply repellents only to exposed skin and/or clothing (as directed on the product label). Do not use under clothing.

- Never use repellents over cuts, wounds, or irritated skin.

- Do not apply to eyes and mouth, and apply sparingly around ears. When using sprays do not spray directly onto face; spray on hands first and then apply to face.

- Do not allow children to handle the products, and do not apply to children's hands. When using on children, apply to your own hands and then put it on the child.

- Do not spray in enclosed areas. Avoid breathing a repellent spray, and do not use it near food.

- Use just enough repellent to cover exposed skin and/or clothing. Heavy application and saturation is unnecessary for effectiveness; if biting insects do not respond to a thin film of repellent, then apply a bit more.

- After returning indoors, wash treated skin with soap and water or bathe. This is particularly important when repellents are used repeatedly in a day or on consecutive days. Also, wash treated clothing before wearing it again.

- If you suspect that you or your child are reacting to an insect repellent, discontinue use, wash treated skin, and then call your local poison control center. If/when you go to a doctor, take the repellent with you.

- Get specific medical information about the active ingredients in repellents and other pesticides by calling the National Pesticide Information Center (NPIC) at 1-800-858-7378. The NPIC website is http://npic.orst.edu.

Important Information on Using Pesticides

EPA recommends the following precautions when using an insect repellent or pesticide:

- Check the container to ensure that the product bears an EPA-approved label and registration number. Never use a product that has not been approved for use by EPA.

- Read the entire label before using a pesticide. Even if you have used it before, read the label again. Don't trust your memory.

- Follow use directions carefully, use only the amount directed, at the time and under the conditions specified, and for the purpose listed. For example, if you need a tick repellent, make sure that the product label lists this use. If ticks are not listed, the product may not be formulated for that use.

- Store pesticides away from children's reach, in a locked utility cabinet or garden shed.

Avoiding Ticks and Lyme Disease

Lyme disease has become the leading tick-borne illness in the United States. In 1999, 16,273 cases of Lyme disease were reported to the Centers for Disease Control and Prevention (CDC). The deer tick, also known as the black-legged tick, is the species that most often transmits Lyme disease. With proper precautions, Lyme disease is preventable.

- Ticks are most active from April through October, so exercise additional caution when venturing into tick country during that time period.

- When in a tick-infested area, a good prevention is an insect repellent; however, consider using a product designed to be applied to clothing rather than your skin.

- Tuck pants cuffs into boots or socks, and wear long sleeves and light-colored clothing which makes it easier to spot ticks.

- Stay to the center of hiking paths, and avoid grassy and marshy woodland areas.

- Inspect yourself and your children for clinging ticks after leaving an infested area. Ticks are hard to see—nymphs are dot-sized; adults, smaller than a sesame seed.

- If you discover a tick feeding, do not panic. Studies indicate that an infected tick does not usually transmit the Lyme organism during the first 24 hours.

- If you suspect Lyme disease or its symptoms, contact your doctor immediately.

Pesticide Emergencies

In case of an emergency, first determine what the person was exposed to and what part of the body was affected before you take action, since taking the right action is as important as taking immediate action. If the person is unconscious, having trouble breathing, or having convulsions, give the indicated first aid immediately. Call 911 or your local emergency service. If these symptoms are not evident, contact your local Poison Control Center, physician, 911, or your local emergency service and follow its directions. The following are general first aid guidelines:

- **Poison in eye.** Eye membranes absorb pesticides faster than any other external part of the body. Eye damage can occur in a few minutes with some types of pesticides. If poison splashes into an eye, hold the eyelid open and wash quickly and gently with clean running water from the tap or a gentle stream from a hose for at least 15 minutes. If possible, have someone contact a Poison Control Center while the victim is being treated. Do not use eye drops, chemicals, or drugs in the wash water.

- **Poison on skin.** If pesticide splashes on the skin, drench area with water and remove contaminated clothing. Wash skin and hair thoroughly with soap and water. Later discard contaminated clothing or thoroughly wash it separately from other laundry.

- **Inhaled poison.** Get the victim to fresh air immediately. Open doors and windows to prevent fumes from poisoning others. Call the fire department.

- **Swallowed poison.** Induce vomiting only if the emergency personnel on the phone tell you to do so. It will depend on what the victim has swallowed; some petroleum products, or caustic poisons can cause serious damage if vomited. Always keep Syrup of Ipecac on hand (1 bottle per household). Be sure the date is current and keep it out of children's reach.

Chapter 25

Fire Safety Tips

In 1999, more than 2,900 people were killed and another 16,425 were injured in home fires in the United States. In a fire, smoke alarms cut the chances of dying in half.

Reduce Your Risk

Residential fires can be dangerous and destructive, but you can reduce your risk for fire-related injuries if you follow a few simple tips.

Install smoke alarms outside each separate sleeping area and on every floor of your home, including the basement.

- CDC suggests using smoke alarms with lithium-powered batteries and a "hush button." A lithium-powered battery lasts up to 10 years, and a hush button allows you to quickly stop nuisance alarms that are caused by such things as steam or oven smoke.

- If 10-year, long-life smoke alarms are not available, install smoke alarms that use a regular 9-volt battery, but be sure to replace the battery every year. (A useful tip to help you remember: when you change your clocks to standard time in the fall,

From "Fire Safety," SafeUSA™, Centers for Disease Control and Prevention, 2002. More information from SafeUSA™ is available online at www.safeusa.org.

change the battery. Or pick a fall holiday like Halloween or Thanksgiving to change the battery.)

- Smoke alarms have a useful life of about 10 years. At that age the entire alarm should be replaced, even if it seems to be working.

- Test smoke alarms every month to make sure they work properly. This can be done by pushing the test button. If the smoke alarm is out-of-reach, you can push the test button with a broom handle or yard stick.

Make a family fire escape plan and practice it every 6 months.

In a typical home fire, people have only about 2 minutes to get outside. It's easy for anyone to panic and be confused during that short time, especially children. During a fire, children often try to hide in a closet or under beds where they feel safe rather than going outside. That's why it's so important to make a fire escape plan for everyone in the family and practice it at least twice a year. However, in a national survey, only 53 percent of respondents said they had a plan to follow if there were a fire in their home, and of these, only 3 of 10 had ever practiced the plan.

- In the plan, discuss at least two different ways to get out of every room and choose a safe place in front of the house or apartment building for family members to meet after escaping a fire. Having a meeting place will let you know that everyone has gotten out safely, and no one will get hurt looking for someone who is already safe.

- Talk with your family about what to do in the event of a fire:
  - Get out as fast as possible and go to your family's designated meeting place.
  - Do not stop to grab photographs or other belongings.
  - Do not go back into a burning house or apartment building.
  - Call the fire or rescue department from a neighbor's house.
  - If there is smoke in the room, stay low or crawl to your exit.
  - If you cannot escape, put wet towels or fabric around doors to block off smoke, crawl to a window, and open it. Yell out the window for help and wave a sheet or cloth for attention. If there is a phone in the room, call for help.

Prevent a fire from starting in your home.

- When cooking, never leave food on a stove or in an oven unat-tended. Avoid wearing clothes with long, loose-fitting sleeves. Do not hang pot holders and towels near burners.

- If you are a smoker, do not smoke in bed, never leave burning cigarettes unattended, do not empty smoldering ashes in a trash can, and keep ashtrays away from upholstered furniture and curtains.

- Keep matches and lighters away from children's reach, safely store flammable substances used around the home, and never leave burning candles unattended.

- Never leave young children alone in the home, even for a short period. Unattended children can start a fire by trying to cook something or by using a heater or electrical appliance in the wrong way.

- Keep space heaters at least 3 feet from anything that can burn, including furniture, bedding, and clothing. Do not leave space heaters on when you are not in the room or when you go to sleep.

Teach children to stop, drop, and roll.

Clothing fires are a major cause of burn injuries to children. Chil-dren can set their clothes on fire by playing with matches or getting too close to open fires or stoves. If this happens, children's natural reaction is to run, which will make the situation worse. Parents should teach their children the "stop, drop, and roll" maneuver to smother the flames. This has saved many lives, and parents should practice the maneuver with their children. The moment clothes start to burn:

- **stop** where you are,
- **drop** to the ground,
- and **roll** over and over with your hands covering your face.

Who Is Affected?

While most of us understand the importance of fire safety, we of-ten forget just how dangerous a fire can be. In 1999, more than 2,900 people were killed and another 16,425 were injured in home fires in the United States. Older adults, children younger than 5 years old, and people in substandard housing or mobile homes are at the highest risk for fire-related deaths. Among children between the ages of 1 and 9 years, fire and burn-related injuries are the third leading cause of injury death.

The most common causes of home fires are cooking and heating equipment. Heating appliances, including portable space heaters, can ignite furniture and other combustibles left too close to the heater. However, smoking is the leading cause of deaths from fires in the home and are often the result of carelessly discarded cigarettes or matches igniting furniture or mattresses. Alcohol use and fires are also a deadly mix. One study found that intoxication contributed to 40 percent of deaths due to home fires.

Most victims of fires die from smoke or toxic gases and not from burns. Fires produce poisonous gases that can spread quickly and far from the fire itself to claim victims who are asleep and not aware of the fire. Even if people awaken, the effects of exposure to these gases can cloud their thinking and slow their reactions so that they cannot escape. That is why it is so important for people to have early warning so they can escape before their ability to think and move is impaired.

One of the most important fire safety devices for the home is one that provides such a warning—the smoke alarm. Studies have shown that in a fire, smoke alarms cut the chances of dying in half. As many as 93 percent of U.S. homes have at least one smoke alarm, but one in four homes with smoke detectors have nonworking alarms. People with nonworking smoke alarms most often report that they disconnected or removed the battery to stop nuisance alarms, or they forgot to replace the old battery.

Additional Resource

Fire Prevention Week

In a typical home fire, people have only about two minutes to get outside safely. Individuals and families should develop a home fire escape plan and practice it. You can learn how at http://www. fire prevention week.org.

Chapter 26

Toy Safety

Statistics on Toy-Related Injuries

In 2001, there were an estimated 255,100 toy-related injuries treated in U.S. hospital emergency rooms. Seventy-nine percent (202,500) of the injuries were to children under 15 years of age and 30 percent (77,100) were to children under 5. Overall, males were involved in 60 percent of the toy-related injuries. Most of the victims (98 percent) were treated and released from the hospital. Riding toys (including unpowered scooters) continued to be associated with more injuries (121,700 or 48 percent) than any other category of toy.

Statistics on Toy-Related Deaths

Twenty-five toy-related deaths involving children under age 15 were reported to the U.S. Consumer Product Safety Commission (CPSC) in 2001. Victims of the 25 fatal incidents ranged in age from 3 months to 12 years old. Twenty-one of the fatalities involved male victims.

Choking or Aspiration Deaths

Nine choking or aspiration deaths occurred with four balloons, a toy building block, a toy dart, a toy ball, and two unspecified toys. These

---

This chapter includes excerpts from "Toy-Related Deaths," U.S. Consumer Product Safety Commission (CPSC), October 2002, "For Kids' Sake: Think Toy Safety," CPSC Document #281, 1995; and "Toy Safety Shopping Tips," CPSC and Kmart Corporation, 1997.

children ranged in age from 3 months to 8 years old. The children involved in the four balloon-related fatalities were 8 months to 4 years old.

Head Injury Deaths

Four of the toy-related deaths were the result of head injuries. All of these deaths involved nonpowered scooters. The ages of the victims ranged from 8 to 12 years. Three of the deaths resulted from a collision with a motor vehicle and one death resulted from a fall on a steep slope.

Deaths Due to Multiple Injuries

Four fatalities were the result of multiple injuries suffered during the toy-related incident. These children ranged in age from 2 to 12 years. Three of the deaths involved non-powered scooters and one death was associated with a toy scooter/kiddie car. The scooter-related fatalities were due to blunt force trauma to the head, neck, and chest; multiple injuries and fractures; and head and chest injuries. The toy scooter/kiddie car-related death was due to multiple blunt trauma injuries. All of these deaths were the result of collisions with motor vehicles (two cars, a van, and a garbage truck).

Deaths Due to Drowning

There were two deaths due to drowning associated with toys, and both deaths involved riding toys. A 1-year-old male rode his tricycle onto a torn swimming pool cover and subsequently drowned in the pool. A 2-year-old male drowned when he fell into a residential spa while riding a tricycle.

Deaths Due to Other Diagnoses

There were three other diagnoses associated with the toy-related deaths, involving three incidents. Two of the fatalities involved toy boxes and one involved two remote controlled toys. A girl (age not specified) was standing on a plastic toy box that tipped over. She fell, striking her neck on the edge of the box. Her death was due to a cervical spinal cord injury. A 3-year-old male apparently got locked inside a toy box and suffocated. A 3-year old male took two remote controlled toys to bed with him and the cords attached to the controllers became wrapped around his neck. He fell asleep and strangled.

Incidents with an Unspecified Cause of Death

There were three fatalities associated with toys where the incident report does not give a specific cause of death. All of these fatal incidents occurred with non-powered scooters and motor vehicles. In two of the scooter-related deaths, the child was struck by a car and in one scooter fatality the child was run over by a van after he fell to the ground. The deceased were two 8-year-olds and a 9-year-old. Given the nature of the incidents, it is likely that the cause of death was some type of blunt force trauma.

Table 26.1. Reported Toy-Related Deaths in Children, 2001.

Type of Toy	Deaths
Total	25
Non-powered Scooters	10
Balloons	4
Riding Toys, Excluding Non-Powered Scooters	3
Toy Boxes	2
Toy Building Block	1
Toy Dart	1
Remote Controlled Toys	1
Toy Ball	1
Toys, Not Specified	2

When Buying Toys

Choose toys with care. Keep in mind the child's age, interests, and skill level. Look for quality design and construction in all toys for all ages. Make sure that all directions or instructions are clear—to you, and, when appropriate, to the child. Plastic wrappings on toys should be discarded at once before they become deadly playthings. Be a label reader. Look for and heed age recommendations, such as "Not recommended for children under three." Look for other safety labels including: "Flame retardant/Flame resistant" on fabric products and "Washable/hygienic materials" on stuffed toys and dolls.

Shopping Tips

Under 3 Years Old

- Children under 3 tend to put everything in their mouths. Avoid buying toys intended for older children which may have small parts that pose a choking danger.

- Never let children of any age play with uninflated or broken balloons because of the choking danger.

- Avoid marbles, balls, and games with balls that have a diameter of 1.75 inches or less. These products also pose a choking hazard to young children.

- Children at this age pull, prod, and twist toys. Look for toys that are well-made with tightly secured eyes, noses, and other parts.

- Avoid toys that have sharp edges and points.

Ages 5 through 5

- Avoid toys that are constructed with thin, brittle plastic that might easily break into small pieces or leave jagged edges.

- Look for household art materials, including crayons and paint sets, marked with the designation "ASTM D-4236." This means the product has been reviewed by a toxicologist and, if necessary, labeled with cautionary information.

- Teach older children to keep their toys away from their younger brothers and sisters.

Ages 6 through 12

- For all children, adults should check toys periodically for breakage and potential hazards. Damaged or dangerous toys should be repaired or thrown away.

- If buying a toy gun, be sure the barrel, or the entire gun, is brightly colored so that it's not mistaken for a real gun.

- If you buy a bicycle for any age child, buy a helmet too, and make sure the child wears it.

Maintaining Toys

New toys intended for children under eight years of age should, by regulation, be free of sharp glass and metal edges. Regulations also prohibit sharp points in new toys and other articles intended for use by children under eight years of age. With use, however, older toys may break, exposing cutting edges, dangerous points, or prongs. Stuffed toys may have wires inside the toy which could cut or stab if exposed. Older toys can also break to reveal parts small enough to be swallowed or to become lodged in a child's windpipe, ears, or nose.

Check all toys periodically for breakage and potential hazards. A damaged or dangerous toy should be thrown away or repaired immediately. Edges on wooden toys that might have become sharp or surfaces covered with splinters should be sanded smooth. When repainting toys and toy boxes, avoid using leftover paint, unless purchased recently, since older paints may contain more lead than new paint, which is regulated by the U.S. Consumer Product Safety Commission (CPSC). Examine all outdoor toys regularly for rust or weak parts that could become hazardous.

Storing Toys

Teach children to put their toys safely away on shelves or in a toy chest after playing to prevent trips and falls. Toy boxes should be checked for safety. Use a toy chest that has a lid that will stay open in any position to which it is raised, and will not fall unexpectedly on a child. For extra safety, be sure there are ventilation holes for fresh air. Watch for sharp edges that could cut and hinges that could pinch or squeeze. See that toys used outdoors are stored after play—rain or dew can rust or damage a variety of toys and toy parts creating hazards.

Loud Noises

Toy caps and some noisemaking guns and other toys can produce sounds at noise levels that can damage hearing. The law requires the following label on boxes of caps producing noise above a certain level: "WARNING — Do not fire closer than one foot to the ear. Do not use indoors." Caps producing noise that can injure a child's hearing are banned.

Projectiles

Projectiles—guided missiles and similar flying toys—can be turned into weapons and can injure eyes. Children should never be permitted to play with adult lawn darts or other hobby or sporting equipment with sharp points. Arrows or darts used by children should have soft cork tips, rubber suction cups, or other protective tips intended to prevent injury. Check to be sure the tips are secure. Avoid dart guns or other toys which might be capable of firing articles not intended for use in the toy, such as pencils or nails.

Electric Toys

Electric toys that are improperly constructed or wired or misused can shock or burn. Electric toys must meet mandatory requirements for maximum surface temperatures, electrical construction, and prominent warning labels. Electric toys with heating elements are recommended only for children over eight years old. Children should be taught to use electric toys properly, cautiously, and under adult supervision.

Keeping Children Safe

Under the Federal Hazardous Substances Act and the Consumer Product Safety Act, the CPSC has set safety regulations for certain toys and other children's articles. Manufacturers must design and manufacture their products to meet these regulations so that hazardous products are not sold.

Protecting children from unsafe toys is the responsibility of everyone. Careful toy selection and proper supervision of children at play is still—and always will be—the best way to protect children from toy-related injuries.

To report a product hazard or a product-related injury, write to the U.S. Consumer Product Safety Commission, Washington, D.C., 20207, or call the toll-free hotline: 800-638-2772. A teletypewriter for the deaf is available at 800-638-8270. For additional information from the CPSC online, visit www.cpsc.gov.

Chapter 27

Holiday and Halloween Safety

Holiday Safety

The holidays are an exciting and busy time, filled with feasting, celebrating, exchanging gifts, and visiting family and friends. But with all the joys of the holiday season come potential safety hazards that can cause injury and even death. Help prevent injuries by following these tips.

Tips for Preventing Injuries during the Holidays

The following tips—provided by the American Academy of Pediatrics, U.S. Consumer Product Safety Commission, National SAFE KIDS Campaign, and other safety organizations—can help you and your family have a safe holiday season.

Deck the Halls...Safely

- Place Christmas trees and other greenery away from fireplaces and radiators. Keep tree stands filled with water—dried out Christmas trees are a fire hazard.

- Check each set of tree lights for frayed wires, broken bulbs, and loose connections. Throw away damaged sets. Never string more

---

From "Holiday Safety" and "Halloween Safety," SafeUSA™, Centers for Disease Control and Prevention (CDC), 2002. For more information from SafeUSA™ visit their website at www.safeusa.org.

than three sets of lights on an extension cord, and never run cords or strings of lights behind drapes or under carpets. Turn lights off when you go to bed or leave the house.

- Place lit menorahs and other candles away from decorations and drapes. Place candles out of children's reach and where pets can't knock them over. Blow out all candles before going to bed or leaving the house.

- If you have small children, avoid sharp or breakable decorations. Keep tinsel and other small trimmings out of children's reach. Avoid using decorations that look like candy or food— they may tempt a child to eat them.

- Use caution when decorating with spun-glass "angel hair" or "bubble lights." They can cause injury if they are swallowed. Only use spray snow that's labeled nontoxic.

- Keep holiday plants away from children and pets. Mistletoe, holly berries, and Christmas cactus are poisonous if swallowed. Poinsettias can cause stomach irritation in humans, and they can make pets very sick.

Shop 'Til You Drop

Help keep your children stay safe while shopping.

- Teach them to go to a store clerk or security guard if you get separated.

- Keep children under age 4 in a stroller or supervise them closely.

- If you place your child in a shopping cart, always use the safety belt. Stay close to the cart. Never let your child stand in or push a shopping cart.

Don't be an easy victim for violent crime.

- Stay alert at all times and pay attention to your surroundings.

- Park in a well-lit space away from decorative bushes. Lock your car, roll up the windows, and hide packages in the trunk or under a blanket. Be especially alert in parking decks and underground garages.

- Don't overload yourself with packages.

- Have your car keys in hand before heading to the parking lot.

Be careful when riding on escalators.

- Make sure no one in your group has loose shoe laces, drawstrings, scarves, or mittens that could get trapped in the escalator.
- Hold your child's hand, face forward, and keep feet away from the edge of the steps.
- Never bring strollers, carts, or walkers on an escalator.

Where possible, cross the street at designated crosswalks. Before you step off the curb, make sure approaching vehicles have come to a complete stop.

The Joy of Giving

- Make sure the toys you give children are safe for them. Read package labels and follow age recommendations.
  1. Do not give children under age 3 toys that contain small or metal parts or toys that break easily.
  2. Do not give children under age 8 toys that have sharp edges, points, or heating elements.
  3. Avoid toys that shoot small objects into the air.
  4. Avoid toys that make loud or shrill noises.
- Include helmets and other protective gear (such as elbow, knee, and wrist pads) when giving bicycles, skates, or skateboards.
- If you're considering buying your child a BB or pellet gun, make sure your child knows the proper way to use it. Supervise your children when they use these guns.
- Do not throw gift wrappings in the fireplace. They can cause a flash fire. Throw away all toy packaging right away so it doesn't become a choking or suffocation hazard.
- Keep batteries away from children. They are toxic if swallowed.

Over the River and Through the Woods

- When you leave the house, turn off all tree lights and blow out all candles.
- Buckle your seatbelt every time you drive or ride in a car. Whether you're traveling by car or plane, make sure your child is buckled in a safety seat, booster seat, or seatbelt.

- Avoid driving in snowy or icy weather. If that's not possible, drive slowly. It takes longer to stop on wet or icy roads.

- Remember that homes you visit may not be child-proofed. Ask to move breakable or dangerous items out of children's reach. If the host's home has stairs, bring a safety gate.

- When staying overnight, bring outlet covers and check that cabinets are free of toxic items or have safety latches.

- When visiting friends or relatives who have a dog, let the dog sniff you before you try to pet it. Do not leave your child alone with the dog.

- Never drive after you drink or use drugs.

Eat, Drink, and Be Safe

- When hosting a holiday party or feast, follow some basic safety tips to prevent injuries.
    1. Turn handles of pots and pans on the stove inward so children can't reach them. Use the back burners, if possible.
    2. Keep knives and other sharp utensils away from children.
    3. Keep hot foods and drinks away from table and counter edges.
    4. Never hold a child while you're carrying hot foods or drinks or while you're cooking.

- Offer plenty of nonalcoholic drink alternatives. Keep all drinks—alcoholic or not—away from children.

- Do not place candy, chocolates, or other treats within children's reach.

- Clean up right after a meal or party. Children can choke on left-over food or be exposed to alcohol or tobacco.

- Don't let any of your guests drive home if they've been drinking.

Who Is Affected?

Many of the deaths and injuries that occur between Thanksgiving and New Year's Day are directly related to holiday festivities.

According to the National Highway Traffic Safety Administration, 598 people died in traffic crashes during Thanksgiving weekend in 1998. On the days surrounding Christmas that year, 364 died; 545 died on or around New Year's Day. About 50 percent of these deaths were related to alcohol. The number of crash-related injuries is much higher. In 1997, in just one state, 920 people were injured in traffic crashes during the Thanksgiving holiday, and 778 were injured at Christmas.

Holiday decorations make a home look festive, but improper use can result in injuries, deaths, and property loss. According to the U.S. Consumer Product Safety Commission (CPSC), approximately 1,300 people are treated each year in emergency departments for injuries related to holiday lights, and another 6,200 are treated for injuries related to holiday decorations and Christmas trees. Holiday lights cause about 510 fires each year, and Christmas trees are involved in about 400 fires. Candles are also a major cause of fire-related deaths. The National Fire Protection Association reported 156 deaths in 1997 from home fires started by candles. In addition to these deaths, more than $170 million in property losses was attributed to candles. About one-sixth of fires started by candles occur in December.

Many injuries occur to both adults and children on shopping trips. Each year, about 21,000 children age 5 and under are treated in emergency departments for injuries associated with shopping carts. Escalators, found in almost every shopping mall, are associated with about 6,000 injuries each year, according to the CPSC. Violent crimes can also result in injuries, and the 1995 National Crime Victimization Survey found that 12 percent of violent crimes occurred in commercial establishments. Eight percent occurred in parking lots and garages.

Toys are the gift of choice for many children, but when they are inappropriate for a child's age, they can be dangerous. In 1996, the CPSC reported 13 toy-related deaths. About 110,000 children under age 15 were treated in emergency departments for toy-related injuries; more than half of them were under age 5. The Child Safety Protection Act requires manufacturers to include safety warnings on toy labels to help prevent injuries. Parents and others buying toys for children must follow these warnings. Some toys are associated with a high injury rate, and parents must provide close supervision and instructions for proper use in order to prevent a toy-related injury. For example, each year about 30,000 people—80 percent of whom are age 19 or under—are treated in emergency departments for injuries related to BB and pellet guns.

Safety on Halloween

Most people think of Halloween as a time for fun and treats. However, roughly four times as many children aged 5–14 are killed while walking on Halloween evening compared with other evenings of the year, and falls are a leading cause of injuries among children on Halloween. Many Halloween-related injuries can be prevented if parents closely supervise school-aged children during trick-or-treat activities.

Safety Tips

Parents can help prevent children from getting injured at Halloween by following these safety tips from the American Academy of Pediatrics, the Centers for Disease Control and Prevention, and the National Safety Council.

Children Should

- Go only to well-lit houses and remain on porches rather than entering houses.
- Travel in small groups and be accompanied by an adult.
- Know their phone number and carry coins for emergency telephone calls.
- Have their names and addresses attached to their costumes.
- Bring treats home before eating them so parents can inspect them.
- Use costume knives and swords that are flexible, not rigid or sharp.

When walking in neighborhoods, they should:

- Use flashlights, stay on sidewalks, and avoid crossing yards.
- Cross streets at the corner, use crosswalks (where they exist), and do not cross between parked cars.
- Stop at all corners and stay together in a group before crossing.
- Wear clothing that is bright, reflective, and flame retardant.
- Consider using face paint instead of masks. (Masks can obstruct a child's vision.)
- Avoid wearing hats that will slide over their eyes.
- Avoid wearing long, baggy, or loose costumes or oversized shoes (to prevent tripping).
- Be reminded to look left, right, and left again before crossing the street.

Parents and Adults Should

- Supervise the outing for children under age 12.

- Establish a curfew (a return time) for older children.

- Prepare homes for trick-or-treaters by clearing porches, lawns, and sidewalks and by placing jack-o-lanterns away from doorways and landings.

- Avoid giving choking hazards such as gum, peanuts, hard candies, or small toys as treats to young children.

- Inspect all candy for safety before children eat it.

Parents and adults should ensure the safety of pedestrian trick-or-treaters:

- Make sure children under age 10 are supervised as they cross the street.

- Drive slowly.

- Watch for children in the street and on medians.

- Exit driveways and alleyways carefully.

- Have children get out of cars on the curb side, not on the traffic side.

And a Few Tips about Pumpkins

- Carve pumpkins on stable, flat surfaces with good lighting.

- Have children draw a face on the outside of the pumpkin, then parents should do the cutting.

- Place lighted pumpkins away from curtains and other flammable objects, and do not leave lighted pumpkins unattended.

Who Is Affected?

A study conducted by the Centers for Disease Control and Prevention (CDC) showed that during 1975–1996, the number of deaths among young pedestrians was four times higher on Halloween evening when compared with the same time period during all other evenings of the year. Halloween poses special risks to young pedestrians. For example, most of the time children spend outdoors is typically during daylight hours. However, Halloween activities often occur after dark. Also, children engaged in "trick or treat" activities frequently cross streets at mid-block rather than at corners or crosswalks, putting them at risk for pedestrian injury.

Many parents overestimate children's street-crossing skills. The pedestrian skills of children are limited by several factors related to their physical size and developmental stage. For instance, young children may lack the physical ability to cross a street quickly, and their small size limits their visibility to drivers. Children are likely to choose the shortest rather than the safest route across streets, often darting out between parked cars. In addition, young children do not evaluate potential traffic threats effectively, cannot anticipate driver behavior, and process sensory information more slowly than adults.

Chapter 28

Preventing Traumatic Brain Injury

Introduction

A traumatic brain injury (often called a TBI) is an injury to the head that disrupts the normal function of the brain. Nearly 1.5 million cases of TBI—some mild, some severe—are reported each year in this country. About 50,000 of the people who have a TBI die, and about 80,000 leave the hospital with a disability. Today, about 5.3 million people in this country live with a disability that was caused by a traumatic brain injury.

Preventing Traumatic Brain Injuries

The following safety tips, provided by the Centers for Disease Control and Prevention (CDC) and the Brain Injury Association, may help reduce the chances that you or your children will have a traumatic brain injury.

• Wear a seatbelt every time you drive or ride in a car.

• Buckle your child into a child safety seat, booster seat, or seatbelt (depending on the child's age) every time the child rides in a car.

From "What You Should Know about Traumatic Brain Injury," SafeUSA™, Centers for Disease Control and Prevention (CDC), 2002. For more information from SafeUSA™ visit their website at www.safeusa.org.

273

- Wear a helmet and make sure your children wear helmets when
  - riding a bike or motorcycle
  - playing a contact sport such as football or ice hockey
  - using in-line skates or riding a skateboard
  - batting and running bases in baseball or softball
  - riding a horse
  - skiing or snowboarding
- Keep firearms and bullets stored in a locked cabinet or safe when not in use.
- Avoid falls by
  - using a step-stool with a grab bar to reach objects on high shelves
  - installing handrails on stairways
  - installing window guards to keep young children from falling out of open windows
  - using safety gates at the top and bottom of stairs when young children are around
- Make sure the surface on your child's playground is made of shock-absorbing material (for example, hardwood mulch, sand).

The following are common symptoms of concussion among adults:

- low-grade headaches or neck pain that won't go away
- having more trouble than usual with mental tasks (for example, remembering, concentrating, making decisions)
- slowness in thinking, speaking, acting, or reading
- getting lost or easily confused
- feeling tired all the time, lacking energy or motivation
- changes in sleeping patterns (sleeping a lot more or having a hard time sleeping)
- feeling light-headed or dizzy, losing your balance
- increased sensitivity to sounds, light, or distractions
- blurred vision, eyes that tire easily

- loss of the sense of smell or taste
- ringing in the ears
- mood changes (for example, feeling sad or angry for no reason)

Some symptoms that may appear in a child with a concussion include the following:

- listlessness or tiring easily
- irritability or crankiness
- changes in eating or sleeping patterns
- changes in the way the child plays
- changes in performance at school
- lack of interest in favorite toys or activities
- loss of new skills, such as toilet training
- loss of balance, unsteady walking

Tips for People with TBI

If you think you or your child may have a brain injury, see a doctor right away. The doctor will tell you what to do to help the healing process. But here are some general tips to aid in recovery:

- While healing, get lots of rest.
- Don't rush back into daily activities like work or school.
- Avoid doing anything that could cause another blow or jolt to the head.
- Ask your doctor when it's safe to drive a car, ride a bike, or use heavy equipment because your ability to react may be slower after a brain injury.
- Take only the drugs your doctor has approved, and don't drink alcohol until your doctor says it's OK.
- If you have a hard time remembering things, write them down.

If the brain injury was severe, the injured person may need therapy to learn skills that were lost, such as speaking, walking, or reading. Your doctor can help arrange rehabilitation services.

Who Is Affected?

Each year in the U.S., nearly 1.5 million cases of TBI are reported. Of those, about 50,000 die and another 80,000 suffer disabilities. Today, about 5.3 million people in this country live with a disability that was caused by a traumatic brain injury.

A TBI can be mild where there is only a brief loss of consciousness (or none at all), and there are no major complications—or it can be severe. Severe TBIs are characterized by a loss of consciousness for days or weeks (called a coma) and bruises (contusions) or blood clots on the brain or damage to the brain's nerve fibers. While mild TBIs—called concussions—cause symptoms that go away in days or weeks, severe TBIs often cause permanent problems related to thinking, speaking, movement, or behavior.

People over 75 years old have the highest rate of TBI. About 191 out of every 100,000 people in that age group have a TBI each year; the most common cause is falls. People age 15–24 have the next highest rate of TBI, with 145 out of every 100,000 persons sustaining a TBI in a given year. The most common cause of TBI for that age group is transportation. Among children under 5 years old, 82 out of 100,000 have a TBI each year, and most of those injuries are caused by falls and motor vehicle crashes.

Among all age groups, the top three causes of TBI are motor vehicle crashes, falls, and violence.

Nearly half of all TBIs are related to transportation (motor vehicles, bicycles, etc.). One-quarter are caused by falls. And about 17 percent are caused by firearms and other assaults. Firearms cause about 10 percent of TBIs, but they cause 44 percent of TBI-related deaths. Nine out of ten people with a firearm-related TBI die.

Chapter 29

Preventing Injuries on the Playground

Chapter Contents

Section 29.1

Playground Safety

This section contains text from "Playground Safety" Centers for Disease Control and Prevention (CDC), SafeUSA website, http://www.cdc.gov/safeusa/playgro/playgrou.htm, page last updated May 24, 2000, and "Public Playground Safety Checklist," U.S. Consumer Product Safety Commission (CPSC) and KaBOOM!, CPSC Doc. No. 327, undated, available online at http://www.cpsc.gov/cpscpub/pubs/327.html.

Playground Safety—Introduction

Every two-and-a-half minutes a child is injured on a playground in the United States. Supervising children as they play on equipment and choosing playgrounds with cushioning materials under the equipment will reduce children's risk of injury.

Safety Tips

You can help keep your child safer from injuries on the playground if you follow a few simple tips. These tips apply to backyard and fast-food restaurant playgrounds, as well as to public or school playgrounds.

- Supervise children at all times, especially when they are on climbing equipment, swings, and slides. Prevent behaviors like pushing, shoving, and crowding around equipment.

- Make sure that children play on playground equipment that is appropriate for their age. For example, don't let young children play on high climbing equipment such as monkey bars. Keep all children off equipment from which they might fall six or more feet.

- Check the surface under playground equipment. Avoid playgrounds with asphalt, concrete, grass, and soil surfaces under the equipment. Look for surfaces of hardwood fiber, mulch chips, pea gravel, fine sand, or shredded rubber—materials that can cushion a fall—with a depth of at least 4–6 inches. The deeper the cushioning material, the better.

- Remove or cut the hood and neck drawstrings from all children's outerwear to prevent entanglement and strangulation. Children have died when hood or neck drawstrings were caught on slides and other playground equipment.

- Make sure spaces that could trap children's heads, such as openings in guardrails or between ladder rungs, measure less than 3.5 inches (so children can't get their heads in) or more than 9 inches (so they can get out).

- Check playground equipment to make sure it is in good repair, without jagged edges or sharp points.

- Check for hot surfaces on metal playground equipment before allowing young children to play on it. Metal equipment can heat up in direct sunlight and cause burn injuries in a few seconds.

- Make sure there are no obvious hazards around the playground, such as broken glass.

- Make sure there is fencing between the playground and the street to prevent children from running in front of cars.

Who Is Affected?

Each year in the United States about 200,000 children in preschools and elementary schools are seen in emergency departments for injuries sustained on playground equipment. That's roughly one injury every two-and-a-half minutes. More than one-third of these injuries are severe, including fractures, internal injuries, concussions, and dislocations.

Nearly all severe playground-related injuries are the result of children falling or jumping from climbing equipment, slides, and swings. Protective surfaces made of energy-absorbing (cushioning) materials under and around equipment can prevent and reduce the severity of injuries related to falling on the playground. Supervising children while they play on equipment is also extremely important.

Public Playground Safety Checklist

Additional safety tips:

1. Make sure play structures more than 30 inches high are spaced at least 9 feet apart.

2. Check for dangerous hardware, like open "S" hooks or protruding bolt ends.

3. Check for sharp points or edges in equipment.

4. Look out for tripping hazards, like exposed concrete footings, tree stumps, and rocks.

5. Make sure elevated surfaces, like platforms and ramps, have guardrails to prevent falls.

6. Check playgrounds regularly to see that equipment and surfacing are in good condition.

Section 29.2

Home Playground Safety Tips

Excerpted from "Home Playground Safety Tips," Consumer Product Safety Commission (CPSC), CPSC Document #323, undated, available online at http://www.cpsc.gov/cpscpub/pubs/323.html.

Each year, about 51,000 children are treated in U.S. hospital emergency rooms for home playground equipment-related injuries. Also, about 15 children die each year as a result of playground equipment-related incidents. Most of the injuries are the result of falls. These are primarily falls to the ground below the equipment, but falls from one piece of equipment to another are also reported. Most of the deaths are due to strangulations, though some are due to falls.

Protective Surfacing

Since almost 60% of all injuries are caused by falls to the ground, protective surfacing under and around all playground equipment can reduce the risk of serious head injury.

Falls on asphalt and concrete can result in serious head injury and death. Do not place playground equipment over these surfaces. Also grass and turf lose their ability to absorb shock through wear and environmental conditions. Always use protective surfacing.

Certain loose-fill surfacing materials are acceptable, such as the types and depths shown in the Table 29.1.

Certain manufactured synthetic surfaces also are acceptable; however, test data on shock absorbing performance should be requested from the manufacturer.

Table 29.1. Fall height in feet from which a life threatening head injury would not be expected.

Type of Material	6" Depth	9" Depth	12" Depth
Double Shredded Bark Mulch	6	10	11
Wood Chips	7	10	11
Fine Sand	5	5	9
Fine Gravel	6	7	10

Use Zones

A use zone, covered with a protective surfacing material, is essential under and around equipment where a child might fall. This area should be free of other equipment and obstacles onto which a child might fall.

Stationary climbing equipment and slides should have a use zone extending a minimum of 6' in all directions from the perimeter of the equipment.

Swings should have a use zone extending a minimum of 6' from the outer edge of the support structure on each side. The use zone in front and back of the swing should extend out a minimum distance of twice the height of the swing as measured from the ground to the swing hangers on support structure.

Swing Spacing

To prevent injuries from impact with moving swings, swings should not be too close together or too close to support structures. Swing spacing should be:

- At least 8 inches between suspended swings and between a swing and the support frame.

- At least 16 inches from swing support frame to a pendulum see-saw.

- Minimum clearance between the ground and underside of swing seat should be 8 inches.

- Swing sets should be securely anchored.

Potential Head Entrapment Hazards

In general, openings that are closed on all sides should be less than 3½" or greater than 9". Openings that are between 3½" and 9" present a head entrapment hazard because they are large enough to permit a child's body to go through, but are too small to permit the head to go trough. When children enter such openings, feet first, they may become entrapped by the head and strangle.

Potential Entrapment and Strangulation Hazards

Open "S" hooks, especially on swings, and any protrusions or equipment component/hardware which may act as hooks or catch-points can entangle with children's clothing and cause strangulation incidents. Close "S" hooks as tightly as possible and eliminate protrusions or catch-points on playground equipment.

Playground Maintenance

Playgrounds should be inspected on a regular basis. Inspect protective surfacing, especially mulch, and maintain the proper depth. If any of the following conditions are noted, they should be removed, corrected or repaired immediately to prevent injuries:

- Hardware is loose or worn, or has protrusions or projections.

- Ropes, and items with cords placed around the neck can get caught on playground equipment and strangle a child. Many children have died when a rope they were wearing got caught on playground equipment, or they became entangled in a rope.

- Supervise, and teach your child safe play. Teach your child not to walk or play close to a moving swing, and not to tie ropes to playground equipment.

- Exposed equipment footings.

- Scattered debris, litter, rocks, or tree roots.

- Rust and chipped paint on metal components.

- Splinters, large cracks, and decayed wood components.

- Deterioration and corrosion on structural components which connect to the ground.

- Missing or damaged equipment components, such as handholds, guardrails, and swing seats.

Other Hazards

- Platforms more than 30" above the ground should have guard-rails to prevent falls.

- There should be no exposed moving parts which may present a pinching or crushing hazard.

Section 29.3

Never Put Children's Climbing Gyms on Hard Surfaces

"Never Put Children's Climbing Gyms On Hard Surfaces, Indoors or Out-doors" Consumer Product Safety Commission (CPSC), CPSC Doc. No. 5119, undated, available online at http://www.cpsc.gov/cpscpub/pubs/5119.html.

The US Consumer Product Safety Commission (CPSC) is warning parents and daycare providers that children's plastic climbing equipment should not be used indoors on wood or cement floors, even if covered with carpet, such as indoor/outdoor, shag, or other types of carpet. Carpet does not provide adequate protection to prevent injuries.

CPSC has reports of two children killed and hundreds injured at home and at day-care centers when they fell from climbing equipment placed indoors on cement, wood or carpeted floors.

Parents and child care-givers should put all climbing equipment outdoors on surfaces such as sand or mulch to prevent children's head injuries. Manufacturers of plastic climbing equipment are labeling their products with warnings to NEVER put the equipment on concrete, asphalt, wood, or other hard surfaces and that carpet may NOT prevent injury.

For more information on child safety, call the Consumer Product Safety Commission at (800) 638-2772.

Section 29.4

Soft Contained Play Equipment Safety Checklist

"Soft Contained Play Equipment Safety Checklist," Consumer Product Safety Commission (CPSC), CPSC Document #328, undated, available online at http://www.cpsc.gov/cpscpub/pubs/328.html.

The Consumer Product Safety Commission staff developed the following checks to help parents and children use soft contained play equipment safely.

Equipment Check

• Check the safety netting for tears or frays. Torn netting could allow a child to climb onto the outer portions of the equipment and fall onto a hard surface.

• Check cargo webbing and rope equipment for tears or frays. Torn rope equipment or loose sewing connections in the cargo webbing may be an entrapment or tripping hazard.

• Check floor surfacing for tears. Floor surfacing should not be torn, in order to prevent trips or ankle sprains. If mats are used outside of the soft contained play equipment, they should be placed tightly together and should not be torn, in order to prevent trips or ankle sprains.

- Check the equipment for general cleanliness. Dirty equipment is an indication that the owner/operator may not have kept up with the routine maintenance and repair. Walkways should be clear of trash and clutter to prevent tripping.

Safe Use Check

- Obey the posted safety guidelines of the soft contained play equipment. Guidelines should explain proper equipment use.

- Follow use and size recommendations. Smaller children are at a disadvantage in a collision with a larger child. If your child meets the size restriction for the toddler section, do not bring him/her into the older children's section. Keep older, larger children from playing in the toddler section.

- Remove clothing strings, necklaces, earrings, and all loose items in pockets before the child enters the soft contained play equipment. Loose hanging strings and jewelry can get caught in play equipment. Items inside pockets can fall into the ball pools.

- Do not allow children to play or linger in front of slide exits or to climb up slides. A child playing in front of a slide exit or climbing up a slide could be struck by a child coming down the slide. Children like to bury themselves under the balls in a ball pool. If a slide exits into the ball pool, a child playing in the balls in front of the exit may be struck.

- Do not allow children to play or linger at the base of climbing equipment in a ball pool. Children jump off equipment such as the mountain climb into the ball pool. A child playing at the base of the equipment could be struck.

Chapter 30

Bike Safety

Bike crashes can result in serious injury. In 1997, more than half a million persons were injured badly enough to need emergency department care as a result of bike crashes in the United States. Wearing a bike helmet reduces the risk of brain injury from a bike crash by as much as 88%.

Bike Safety Tips

You greatly reduce the chances of having a bike-related injury if you follow these simple tips:

- Children and adults should always wear a bike helmet every time they ride a bike. Think of a bike helmet as a necessity, not an accessory.

- Adults are important role models for children. If you wear a bike helmet, your children are more likely to wear helmets, too.

- If your child doesn't want to wear a helmet, find out why. Some children don't like to wear helmets because they fear they will be teased by peers or because they think bike helmets are unattractive. Talk about these concerns with your child and choose a helmet he or she will want to wear.

From "Bike Safety," SafeUSA™, Centers for Disease Control and Prevention (CDC), 2002. For more information from SafeUSA™ visit their website at www.safeusa.org.

- Buy a bike helmet that meets the national safety standards. When choosing a helmet:
  - get one that is the right size;
  - make sure it sits on top of the head in a level position, not tilted back on the head;
  - adjust the straps for a snug and comfortable fit. Teach children always to keep the helmet straps buckled when riding.
- Model and teach children to follow the rules of the road:
  - ride on the right side of the road with the traffic flow, not against it;
  - obey traffic signs and signals;
  - use correct hand signals;
  - stop at all intersections and crosswalks, both marked or unmarked;
  - stop and look both ways before entering a street;
  - yield the right-of-way to pedestrians and skaters.
- Have children ride on sidewalks and paths until they are at least 10 years old, are able to show good riding skills, and are able to observe the basic rules of the road.
- If riding at dawn, at dusk, or at night, wear reflective clothing (not just light-colored clothing) and make sure that the bike has a headlight and a rear reflector.
- Make sure the bike is in good working order, especially the brakes.
- Encourage your community to build bike paths to separate bike riders from traffic.

Who Is Affected?

Bike riding is both fun and a great way to exercise. But it also can be a risky activity. In 1997, 813 persons were killed and an estimated 567,000 persons were injured badly enough to need emergency department care as a result of bike crashes in the United States. The toll on young people is especially high: 31% of bike-related deaths were among riders younger than age 16, and two-thirds of those injured were children or young teens.

Many people don't realize the risk of serious injuries from bike crashes. Injuries to the head are particularly dangerous and are the leading cause of death and permanent disability in bike crashes. Each year an estimated 140,000 children are treated in emergency departments for head injuries sustained while riding bikes.

However, many bike-related injuries and deaths could be avoided if riders wore helmets. Wearing a bike helmet reduces the risk of brain injury by as much as 88%, and reduces the risk of injury to the face by 65%. Unfortunately, only about 25% of children aged 4-15 years wear a bike helmet when riding, and teen use of helmets is nearly zero. The main reasons children don't wear helmets are because they aren't fashionable ("cool"), their friends don't wear them, and helmets are thought to be uncomfortable (usually too hot). Another important reason is that the parents or the child never knew about the need to protect oneself from bike-related injury or how effective helmets are in preventing head injuries.

Chapter 31

Children and Sports

Chapter Contents

Section 31.1

When Should Kids Start Sports

When Should Kids Start Sports?

It's not easy to determine how early to start children in organized sports. Children of the same age vary considerably in their physical and psychological maturation, and there is no practical method of measuring maturity. Assuming the child has shown interest, five or six is the generally accepted earliest starting age for organized team sports. At the early ages participation should be limited to sports that involve a lot of physical activity and encourage the development of major motor muscles.

Children in grades 1–4 can benefit most from games that are modified to meet their needs and abilities. Play and fun are more important to this age group than highly structured sports that emphasize the outcome rather than the process. Parents and coaches are usually the ones concerned about winning and losing. When helping your child select a sport, keep balance in mind. Encourage your children to try many sports and activities when young and not to think of specializing or playing competitively until they reach middle school. Make sure a balance also occurs between adult organized activities and free playtime. Children need time to just be kids and to play with other kids without a set of rules or adult involvement.

The most important decisions to make are which youth sports organizations and which coaches are best for your child. Make sure that you take the time to find out about the league, its leaders, and coaches. Better yet, get involved and volunteer to coach. Participating in sports is a healthy way, both physically and socially, for your children to channel their youthful energy in a positive direction. Make sure your children's first experience encourages them to begin a lifelong interest in physical activities and good health.

There are many other options besides team sports available to a child who wants to participate in sports. Parents should also encourage their children to become involved in individual and lifetime sports such as bowling, golf, swimming, tennis, gymnastics, and martial arts. You can find information about these sports by visiting the facilities or through the yellow pages of the phone book.

Questions Parents Should Ask

There are a number of key questions parents should ask about a youth sports program before enrolling their child. You always have the right to ask questions, even when volunteers run the league. The following thoughts and questions can help you evaluate a youth sports program.

Program organization: Who is in charge of the program? Who can you contact if you have a problem or question? Who sponsors the league (YMCA, private organization, etc.)? Do they have a written set of goals and program guidelines? How much are registration fees? Were does the money go? Do they have a written budget for you to see? Is it a developmental or competitive league? (Programs for kids 12 and under should concentrate on skill development, exercise, and fun.) How long is the season? How frequent are practices and games? What kind of equipment is used and who is responsible for providing it?

Safety: Is protective equipment necessary and is it used properly? Is a medical exam required to participate? Is the playing area safe for practices and games? Does the league have injury insurance? Is someone trained in Red Cross or emergency procedures? (Coaches should have some basic first aid training.) Is physical conditioning important for the sport and is it provided?

Psychological and developmental factors: Is emphasis placed on enjoyment and participation? Are there separate divisions for different skill levels? Will kids be cut from a team? (Tryouts that involve cuts should be permitted only above the age of 12 and then only if the child has the option of playing on a less competitive team.) Are opponents thought of as the enemy? Are game rules adapted to the child's skill development, age and size?

Quality of adult leadership: How are coaches selected? What kind of training has the coach received? (He/she should understand the psychology of working with the kids in sports, basic injury prevention and treatment techniques, team and practice organization, and how to teach sports fundamentals to kids.) Are referees trained and evaluated? Were background checks conducted on coaches and referees before they were accepted?

Measures of success: How is success measured? (There should be ways other than winning for children to achieve success.) Are all team members rewarded in some way for their success or the progress they have made? How much emphasis is placed on making the all-star team, play-offs, or receiving a trophy?

Conclusions: You don't have to ask all of these questions and you may have others that you feel are more important. As your questions are answered you will develop a "feel" for the organization. If you are uncomfortable with what they have told you, look for another organization. Kids deserve a fun and rewarding sports experience and it's a parent's job to see that they receive it.

Financing Your Child's Sports Expenses

Just like everything else in life, it costs money to operate a youth sports program. Youth leagues usually pay for the use of the playing fields and courts, as well as their upkeep, electricity, water, etc. In addition, referees must be paid, uniforms and equipment purchased, and if the league is affiliated with a national organization, they must pay insurance and other fees to their national office.

Thus, to some extent, all leagues must develop revenue sources. These sources include fund-raisers, concession stand sales and registration fees. Fees for an 8- to 10-week sports league could range from as little as $10 per child to over $100. Most youth leagues have a scholarship policy that permits parents to obtain free or reduced price registration. This is usually based on a written petition from the parents. If you have an honest need for financial support, you should always inquire about scholarships before you decide not to register your child in a sports league. You'd be surprised how often the league will assist.

Always ask about fees before you register. You deserve to know what the registration fees are and if there are any hidden costs that will surface later. For example, some leagues charge a low registration fee but require each team to purchase its own uniforms. And finally, remember that it's the leadership of the program and not the registration fees that usually determines the quality of your child's sports experience.

Section 31.2

Tips for Preventing Sports Injuries

Excerpted from SafeUSA™ fact sheets on individual sports, Centers for Disease Control and Prevention, 2002. For the complete text or for more information from SafeUSA™, visit their website at www.safeusa.org.

For All Sports

- Before your child starts a training program or plays in a competition, take him or her to the doctor for a physical exam. The doctor can help assess any special injury risks your child may have.

- **Make sure your child wears all the required safety gear every time he or she plays and practices.**

- Insist that your child warm up and stretch before playing.

- Teach your child not to play through pain. If your child gets injured, see your doctor. Follow all the doctor's orders for recovery, and get the doctor's OK before your child returns to play.

- Make sure first aid is available at all games and practices.

Tips for Preventing Baseball and Softball Injuries

To help your child avoid injuries while playing baseball or softball, follow these safety tips from the American Academy of Pediatrics, the Centers for Disease Control and Prevention (CDC), the Consumer Product Safety Commission, and other sports and health organizations.

- Insist that your child wear a helmet when batting, waiting to bat, or running the bases. Helmets should have eye protectors, either safety goggles or face guards. Shoes with molded cleats are recommended (most youth leagues prohibit the use of steel spikes). If your child is a catcher, he or she will need additional safety gear: catcher's mitt, face mask, throat guard, long-model chest protector, and shin guards.

295

- If your child is a pitcher, make sure pitching time is limited. Little League mandates time limits and requires rest periods for young pitchers.

- Talk to and watch your child's coach. Coaches should enforce all the rules of the game, encourage safe play, and understand the special injury risks that young players face. Make sure your child's coach teaches players how to avoid injury when sliding (prohibits headfirst sliding in young players), pitching, or dodging a ball pitched directly at them.

- Above all, keep baseball and softball fun. Putting too much focus on winning can make your child push too hard and risk injury.

Encourage your league to use breakaway bases. These bases, which detach when someone slides into them, can prevent many ankle and knee injuries in both children and adults. Leagues with players 10 years old and under should alter the rules of the game to include the use of adult pitchers or batting tees. Remember, you don't have to be on a baseball diamond to get hurt. Make sure your child wears safety gear and follows safety rules during informal baseball and softball games, too.

Tips for Preventing Basketball Injuries

To help your child avoid sports injuries, follow these safety tips from the American Academy of Orthopaedic Surgeons, the National SAFE KIDS Campaign, and other sports and health organizations. (Note: These tips apply to adults, too.)

- Knee and elbow pads protect against scrapes and bruises, and mouth guards prevent serious dental injuries. Eye protection is recommended (eye injuries account for about 2 percent of injuries, according to the National Collegiate Athletic Association). If your child wears glasses, talk to the eye doctor about sports eyewear.

- If your child is under age 7, encourage the league to use smaller, mini-foam or rubber balls. These balls are lighter weight and easier for young players to handle.

- Talk to and watch your child's coach. Coaches should enforce all the rules of the game, encourage safe play, and understand the special injury risks that young players face. They should never allow players to hold, block, push, trip, or charge opponents.

- Inspect the court for safety. Baskets and boundary lines should not be close to walls, fences, bleachers, or water fountains. The goals and the walls behind them should be padded. If your child plays outside, make sure the court is free of holes and debris.

- Above all, keep basketball fun. Putting too much focus on winning can make your child push too hard and risk injury.

Tips for Preventing Football Injuries

To help your child avoid injury while playing football, follow these safety tips from the American Academy of Pediatrics, the American Academy of Orthopaedic Surgeons, the Centers for Disease Control and Prevention, and other sports and health organizations. (Note: Adults should heed this safety guidance, too.)

- All tackle football players must wear: a helmet; pads for the shoulders, hips, tailbone, and knees; thigh guards; and a mouth guard with a keeper strap. Talk to your child's coach to find out what kind of cleats are recommended or required in your child's league. If your child wears glasses, talk to your eye doctor about special eyewear for sports.

- If your child gets injured, see your doctor. Follow all the doctor's orders for recovery, and get the doctor's OK before your child returns to play. This is especially important for brain injuries— getting a second brain injury before the first one has healed can be fatal.

- Talk to and watch your child's coach. Coaches should enforce all the rules of the game. They should never allow illegal blocking (pulling a player down by the knees or grabbing the face mask), tackling from behind, or "spearing" (using the top of the helmet to tackle). Coaches should also encourage safe play and understand the special injury risks that young players face.

- Above all, keep football fun. Putting too much focus on winning can make your child push too hard and risk injury.

Whether your child plays football on an organized team or with a few friends in the park, there are still injury risks. Unfortunately, few children who play in backyard football games follow the safety rules observed in league play. As a parent, set rules for informal play, including these:

- Wear helmets and pads.
- Play only with children of similar size and age.
- Play on grass, never in the street or in a parking lot.
- Stick to touch or flag football—they can be less dangerous than tackle.

You can help reinforce these rules by setting a good example. When you play football—or any other sport—always follow the rules and wear appropriate safety gear.

Tips for Preventing Gymnastics Injuries

To help your child avoid gymnastics injuries, follow these safety tips from the American Academy of Pediatrics, the American Academy of Orthopaedic Surgeons, the National SAFE KIDS Campaign, and other sports and health organizations.

- Gymnasts may need wrist guards and hand grips; special footwear and pads may also be required.
- Talk to and watch your child's coach. Coaches should emphasize safety and understand the special injury risks that young gymnasts face.
- Inspect the facilities where your child trains and competes. Equipment should be in good condition and spaced far enough apart to avoid collisions. Floors should be padded, and mats should be secured under every apparatus. Safety harnesses should be used when your child does new or difficult moves.
- Insist that your child have spotters when learning new skills or doing difficult moves. Spotters should be present during practice and competition—they can help catch your child if he or she falls.
- Encourage your child to express concern about doing difficult moves. Don't let the coach push your child to do things he or she is not ready for.
- Above all, keep gymnastics fun. Putting too much focus on winning can make your child push too hard and risk injury.

Tips for Preventing Ice Hockey Injuries

To help your child avoid injury while playing ice hockey, follow these safety tips from the American Academy of Pediatrics, the American Academy of Orthopaedic Surgeons, USA Hockey, and other sports and health organizations. (Note: Adults should follow this guidance, too.)

- All youth, high school, and college ice hockey leagues require players to wear the following gear: a helmet with foam lining and full face mask; a mouth guard; pads for the shoulders, knees, elbows, and shins; and gloves. Some leagues recommend neck guards. All equipment should be certified by the HECC (Hockey Equipment Certification Council), the CSA (Canadian Standards Association), or the ASTM (American Society for Testing and Materials).

- Make sure your child's equipment fits properly. The helmet should fit snugly with a strap that gently cradles the chin when it's fastened.

- Insist that your child warm up and stretch before playing. Exercises that strengthen the neck and increase flexibility may help prevent injuries.

- Talk to and watch your child's coach. Coaches should enforce all the rules of the game, encourage safe play, and understand the special injury risks that young players face. Coaches should limit body checking (some youth leagues prohibit it). Checking from behind should never be allowed. This move, which is an illegal play, has been associated with a high rate of injury.

- Teach your child to avoid head contact with the boards or other players. Serious head and neck injuries can occur from this kind of contact.

- Above all, keep ice hockey fun. Putting too much focus on winning can make your child push too hard and risk injury.

Injury Prevention Tips for In-line Skaters and Skateboarders

To help your child avoid injuries while in-line skating and skateboarding, follow these safety tips from the American Academy of Pediatrics, the Centers for Disease Control and Prevention (CDC), the U.S.

299

Consumer Product Safety Commission, and other sports and health organizations. (Note: Adult skaters should heed this advice, too.)

• Make sure your child wears all the required safety gear every time he or she skates. All skaters should wear a helmet, knee and elbow pads, and wrist guards. If your child does tricks or plays roller hockey, make sure he or she wears heavy-duty gear.

• Check your child's helmet for proper fit. The helmet should be worn flat on the head, with the bottom edge parallel to the ground. It should fit snugly and should not move around in any direction when your child shakes his or her head.

• Choose in-line skates or a skateboard that best suits your child's ability and skating style. If your child is a novice, choose in-line skates with three or four wheels. Skates with five wheels are only for experienced skaters and people who skate long distances. Choose a skateboard designed for your child's type of riding—slalom, freestyle, or speed. Some boards are rated for the weight of the rider.

• Find a smooth skating surface for your child; good choices are skating trails and driveways without much slope (but be careful about children skating into traffic). Check for holes, bumps, and debris that could make your child fall. Novice in-line skaters should start out in a skating rink where the surface is smooth and flat and where speed is controlled.

• Don't let your child skate in areas with high pedestrian or vehicle traffic. Children should not skate in the street or on vehicle parking ramps.

• Tell your child never to skitch. Skitching is the practice of holding on to a moving vehicle in order to skate very fast. People have died while skitching.

• If your child is new to in-line skating, lessons from an instructor certified by the International In-line Skating Association may be helpful. These lessons show proper form and teach how to stop. Check with your local parks and recreation department to find a qualified instructor.

Tips for Preventing Martial Arts Injuries

To help your child avoid injuries while practicing martial arts, follow these safety tips from the American Academy of Pediatrics, the

American Academy of Orthopaedic Surgeons, and other sports and health organizations.

- Keep martial arts fun. Putting too much emphasis on winning can make your child push too hard and sacrifice good technique, which can increase the risk of injury.

Tips for Preventing Soccer Injuries

To help your child avoid injury while playing soccer, follow these safety tips from the American Academy of Pediatrics, the American Academy of Orthopaedic Surgeons, the U.S. Consumer Product Safety Commission, and other sports health organizations. (Note: Adults should heed this safety guidance, too.)

- Your child should wear shin guards during every game and every practice. Shoes with molded cleats or ribbed soles are recommended.

- Don't allow your child to shoot goals before warming up.

- Insist that your child follow and that coaches and referees enforce all the rules of the game. For example, most leagues prohibit sliding tackles from behind, which can result in serious injury to players.

- Talk to and watch your child's coach. Coaches should enforce all the rules of the game, encourage safe play, and understand the special injury risks that young players face.

- Ask your child's doctor and coach whether it's safe for your child to "head" the ball and, if so, make sure your child knows how to head the ball correctly to avoid head and neck injury.

- Don't let your child climb on the goal posts or hang or swing from the crossbar.

- Above all, keep soccer fun. Putting too much focus on winning can make your child push too hard and risk injury.

Make sure the field and equipment are safe. Work with coaches, city officials, and other parents to improve safety.

- Encourage your child's league to use waterproof, synthetic balls instead of leather ones. Leather balls can become waterlogged and very heavy, making them dangerous for play.

301

- Make sure movable soccer goals are anchored to the ground at all times, not just during play. Goals have been known to tip over in strong winds or when climbed on, causing severe injuries.

- If the goal posts on your field(s) don't have padding, talk to school or park authorities about adding pads. Studies have shown that padding on goal posts greatly reduces the risk of serious injury caused by a player's head hitting the post.

Tips for Preventing Trampoline Injuries

A trampoline is not a toy. The American Academy of Pediatrics offers this advice for parents:

- Never buy a trampoline for use at home.

- Never allow your child to use a trampoline at someone else's home.

Section 31.3

Safety Concerns for Winter Sports

Excerpted from "Winter Sports Injury Prevention: Safety on the Slopes," SafeUSA™, Centers for Disease Control and Prevention (CDC), 2002. For more information from SafeUSA™, visit their website at www.safeusa.org.

Millions of persons ski, snowboard, and sled each year in the United States. These cold weather activities, which can be exhilarating, also result in many injuries each year. By developing skills with a qualified instructor and supervising young children while they participate in these activities, you can help reduce the risk of injury.

You can reduce the chance of becoming injured while skiing, snowboarding, and sledding if you follow these safety tips from the American Academy of Orthopaedic Surgeons, the National Ski Areas Association, SAFE KIDS, and the U.S. Consumer Product Safety Commission.

Skiing and Snowboarding

Preparation

- Before you get out on the slopes, be sure you're in shape. You'll enjoy the sports more and have lower risk of injury if you're physically fit.

- Take a lesson (or several) from a qualified instructor. Like anything, you'll improve the most when you receive expert guidance. And be sure to learn how to fall correctly and safely to reduce the risk of injury.

- Don't start jumping maneuvers until you've had proper instruction on how to jump and have some experience. Jumps are the most common cause of spinal injuries among snowboarders.

- Obtain proper equipment. Be sure that your equipment is in good condition and have your ski or snowboard bindings adjusted correctly at a local ski shop. (Extra tip for snowboarders: wrist guards and knee pads can help protect you when you fall.)

- Wear a helmet to prevent head injuries from falls or collisions. (One study showed that helmet use by skiers and snowboarders could prevent or reduce the severity of nearly half of head injuries to adults and more than half of head injuries to children less than 15 years old.) Skiers and snowboarders should wear helmets specifically designed for these sports.

- When buying skiwear, look for fabric that is water- and wind-resistant. Look for wind flaps to shield zippers, snug cuffs at wrists and ankles, collars that can be snuggled up to the chin and drawstrings that can be adjusted for comfort and to keep the wind out.

- Dress in layers. Layering allows you to accommodate your body's constantly changing temperature. For example, dress in polypropylene underwear (top and bottoms), which feels good next to the skin, dries quickly, absorbs sweat and keeps you warm. Wear a turtleneck, sweater, and jacket.

- Be prepared for changes in the weather. Bring a headband or hat with you to the slopes (60 percent of heat loss is through the head) and wear gloves or mittens.

- Protect your skin from the sun and wind by using a sun screen or sun block. The sun reflects off the snow and is stronger than you think, even on cloudy days.

- Always use appropriate eye protection. Sunglasses or goggles will help protect your vision from glare, help you to see the terrain better, and help shield your eyes from flying debris.

When You're on the Slopes

- The key to successful skiing and snowboarding is control. To have it, you must be aware of your technique and level of ability, the terrain, and the skiers and snowboarders around you.

- Take a couple of slow ski or snowboard runs to warm up at the start of each day.

- Ski or snowboard with partners and stay within sight of each other, if possible. If one partner loses the other, stop and wait.

- Stay on marked trails and avoid potential avalanche areas such as steep hillsides with little vegetation. Begin a run slowly. Watch out for rocks and patches of ice on the trails.

- Be aware of the weather and snow conditions and how they can change. Make adjustments for icy conditions, deep snow powder, wet snow, and adverse weather conditions.

- If you find yourself on a slope that exceeds your ability level, always leave your skis or snowboard on and side step down the slope.

- If you find yourself skiing or snowboarding out of control, fall down on your rear end or on your side, the softest parts of your body.

- Drink plenty of water to avoid becoming dehydrated.

- Avoid alcohol consumption. Skiing and snowboarding do not mix well with alcohol or drugs.

- Beware of medicines or drugs that impair the senses or make you drowsy.

- If you're tired, stop and rest. Fatigue is a risk factor for injuries.

The National Ski Areas Association endorses a responsibility code for skiers. This code can be applied to snowboarders also. The following are the code's seven safety rules of the slopes:

1. Always stay in control and be able to stop or avoid other people or objects.

2. People ahead of you have the right of way. It is your responsibility to avoid them.

3. You must not stop where you obstruct a trail or are not visible from above.

4. Whenever starting downhill or merging into a trail, look uphill and yield to others.

5. Always use devices to help prevent runaway equipment.

6. Observe all posted signs and warnings. Keep off closed trails and out of closed areas.

7. Prior to using any lift, you must have the knowledge and ability to load, ride, and unload safely.

Sledding

The American Academy of Orthopaedic Surgeons recommends the following safety guidelines to improve sledding safety for children:

Essential

- Sled only in designated areas free of fixed objects such as trees, posts, and fences.

- Children in these areas must be supervised by parents or adults.

- All participants must sit in a forward-facing position, steering with their feet or a rope tied to the steering handles of the sled. No one should sled head-first down a slope.

- Do not sled on slopes that end in a street, drop off, parking lot, river, or pond.

Preferred

- Children under 12 years old should sled wearing a helmet.

- Wear layers of clothing for protection from injuries.

- Do not sit/slide on plastic sheets or other materials that can be pierced by objects on the ground.

- Use a sled with runners and a steering mechanism, which is safer than toboggans or snow disks.

- Sled in well-lighted areas when choosing evening activities.

Chapter 32

Preventing Frostbite and Heat Illness

Chapter Contents

Section 32.1

What You Should Know about Frostbite

Information in this section is reprinted from "Frostbite," a brochure published by the University of Rochester Health Service, Rochester, New York. © 2001 University of Rochester. Reprinted with permission.

What Is Frostbite?

Frostbite is a thermal injury to the skin which can result from prolonged exposure to moderate cold or brief exposure to extreme cold. When skin is exposed to the cold, blood vessels in the skin clamp down or constrict. As a result of a decreased blood flow to the skin, the fluid in and around skin cells develops ice crystals. This causes frostbite to occur. Areas of the body most prone to frostbite are fingers, toes, hands, feet, nose, ears, and cheeks.

Signs and Symptoms

The signs and symptoms of frostbite vary depending on the severity of the case. A person may experience any of the following:

- pain in the affected area
- numbness in the affected area
- prickly sensations
- firm, whitened skin areas
- peeling or blistering
- itching
- swelling
- mottled skin (blotchy, red and white)
- hard, glossy, grayish, yellow skin

Treatment of Frostbite

The treatment of frostbite will depend on the severity of skin damage. Hospitalization may be necessary in some severe cases. Therefore, it is important to seek an evaluation by your health care provider or nearest medical care practitioner as soon as possible.

All types of frostbite require re-warming of the affected area. This is usually achieved by gently warming the exposed skin in lukewarm water. An antibiotic ointment may be prescribed for application to the affected area.

If blisters occur, they should be left intact whenever possible. Some skin peeling and "sponginess" may occur in the affected area as well. Elevating the affected part may be necessary if swelling occurs. Most importantly, the skin area must be protected from cold and sunlight for an indefinite period after the frostbite, as it will be more vulnerable to thermal injury in the future.

If You Think You Have Frostbite

- Move indoors to a warm environment as soon as possible.

- Do not rub the affected area as this can cause further damage due to the presence of ice crystals in the skin cells.

- Gently re-warm the affected body part by placing it against a warm body part (for example, placing hands under arms), or warming with lukewarm water or warm blankets.

- See your health care provider for evaluation as soon as possible.

Prevention

Prevention is the key to avoiding frostbite and its recurrence. Ways to avoid frostbite injury are:

- Do not go outdoors for prolonged periods in severely cold weather.

- Cover vulnerable body parts such as cheeks and nose with a scarf.

- Wear loose fitting, warm, layered clothing when out in the cold.

- Avoid caffeine, tobacco, and alcohol when going out in the cold, as these leave the skin more prone to thermal injury.

- Change any wet clothing immediately!

- Check skin every 10-20 minutes for signs of frostbite.

- Wear mittens instead of gloves. Wear wool or insulated type socks. Wear a hat and scarf to cover ears.

In Summary

- Frostbite can occur anytime skin is exposed to prolonged or severe cold.

- If frostbite is suspected, it should be evaluated as soon as possible.

- Symptoms of frostbite can include pain, prickling sensations, white, hard skin, numbness, mottled skin, blisters and skin peeling.

- Frostbitten skin needs to be gently re-warmed.

- Once skin has been frostbitten, it remains vulnerable to thermal injury for an indefinite period.

- Prevention is the best treatment.

Section 32.2

Heat Stress in Children

From "Preventing Heat Stress in Children and Adolescents," *HealthLink*, © 2001 Medical College of Wisconsin. Reprinted with permission of the Medical College of Wisconsin/MCW HealthLink http://healthlink.mcw.edu.

Kids love summer. When adults are wilting through the sweltering days, kids seem to breeze through July and August with barely a dent in their energy levels. But children are in fact much more susceptible to heat stress than adults.

Heat stress, or heat exhaustion, is characterized by dizziness, weakness, nausea, headache, and cramps. The skin feels cold and damp, and blood pressure may be low. (Heatstroke is a much more acute and dangerous reaction to prolonged or excessive exposure to heat, when the body temperature is above 105 degrees, the individual stops sweating, any may be paralyzed or lose consciousness—all symptoms signaling a failure of the body's heat regulating system).

Parents, coaches, camp counselors, and kids themselves need to be aware that when the temperature is above 95 degrees children and adolescents have markedly lower exercise tolerance than adults. And the hotter the air temperature and higher the humidity, the more susceptible children and adolescents are to heat stress.

High humidity can be a factor even without extremely high air temperatures; 70% of heat stress is due to humidity, 20% due to solar radiation, and only 10% to air temperature.

Children's bodies have greater surface area to body mass ratio, so they absorb more heat on a hot day (and lose heat more rapidly on a cold day). Also, children have considerable lower sweating capacity than adults, and so they are less able to dissipate body heat by evaporative sweating and cooling.

Children are less likely to feel thirsty during prolonged play and exercise, and sometimes they just don't want to be interrupted. They need to be reminded to drink water or another beverage. Salt tablets are not recommended.

To prevent heat-induced illness in children and adolescents, the Committee on Sports Medicine and Fitness of the American Academy of Pediatrics (in *Pediatrics*, Volume 106, July 2000 pages 158–159), emphasizes that:

- Children need time to become acclimated to a warmer climate by gradually increasing their level of exposure and of exercise.

- The duration of exercise and rest periods should be adjusted according to the humidity, air temperature, and degree of sun exposure experienced by the players.

- Children should be well hydrated before starting prolonged physical activity.

- They should drink liquids periodically during activities even if they do not feel thirsty: 5 ounces of cold water or a flavored salted beverage like a sports drink each 20 minutes for a child weighing 40 lbs.; 9 ounces every 20 minutes for an adolescent weighing 132 lbs.

- Clothing should be light colored, lightweight and limited to one layer of absorbent fabric to facilitate the evaporation of sweat. If clothes become wet, they should be changed for dry ones.

Note

Medical knowledge changes rapidly. In view of the possibility of human error or changes in the field of medicine, the authors, editors, the Medical College of Wisconsin, and any other party involved in the preparation or publication of *HealthLink* cannot guarantee that the information contained herein is in every respect accurate and complete. The are not responsible for any errors or omissions or for the results obtained from the use of this information. Readers are encouraged to confirm the information found in *HealthLink* with other sources.

Chapter 33

Water Safety

In 1996, nearly 1,000 children younger than 15 years of age drowned in the United States. It is surprising to many parents that young children tend not to splash or make noise when they get into trouble in the water and thus usually drown silently. An adult should always be watching young children playing, swimming, or bathing in water.

Tips for General Water Safety

You can greatly reduce the chances of you and your children becoming a drowning victim or being injured if you follow a few simple safety tips:

1. Make sure an adult is constantly watching young children swimming, playing, or bathing in water. Do not read, play cards, talk on the phone, mow the lawn, or do any other distracting activity while supervising children around water.

2. Never swim alone or in unsupervised places. Teach your children to always swim with a buddy.

3. Keep small children away from buckets containing liquid: 5-gallon industrial containers are a particular danger. Be sure to

From "Water Safety," SafeUSA™, Centers for Disease Control and Prevention (CDC), 2002. For more information from SafeUSA™ visit the website at www.safeusa.org.

empty buckets of all liquid when household chores are done. An infant or toddler can drown in as little as one inch of water.

4. Never drink alcohol before or during swimming, boating, or water skiing. Never drink alcohol while supervising children around water. Teach teenagers about the danger of drinking alcohol and swimming, boating, or water skiing.

5. To prevent choking, never chew gum or eat while swimming, diving, or playing in water.

6. Learn to swim. Enroll yourself and your children aged 4 and older in swimming classes. Swimming classes are not recommended for children under age 4.

7. Learn CPR (cardio-pulmonary resuscitation). This applies particularly to pool owners and water sports enthusiasts.

8. Do NOT use air-filled swimming aids (such as "water wings") in place of life jackets or life preservers with children. Using air-filled swimming aids can give parents and children a false sense of security, which may increase the risk of drowning. These air-filled aids are toys and are not designed to be personal flotation devices (life jackets). Air-filled plastic tubes can deflate because they become punctured or unplugged.

9. Check the water depth before entering. The American Red Cross recommends nine feet as a minimum depth for diving or jumping.

If you have a swimming pool at your home:

1. Install a four-sided, isolation pool-fence with self-closing and self-latching gates around the pool. Such a fence should be at least four feet tall and should completely separate the pool from the house and play area of the yard.

2. Prevent children from having direct access to the swimming pool.

3. Install a telephone near the pool. Know how to contact local emergency medical services. Post the emergency number, 911, in an easy-to-see place.

4. Remember always to closely supervise children using the pool and insist that others do too.

Additional Tips for Open Water

1. Know the local weather conditions and forecast before swimming or boating. Thunderstorms and strong winds are dangerous to swimmers and boaters.

2. Restrict activities to designated swimming areas, usually marked by buoys.

3. Use U.S. Coast Guard-approved personal flotation devices (life jackets) when boating, regardless of distance to be traveled, size of boat, or swimming ability of boaters.

4. Remember that open water usually has limited visibility, and conditions can sometimes change from hour to hour. Currents are often unpredictable, moving rapidly and quickly changing direction. A strong water current can carry even expert swimmers far from shore.

5. Watch for dangerous waves and signs of rip currents—water that is discolored, unusually choppy, foamy, or filled with debris.

6. If you are caught in a rip current, swim parallel to the shore. Once you are out of the current, swim toward the shore.

Who Is Affected?

Water sports—like swimming, wading, boating, and water skiing—are fun and exciting. But they can also be dangerous for people of all ages. In 1996, nearly 4,000 people drowned in the United States, including almost 1,000 children younger than 15 years of age. Among children aged 1–9, drowning is the second leading cause of death from injuries. Near-drownings can result in brain damage.

Childhood drownings and near-drownings often occur when a child is left alone, even for a few seconds. It is surprising to many parents that young children tend not to splash or make noise when they get into trouble in the water and thus usually drown silently. Most children who drown in pools were last seen inside the home, had been out of sight less than five minutes, and were in the care of one or both parents at the time.

How young children drown tends to vary by age. For example:

*   Children under age one most often drown in bathtubs, buckets, and toilets.

315

- Children aged 1–4 most often drown in swimming pools, hot tubs, and spas.

- Children aged 5–14 most often drown in swimming pools and open water, such as lakes and rivers.

Many people don't realize that alcohol use is involved in many drownings: 25–50% of adolescent and adult drownings involve alcohol use. In 40–50% of drownings among adolescent boys, alcohol is a major contributing factor.

Chapter 34

Car Safety and Children

Chapter Contents

317

Section 34.1

Child Passenger Safety

Excerpted from "Child Passenger Safety," SafeUSA™, Centers for Disease Control and Prevention (CDC), 2002. For more information from SafeUSA™ visit their website at www.safeusa.org.

Safety Tips

You can reduce the risk of children being killed or injured in a motor vehicle crash if you follow a few simple safety tips.

- All children aged 12 years and younger should ride in the back seat for two important reasons. First, the back seat is generally the safest place in a vehicle during a crash. Second, children sitting in the front seat have been injured and killed by passenger air bags as they inflate in a crash. If your vehicle has a passenger air bag, children aged 12 years and younger should always ride in the back.

- Infants should ride in rear-facing child safety seats until they weigh 20 pounds and are one year old. Never place a rear-facing child safety seat in front of an air bag.

- Toddlers and preschoolers aged 1 to 4 years should ride in a forward-facing child safety seat until they weigh about 40 pounds (usually around age four), or until their ears reach the top of the back of the child safety seat, or their shoulders are above the top seat-strap slots.

- Children who have outgrown their child safety seats should ride in a booster seat that positions the shoulder belt across the chest and the lap belt low across the upper thighs. Children should use a booster seat until the lap and shoulder belts in the car fit properly—usually when they are at least 4 feet, 10 inches tall and weigh at least 80 pounds. To ride comfortably and safely, children must be able to bend their knees over the edge of the seat while sitting with their backs firmly against the seat back (without slouching). In most cases, this means that children 4 to 8 years old should ride in a booster seat.

- Children who have outgrown their booster seats should always use a safety belt. The child must be tall enough to sit without slouching, with knees bent at the edge of the seat, with feet on the floor. The lap belt must fit low and tight across the upper thighs. The shoulder belt should rest over the shoulder and across the chest. Never put the shoulder belt under the child's arm or behind the child's back.

- Teens and adults should never drink and drive. They should always wear a safety belt.

Section 34.2

Quick Safety Seat Checkup

Excerpted from "Quick Safety Seat Checkup," National Highway Traffic Safety Administration (NHTSA), U.S. Department of Transportation, revised October 1998. Additional information is available from NHTSA at www.nhtsa.dot.gov.

Does Your Child Ride in the Back Seat?

- The back seat is generally the safest place in a crash.

- If your vehicle has a passenger air bag, it is essential for children 12 and under to ride in back.

- Does your child ride facing the right way? Infants should ride in rear facing restraints, preferably in the back seat. Children over age one and at least 20 pounds may ride facing forward.

Does the Safety Belt Hold the Seat Tightly in Place?

- Put the belt through the right slot. If your safety seat can be used facing either way, use the correct belt slots for each direction.

• The safety belt must stay tight when securing the safety seat. Check the vehicle owner's manual for tips on using the safety belts.

Is the Harness Buckled Snugly around Your Child?

• Keep the straps over your child's shoulder. The harness should be adjusted so you can slip only one finger underneath the straps at your child's chest. Place the chest clip at armpit level.

Does Your Child Over 40 Pounds Have the Best Protection Possible?

• Keep your child in a safety seat with a full harness as long as possible, at least until 40 pounds. Then use a belt-positioning booster seat which helps the adult-sized lap belt and shoulder belt fit the child better.

• A belt-positioning booster seat is preferred for children between 40–80 pounds. It is used with the adult lap and shoulder belt. Check on special products for heavy children too active to sit still in a booster.

How Should a Safety Belt Fit an Older Child?

• The child must be tall enough to sit without slouching, with knees bent at the edge of the seat, with feet on the floor. The lap belt must fit low and tight across the upper thighs. The shoulder belt should rest over the shoulder and across the chest. Never put the shoulder belt under the arm or behind the child's back. The adult lap and shoulder belt system alone will not fit most children until they are at least 4'9" tall and weigh about 80 pounds.

Section 34.3

Where Should Your Child Ride?

Excerpted from "Where Should Your Child Ride?" National Highway Traffic Safety Administration (NHTSA), U.S. Department of Transportation, revised October 1998. Additional information is available from NHTSA at www.nhtsa.dot.gov.

Basic Safety Facts to Remember

- Everybody needs a safety belt or safety seat.

- Anyone who rides loose can hurt those who are buckled up by being thrown against them. People riding without belts or safety seats can be hurled out of the car and seriously hurt.

- The back seat usually is safer than the front, because head-on crashes are the most common kind.

- There must be one belt for each person. Buckling two people, even children, into one belt could injure both. Each child safety seat needs a safety belt to hold it in place.

- If no shoulder belt is available, it's much safer for anyone (except small babies who can't sit up) to use just a lap belt than to ride loose. Keep the lap belt low and snug across the thighs. Other options should be pursued, such as having shoulder belts installed or using harness/vest devices for children.

- Children who have outgrown safety seats are better protected by lap/shoulder belts than by lap belts alone. So if several children are riding in back, and there are shoulder belts there, let the older ones use the shoulder belts. Put the child riding in the car seat in the middle where there is only a lap belt.

- Infants must ride facing the rear of the car, even if they are out of the driver's view in the back seat. Parents should feel just as comfortable in this situation as they do when they put their babies down for a nap and leave the room. If a baby has special health needs that require full-time monitoring, ask another

321

adult to ride with the baby in the back seat and travel alone as little as possible.

• Always read the instructions that come with the safety seat. Also read the section on safety belts and child seat installation in your vehicle owner's manual.

Does Your Car Have an Air Bag for the Front Passenger Seat?

A passenger air bag can seriously harm a child riding in the front seat of the car. Many new cars have air bags for the right front seat. Air bags work with lap/shoulder belts to protect teens and adults. To check if your vehicle has air bags, look for a warning label on the sun visor or the letters "SRS" or "SIR" embossed on the dashboard. The owner's manual will also tell you.

An inflating passenger air bag can kill a baby in a rear-facing safety seat. An air bag also can be hazardous for children age 12 and under who ride facing forward. This is especially true if they are not properly buckled up in a safety seat, booster seat, or lap and shoulder belt.

In a crash, the air bag inflates very quickly. It would hit a rear-facing safety seat hard enough to kill the baby. Infants must ride in the back seat, facing the rear. Even in the back seat, do not turn your baby to face forward until he or she is about one year of age and weighs at least 20 pounds. Look for a seat that meets the higher rear-facing weight limit for heavier babies not yet one year of age.

If there is no room in back and you have no alternative, a child over age one who is forward facing may have to ride in front. Make sure the child is correctly buckled up for his or her age and size and that the vehicle seat is moved as far back as possible. Fasten the harness snugly, and make sure a child using a lap and shoulder belt does not lean toward the dashboard. Read your vehicle owner's guide about the air bags in your car. WARNING: If the front right seat has an air bag, a baby in a rear-facing safety seat must ride in the back seat. All children age 12 and under should ride in back.

Remember: One Person—One Belt

• Never hold a child on your lap because you could crush him in a collision. Even if you are using a safety belt, the child would be torn from your arms in a crash.

• Never put a belt around yourself and a child on your lap.

- Two people with one belt around them could injure each other.

- The cargo area of a station wagon, van, or pickup is a very dangerous place for anyone to ride. Anyone riding in the bed of a pickup truck, even under a canopy, could be thrown out.

Section 34.4

How Should Preschool and School Children Ride Safely?

Excerpted from "How Should Preschool and School Children Ride Safely?" National Highway Traffic Safety Administration (NHTSA), U.S. Department of Transportation, revised October 1998. Additional information is available from NHTSA at www.nhtsa.dot.gov.

Your child should stay in a car safety seat with a full harness until the seat is outgrown, usually at about 40 pounds. When a child's shoulders are above the top set of strap slots, it is time for a booster seat.

Booster seats protect the child's upper body with either the shoulder belt or with a shield. The booster also raises the child so the vehicle lap/shoulder belt fits well.

Why Use a Booster Seat Instead of a Safety Belt?

- Most 40-pound children are not big enough to fit lap and shoulder belts properly.

- A belt that rides up on the tummy could cause serious injury.

- The adult lap and shoulder belt normally does not fit a child until they are about 4'9" tall and weigh approx. 80 lbs.

- Many young children do not sit still enough or straight enough to keep lap belts low across their thighs.

- Boosters are comfortable for children because they allow their legs to bend normally. This also reduces slouching, one cause of poor lap belt fit.

323

Three Kinds of Booster Seats

1. Boosters without shields, for use only with the vehicle lap/ shoulder belt. Because raising the child improves belt fit, these are called "belt-positioning boosters." Some have a high back that gives head support for taller children. Some boosters of this type are built into vehicle seats.

2. Boosters with removable shields. Use without the shield to make lap and shoulder belts fit right. Shield boosters are not currently approved for children weighing over 40 pounds. A child who has outgrown their convertible seat, yet weighs less than 40 pounds can be moved into a high-back booster with a harness. Once the child reaches 40 pounds, the harness is removed and the seat is used with the adult lap and shoulder belt as a belt-positioning booster.

3. High-backed boosters, used as belt-positioning boosters. Most have a clip or strap to hold the shoulder belt in place. Some high-backed boosters have removable harnesses. This type can be used with the harness for a child under 40 lbs. Children who reach 40 pounds before age 3 may not be mature enough to stay seated properly in a belt-positioning booster. A vest that uses the belt system and a tether strap would be an option in this situation.

Which Booster Is Best?

*   The belt-positioning booster is the best choice if your car has combination lap/shoulder belts in the rear seat.

*   Use a booster with a high back if there is no head restraint for the child.

*   The booster with a high back and a removable harness provides the most options in many vehicles. Check the label for the weight limit on the harness.

How Long Should the Booster Be Used?

*   Try the vehicle belts on your child as he or she grows taller. When the child sits comfortably without slouching, with the lap belt low on the hips and the shoulder belt across the shoulder, use the belts without the booster.

- Lap belt fit is most important. A child is usually ready for the adult lap and shoulder belt when the child can sit with their back against the vehicle seat back cushion with knees bent over the vehicle seat edge with feet on the floor.

- Do your child's ears come above the top of the vehicle seat back? If so, a high-back booster will improve neck protection.

- Always follow manufacturer instructions.

How Should a Lap Belt Fit?

The lap belt should fit low over a child's upper thighs. Make sure the child sits straight against the seat back. Keep the belt snug. If the lap belt rides up onto the tummy, it could cause serious injuries in a crash.

How Can You Make a Shoulder Belt Fit Better?

- The shoulder belt should stay on the shoulder and be close to the child's chest.

- If you have the kind of shoulder belt that stays loose when it is pulled out, make sure there is no more than one inch of slack. Too much slack will prevent the belt from working well. Teach your child to tug at the shoulder belt to take up excess slack.

- If the shoulder belt fits so poorly that it goes across the neck or face, raise the child with a belt-positioning booster.

- Never put a shoulder belt under the child's arm or behind the back. Either of these kinds of misuse could cause serious injury in a crash.

- Warning: Some devices advertised to improve belt fit for older children and adults are not covered by government standards. They may help with shoulder belt comfort but may put too much slack in the shoulder belt or cause the lap belt to ride up. Boosters are a better solution for children who fit in them.

Section 34.5

Air Bag Safety

Excerpted from "Air Bag Safety: Buckle up Everyone! Children in Back!" National Highway Traffic Safety Administration (NHTSA), U.S. Department of Transportation, revised October 1998. Additional information is available from NHTSA at www.nhtsa.dot.gov.

An infant or child riding in the front seat can be seriously injured or killed by the inflating air bag. An air bag is not a soft pillow. To do its important job, an air bag comes out of the dashboard very fast—faster than the blink of an eye. Many people's lives have been saved by air bags.

The force of an air bag can hurt people who are too close to it. Drivers can prevent injuries to adults and children from air bags by following these safety steps.

Air Bag Safety Steps

- Infants in rear-facing child safety seats must never ride in the front seat of a vehicle with a passenger air bag.

- Children 12 and under should ride buckled up in the rear seat. They should use child safety seats, booster seats, or safety belts appropriate for their age and size.

- Everyone should buckle up with both lap and shoulder belts on every trip. Driver and front passenger seats should be moved as far back from the dashboard as practical.

- Infants under age one must ride facing the rear of the car in the rear seat. Parents should feel just as comfortable in this situation as they do when they put their babies down for a nap and leave the room.

- If a baby has special health needs and requires full-time supervision, ask another adult to ride with the baby in the back seat and travel alone as little as possible until the health problem is resolved.

• Check your vehicle owner's manual and the instructions provided with your child safety seat for information on air bags and safety seat use.

What about Sports Cars and Pickup Trucks?

If there is no rear seat and no air bag shut-off switch, a child is at high risk from a passenger air bag.

Some pickup trucks made since model year 1996 have switches to shut off the passenger air bag. Other vehicles may have them in future years. Turning off the switch is the best way to protect an infant riding in a rear-facing safety seat or an older child using a safety seat, booster, or safety belt.

What If You Have No Alternative Except Putting a Child in Front?

If there is no room in back, a child over age one may have to ride in the front seat. Here's how to reduce the risk:

• Make sure the child is correctly buckled up with the vehicle seat moved as far back as possible. A toddler/preschooler should use a forward-facing child safety seat; an older child should use a belt-positioning booster or lap/shoulder belt.

• Fasten the harness or lap/shoulder belt securely.

• Make sure an older child does not slip out of the shoulder belt or lean toward the dashboard.

Vehicle owners and lessees can obtain an on-off switch for one or both of their air bags only if they can certify that they are—or a user of their vehicle is—in one of the four risk groups: infants in rear-facing infant seats, drivers or passengers with unusual medical or physical conditions, children ages 1 to 12, or drivers who cannot get back 10 inches from the air bag cover. To be considered eligible for an on-off switch, a National Highway Traffic Safety Administration (NHTSA) request form must be filled out and returned to NHTSA. Forms are available from state motor vehicle offices and may be available from automobile dealerships and repair facilities. Forms can also be requested by contacting NHTSA's Auto Safety Hotline at 1-888-DASH-2-DOT or visiting the NHTSA Web site at http://www.nhtsa.dot.gov.

Chapter 35

Streets, Driveways, and Traffic

Chapter Contents

Section 35.1

Walking and Biking Safety for Children on the Move

This section includes excerpts from "Tip #10—Play It Safe: Walking and Biking Safely," and "Tip #11—Kids on the Move: Walking and Biking Safely," National Highway Traffic Safety Administration, U.S. Department of Transportation, October 1998. Despite the date of these documents, the suggestions are still current. The full text of these documents and additional tips are available online at www.nhtsa.dot.gov/people/injury/childps/tips/.

Toddlers and Preschoolers

Children hit by cars can be hurt or killed, even when cars are moving slowly. Toddlers (one and two year olds) are most often hurt by a backing vehicle. If a child is playing in a driveway or parking area, a driver may not see him. Preschoolers (three and four year olds) are most often hit when dashing across a street near home.

Falls from tricycles or other play vehicles can cause serious head and brain injury. These injuries to young children can be as serious as injuries to older children falling from bikes.

Toddlers and preschoolers:

- move quickly and can run into the street without warning.
- don't know safety rules and expect adults to watch out for them.
- are small and hard for drivers to see.
- cannot judge speed or distance of vehicles moving toward them.

Safety Steps for Parents of Toddlers and Preschoolers

- **Supervise, supervise, supervise:** Parents and caregivers must watch toddlers and preschoolers closely when they are near parked or moving vehicles. To supervise properly, you must be near your child, not watching from a distance. Hold your child's hand when you walk together along the street.

- **Find safe places to play:** Keep children away from traffic. Fenced yards, parks, or playgrounds are good places for your child to ride and play.

- **Set a safe example:** Young children learn by watching adults. Show them safe ways to cross streets and always wear a helmet when you ride a bike.

- **Get them in the habit of looking for cars:** When walking, talk to your child about street safety. Show him/her how to stop at the edge of the street and look for cars. Don't expect your young child to do this by herself.

Biking Safety for Toddlers and Preschoolers

Wearing a bike helmet is the most important way for your child to stay safe on a play vehicle, tricycle, or bike. A helmet can reduce the risk of head injury by 85 percent when worn correctly. Start children wearing helmets with their first tricycles or play vehicles. When children begin helmet use early, they are more likely to keep the habit in later years.

Toddler helmets are lightweight, because a toddler's neck is not strong enough for a regular helmet. Also, these helmets come down low around the back of the head for more coverage. Choose a helmet that meets current safety standards set by the Consumer Product Safety Commission (CPSC). Look for a sticker inside the helmet to verify that the helmet meets current standards.

These suggestions will help ensure the correct fit:

- Make sure the helmet covers the upper part of the forehead and sits level on the head.

- Use the foam pads inside to fit the helmet snugly so it doesn't slip around.

- Adjust the chin strap tightly enough so the helmet pulls down when the child opens his mouth.

Insist that your child wear a helmet whenever she rides. If your child's preschool uses tricycles, work with the school to make helmets available. Urge the school to have a policy requiring helmet use.

Carrying Your Child Safely on a Bike

Never carry a baby under age one on a bicycle. A baby does not have the neck strength to wear a helmet. Her back is not strong enough to sit straight with the motion of the bike.

331

When a child is old enough to ride on an adult's bike, only a skilled rider should carry him. Ride only in safe areas like parks, bike paths, or quiet streets.

- Make sure both adult and child wear properly fitting helmets.

- Make sure the child carrier has a high back, a lap and shoulder harness, and foot guards to keep feet away from the spokes.

- Check that the carrier is fastened firmly to the bike.

- Buckle the harness snugly around the child.

Children in Kindergarten through Third Grade

Children in kindergarten through third grade are learning to become independent. They enjoy walking, riding bikes, and playing outside. They don't have the judgment to cope with traffic by themselves yet, but they can begin to understand safety rules.

Nearly one third of the five- to nine-year-old children killed by motor vehicles are on foot. They are hit by cars most often when playing near home. They tend to run into the street in the middle of the block, where drivers don't expect them.

What Parents Need to Know

- Parents often think their children are able to handle traffic safely by themselves before they actually are ready.

- Children don't have the skills to handle these risky situations until at least age ten.

- Boys are much more likely than girls to be injured or killed in traffic.

- Bicycles are vehicles. Children should not ride bikes in the road until they fully understand traffic rules and show they can follow them.

Young children:

- often act before thinking and may not do what parents or drivers expect.

- assume that if they see the driver, the driver sees them.

- can't judge speed and they think cars can stop instantly.

- are shorter than adults and can't see over cars, bushes, and other objects.

Safety Steps for Parents of Young Children

- **Set limits for your child:** As your children grow, set appropriate limits on where they can walk or bike safely. Don't expect them to be responsible or to start to behave safely until age ten.

- **Find safe places for riding and walking:** Find places away from streets, driveways, and parking lots. Good choices are fenced yards, parks, or playgrounds.

- **Teach safe walking habits:** Begin to teach your child about how to cross streets safely. Give them plenty of chances to practice when you are with them.

- **Set an example:** Young children learn by watching their parents and other adults. Cross streets properly and always wear a helmet when you ride a bike. When you are driving, obey speed limits and watch for children.

Teach the "Safe Street Crossing" Method

Teach your child to:

- Cross with an adult or older friend. (Young children still need supervision around traffic up to at least age ten.)

- Cross at a signalized intersection, when possible.

- Use the crosswalk when crossing near a corner.

- Watch for turning vehicles.

- Stop at the curb. Look left, right, left, and over your shoulder for traffic. Continue to look as you cross.

- Stop to look around parked cars or other objects that block the view of traffic. Let oncoming traffic pass, then look again before crossing.

- Make eye contact with drivers to make sure they see you.

Help Your Child Bike Safely

A big bike "to grow into" is not easy to learn on or to ride safely. A child should be able to sit on the seat with knees straight and feet flat on the ground. Also make sure he can straddle the bike with at least one or two inches between the top bar and crotch.

Children can be hurt riding on or off the road. Many children who are killed in bike crashes are 7 to 12 years old. The most serious injuries children get while biking are head and brain injuries. Head injuries can cause death or lifelong disability.

Insist on bike helmet use. A brain injury cannot be cured. Bike helmet use can reduce the risk of head injury by 85 percent when worn correctly. Make it clear to your child that she must wear a helmet on every ride. It also is important to wear a helmet when doing other sports, like in-line skating and skateboarding.

Selecting and Fitting a Bike Helmet

Choose a bike helmet that meets current safety standards. Every new bike helmet must meet the CPSC standard. Look for a sticker inside the helmet to confirm that it meets current standards.

Follow these guidelines to fit a bike helmet:

- Use foam pads inside to fit the helmet snugly so it doesn't move on the head.

- Fit the helmet so the front is just above the top of the eyebrows. Teach your child to wear it this way.

- Adjust the two side straps so they meet in a "V" right under each ear.

- Adjust the chin strap snugly under the chin. Make it tight enough so the helmet pulls down when the child opens his mouth.

- Check often to make sure straps stay snug and the helmet stays level on the head.

The following suggestions may help encourage your child to wear his helmet:

- Let your child help choose the helmet.

- Explain that a helmet is "just part of the gear," as it is with football, race car driving, or hockey.

- Praise your child for wearing his helmet.

- Talk to other parents, so that all neighborhood families encourage the same safety rules.

For more information, call the National Highway Traffic Safety Administration Auto Safety Hotline: 888-DASH-2-DOT or visit the NHTSA website, www.nhtsa.dot.gov.

Section 35.2

Tips for Parents about Pedestrian Safety

This section includes text from "Walking Safely," SafeUSA™, Centers for Disease Control and Prevention, updated July 2002, and "Pedestrian Signal Quiz," an undated quiz produced by the Federal Highway Administration, available online at http://safety.fhwa.dot.gov/pedestrian_signal_quiz.pdf, cited May 2003.

Adults should supervise children as they cross the street and teach them to look left-right-left again before crossing a street and to keep looking as they cross.

Walking Safety Tips

You greatly reduce the chances of getting injured as a pedestrian if you follow these simple safety tips:

- Supervise young children and do not leave them alone to play, especially near a street or the driveway.

- Make sure that the children's play area is at least 200 feet from any dangerous area (such as a street, driveway, a vacant lot, or water). If it is within 200 feet, the play area should be fenced.

- Obey the school safety patrol, crossing guard, or police officer when walking near a school.

- Teach children to cross streets at a corner, use crosswalks (whenever possible), and obey the traffic signals. Teach them to check for approaching vehicles before crossing even with the green light or "walk" sign on.

- Make sure children under age 10 are supervised when crossing the street. You may also need to supervise older children, especially when they cross streets with heavy traffic or more than two lanes.

- Teach children to look left-right-left again before crossing a street and to keep looking as they cross. Practice this behavior with them until they master it.

- Teach children to walk facing on-coming traffic if no sidewalks are available.

- Wear light-colored clothing if walking at dawn, at dusk, or after dark. Even better, wear reflective tape (placed diagonally across the back) and carry a flashlight.

- Make sure that doors leading to the outside of the house, including garage doors, cannot be opened by young children. This is to prevent children from getting out of the house unnoticed by their parents and being injured in traffic.

Teaching Young Children about Pedestrian Signals

Young children often cannot judge the speed, distance, and size of oncoming vehicles. Teach them that its best to allow an oncoming vehicle to pass, and then wait for a new green light or **WALK** signal. The green light or **WALK** signal means that children should stop at the curb or edge of the road, look both ways for oncoming traffic, and then—if its safe—they can go. It does not mean that they have the right of way. Having the **WALK** signal or green light does not guarantee that cars will stop.

Always stop at the curb and look for cars in all directions before entering the road. When looking left-right-left, make sure to look for turning vehicles, too.

Before crossing the street, children may want to wait for a fresh green light. This means that they wait for the next new **WALK** signal. Doing this gives them the most time to cross.

If children are in the middle of the street and the **DON'T WALK** signal flashes, they shouldn't stop or return to the curb or edge of the road. They should continue to walk at their maximum comfortable pace until they reach the other side. Teach them not to run; they might fall.

And remember: Children crossing the street should be accompanied by an adult whenever possible.

Pedestrian Quiz

*1. What does the green light or **WALK** signal mean?*

It means that you should get ready to cross the street.

*2. Before you step off the curb or the edge of the road to cross the street, what do you **always** do?*

Look to the left, then to the right, then left again for oncoming cars. If a car is approaching, make sure that you can see the driver's eyes, and that he/she has seen you before you step off the curb. Do not run.

*3. What do you do if you are in the middle of the street and the **WALK** signal starts to blink or the **DON'T WALK** signal comes on?*

Continue to walk. Do not run.

*4. If the **WALK** signal is blinking when you get to the curb or edge of the road, what should you do?*

Stop! Do not try to cross the street. Wait for the next **WALK** signal.

*5. If the **DON'T WALK** signal is blinking when you get the curb or edge of the road, but the traffic signal is green, what should you do?*

Stop! Do not try to cross the street. Wait for the next **WALK** signal.

Section 35.3

Creating Safer Streets and Play Places

"Tip #14—Beyond the Front Yard: Creating Safer Streets and Play Places for Children," National Highway Traffic Safety Administration (NHTSA), U.S. Department of Transportation, October 1998. Despite the date of this document, the suggestions are still current. Additional information from NHTSA is available online at www.nhtsa.dot.gov/people/injury/childps/tips.

Crawling... walking... bike riding... in-line and roller skating. As babies grow into school kids, they move farther and faster. They love to be on the move—to the neighbor's house, the school yard, the park, or the store. These activities are great for your children, if your neighborhood has safe playgrounds, sidewalks, and streets.

- Young children need safe places for active play, yet many communities today are not kid-friendly.

- Children over ten years old need safe ways to get themselves to school, sports events, and stores. When they walk or cycle, you— the parent—help your children learn responsibility and independence.

There are things you can do to make these outings safer. Slower traffic, nearby parks, and better sidewalks help everyone in the neighborhood. Older people and those with limited mobility will also appreciate these improvements.

Pedestrian-Friendly Neighborhood Streets

How pedestrian-friendly are your neighborhood streets? Take a walk in your neighborhood with your child. Look at the conditions along the way, and as you walk, ask yourself these questions:

- Are there places for people to walk (or for children to bicycle) off the street?

- Are there places to cross streets easily and safely?

- Are there crossing guards near schools?
- Are the drivers courteous? Do they obey speed limits?
- Was your walk pleasant? Would you do it again?

Note any problems that you find. Here are some examples:

- Traffic speeds are too high.
- No sidewalks or wide shoulders for walking.
- Roadside obstructions make walking difficult (parked cars, trash bins, overgrown bushes, ditches).
- No crosswalks or traffic signals where we want to cross busy streets.
- Drivers do not stop for pedestrians.
- No place for children to play.
- Playgrounds, library, and schools are too far away.

If you want to make your streets friendlier for kids, there are some things that you can do yourself:

- As a driver, set an example by slowing down and giving pedestrians the right of way when crossing. Share the road with bicyclists.
- Obey speed limits, especially in neighborhoods where children play. Be extra careful in school zones.
- If buses or trains run in your area, use them with your child when practical.

Some things to make streets more pedestrian friendly can be done with the cooperation of others. Talk with your neighbors about the problems you see. They may want changes, too. Find others in your community who are concerned with child safety: traffic engineers, police traffic officers, school transportation directors, and parent-teacher associations. Write letters to your newspaper and speak up at public meetings for:

- playgrounds near homes so kids can play out of streets and parking areas;
- "traffic calming" improvements to slow down traffic on neighborhood streets, including traffic circles, speed bumps, and other engineering methods;

- construction of sidewalks or bike/pedestrian paths;

- a neighborhood crime watch, if needed. If playgrounds are being used for other activities, work with community groups to make them child-friendly.

A "Walkability Checklist" (which is also available in Spanish) and other child traffic safety information, is available on the NHTSA website, www.nhtsa.dot.gov. For additional information, you can also call the NHTSA Auto Safety Hotline: 888-DASH-2-DOT.

Chapter 36

Safety on the School Bus

Chapter Contents

Section 36.1

Facts about School Bus Safety

This section includes text from "School Bus Safety," and "School Bus Safety Fact Sheets," undated documents produced by the National Highway Traffic Safety Administration (NHTSA). Additional information from NHTSA is available online at www.nhtsa.dot.gov.

School Bus Safety

Twenty-three million students nationwide ride a school bus to and from school each day. Wherever you live, the familiar yellow school bus is one of the most common motor vehicles on the road. It is also the safest. School buses manufactured after January 1, 1977 must meet more federal motor vehicle safety standards than any other type of motor vehicle. In fact, during normal school transportation hours over the past 10 years, school buses are 87 times safer than passenger cars, light trucks, and vans, according to the Fatality Analysis Reporting System at the U.S. Department of Transportation. But school bus transportation is not without its hazards. Between 1989 and 1999, an average of 30 school age children (ages 5 through 18) were fatally injured each year in school bus-related crashes. Pedestrian fatalities while loading and unloading school buses accounted for nearly three out of every four of those fatalities; more than half of the pedestrian fatalities were young children between 5 and 7 years old.

Facts about School Buses

- Every year, approximately 440,000 public school buses travel more than 4 billion miles and daily transport 24 million children to and from schools and school-related activities. School buses account for an estimated 10 billion student trips each year.

- By all measures, school buses are the safest motor vehicles on the highways.

- When comparing the number of fatalities of children ages 5 through 18 during "normal school transportation hours," in the

1989 through 1999 school years, school buses are 87 times safer than passenger cars, light trucks, and vans.

- From 1989 to 1999, an average of 10 passengers were killed each year in school bus crashes.

- Most of the school bus fatalities were in non-survivable situations (the fatality occurred at the point of maximum damage to the school bus).

- From 1989 to 1999, an average of 30 pedestrians were killed each year while getting on or off school buses, 23 of which were children struck by the school bus. The other 7 pedestrians were struck by another vehicle.

- More than half of the pedestrian fatalities in school bus-related crashes were children between 5 and 7 years old.

- Most student pedestrian fatalities in school bus-related crashes occur when coming home from school during daylight hours.

- School buses manufactured after January 1, 1977, must meet a series of strict Federal Motor Vehicle Safety Standards which have proven to greatly enhance the safety of school buses.

- School buses are required to meet more Federal Motor Vehicle Safety Standards than any other type of motor vehicle.

Getting on and off the Bus Safely

Because getting on and off the bus is the most dangerous part of the school bus ride, the loading and unloading area is called the "Danger Zone." This area—which extends ten feet in front of the bus, ten feet on each side of the bus, and behind the bus—is where children are at greatest risk of not being seen by the bus driver. Throughout the year, especially at the start of school, children need to be taught how to get on and off the school bus safely. Parents should help their children learn and follow these common-sense practices:

- Get to the bus stop at least five minutes before the bus is scheduled to arrive. Running to catch the bus is dangerous and can lead to injuries.

- When the bus approaches, stand at least five giant steps (10 feet) away from the curb, and line up away from the street.

- Wait until the bus stops, the door opens, and the driver says that it's okay before stepping onto the bus.

- If you have to cross the street in front of the bus, walk on the sidewalk or along the road to a point at least five giant steps ahead of the bus before you cross. Be sure that the bus driver can see you and you can see the bus driver when crossing the street. Stop at the edge of the bus and look left-right-left before crossing.

- Use the handrails to avoid falls. When getting off the bus, be careful that clothing with drawstrings and book-bags and back-packs with straps don't get caught in the handrails or door.

- Never walk behind the bus.

- Walk at least five giant steps away from the side of the bus.

- If you drop something near the bus, tell the bus driver. Never try to pick it up, because the driver might not be able to see you.

Riding Safely

Students also need to behave safely during the school bus ride. Basic safety rules include the following:

- Always sit fully in the seat and face forward.

- Never distract the driver.

- Never stand on a moving bus.

- Obey the driver.

- Speak in a low voice, no screaming or shouting.

- Never stick anything out the window (arms, legs, head, book-bags, etc.).

Section 36.2

School Bus Stops: A Risky Part of the Ride

"Tip #12—School Bus Stops: A Risky Part of the Ride," National High-way Safety Administration (NHTSA), U.S. Department of Transportation, October 1998. Despite the date of this document, the suggestions are still current. Additional information from NHTSA is available online at www.nhtsa.dot.gov/people/injury/childps/tips.

Why Students Are in Danger

Millions of children in the United States ride safely to and from school on school buses each day. Although school buses are the safest way to get them to school, an average of 33 school-age children die in school bus-related traffic crashes each year.

Most of those killed are pedestrians, five to seven years old. They are hit in the danger zone around the bus, either by a passing vehicle or by the school bus itself. It is illegal for a car to pass a bus with its red light flashing.

Young children are most likely to be hit because they:

- hurry to get on or off the bus,
- act before they think and have little experience with traffic,
- assume motorists will see them and will wait for them to cross,
- don't always stay within the bus driver's sight.

Safety Steps You Can Take

- Supervise children to make sure they get to the stop on time, wait far away from the road, and avoid rough play.

- Teach your child to ask the driver for help if he drops something near the bus. If a child stoops to pick up something, the driver cannot see him. Then he could be hit by the bus. A book-bag or backpack helps keep loose items together.

- Make sure clothing has no loose drawstrings and backpack straps are short, so they don't get caught in the handrail or bus door.

- Encourage safe school bus loading and unloading.

- If you think a bus stop is in a dangerous place, talk with your school office or transportation director about changing the location.

Teach Your Child to Get on and off the Bus Safely

1. When loading, stay away from the danger zone and wait for the driver's signal. Board the bus in single file.

2. When unloading, look before stepping off the bus to be sure no cars are passing on the shoulder (side of the road). Move away from the bus.

3. Before crossing the street, take five "giant steps" out from the front of the bus, or until the driver's face can be seen. Wait for the driver to signal that it's safe to cross.

4. Look left-right-left when coming to the edge of the bus to make sure traffic is stopped. Continue to watch for traffic when crossing.

Risky Business for Motorists: Passing a Stopped School Bus

What is the most dangerous part of the school bus ride? The bus stop!

Children are at greatest risk when they are getting on or off the school bus. Most of the children killed in bus-related crashes are pedestrians, five to seven years old, who are getting on or off the bus. They are hit by the school bus or by motorists illegally passing a stopped bus.

In neighborhoods, near schools, and at bus stops, drivers need to take special care because children do not behave like adults. Elementary school children:

- Become easily distracted and may start across the street without warning

- Don't understand the danger of moving vehicles

- Can't judge vehicle speed or distance

- May be blocked from view by the bus

Most importantly, children expect vehicles to stop for them at the school bus stop.

Standard School Bus Stop Laws

Learn and follow the school bus laws for motorists in your state. Laws exist to protect children getting on and off the bus AND to protect you from a tragedy. Check with your school transportation office or police department for more information on your state's laws. Here are standard rules:

- Motorists coming to a school bus from either direction must stop when the bus displays flashing red warning lights and extends the stop signal arm. These signals show that children are getting on or off the school bus.

- Vehicles may not pass until the flashing red lights and signals are turned off.

- Drivers traveling in the same direction as the bus are always required to stop.
  - In some states, drivers moving in the opposite direction on a divided roadway are also required to stop. Check the law in your state.

- Never pass on the right side of the bus, where children enter or exit. This is illegal and can have tragic results.

Violation of these laws can result in a citation and fine. In many places, school bus drivers can report passing vehicles.

Section 36.3

Handrails and Drawstrings: Clothing Causes School Bus Hazard

"Tip #13—Handrails and Drawstrings: Clothing Causes School Bus Hazard," National Highway Safety Administration (NHTSA), U.S. Department of Transportation, October 1998. Despite the date of this document, the suggestions are still current. Additional information from NHTSA is available online at www.nhtsa.dot.gov/people/injury/childps/tips/.

Drawstrings Can Be Dangerous

Current styles and fads of children's clothing, especially drawstrings, have brought new injury risks. Some clothing can cause deaths and injuries by catching on bus doors or handrails, playground equipment, and cribs.

Items that can catch in these areas:

- Jackets, sweatshirts, and clothing with drawstrings at the neck or waist;

- Backpack straps, dangling key chains, scarves, belt buckles, and other loose clothing.

How Can a Drawstring Hurt a Child?

A drawstring at the waist, hood, or neck on clothing can catch in a small gap in playground equipment, a bus handrail, or on a bolt. A drawstring with a large toggle or knot at the end is most likely to get caught.

As a child gets off the school bus, a dangling drawstring or loose object may catch in the handrail. If the bus doors close and the child isn't seen, she could be dragged and run over by the wheels.

School Bus Improvements Help Reduce Danger

While clothing changes are very important, school bus manufacturers and school districts are working to change handrails. New handrails are made so they won't catch drawstrings. Older buses are being repaired.

Bus drivers are trained to watch children as they get off the bus. Your child's bus driver should make sure each child has completely cleared the bus when leaving. He also should look for clothing that could get caught.

Simple Steps Make Clothing Safer

- Choose clothes without drawstrings; snaps, Velcro, buttons, or elastic are better choices.

- Remove hood and neck strings.

- Remove drawstrings from the waist and bottom of coats.

- Warn children about dangling key rings, large buckles, and other objects hanging from their backpacks.

Learn More

For a flyer on how to test for handrail snagging or for other school bus safety information (including vehicle recalls), call the NHTSA Auto Safety Hotline: 888-DASH-2-DOT or visit the NHTSA website, www.nhtsa.dot.gov.

Part Five

Food, Nutrition, and Exercise

Chapter 37

Help Your Children Eat Well and Be Physically Active

Eating well and being physically active are key to your child's well-being. Eating too much and exercising too little can lead to overweight and related health problems that can follow children into their adult years. You can take an active role in helping your child—and your whole family—learn healthy eating and physical activity habits.

How are my child's eating and activity habits formed?

Parents play a big role in shaping children's eating habits. When parents eat a variety of foods that are low in fat and sugar and high in fiber, children learn to like these foods as well. It may take 10 or more tries before a child accepts a new food, so do not give up if your child does not like a new food right away.

Parents have an effect on children's physical activity habits as well. You can set a good example by going for a walk or bike ride after dinner instead of watching TV. Playing ball or jumping rope with your children shows them that being active is fun.

With many parents working outside the home, child care providers also help shape children's eating and activity habits. Make sure your child care provider offers well-balanced meals and snacks, as well as plenty of active play time.

If your child is in school, find out more about the school's breakfast and lunch programs and ask to have input into menu choices, or

From "Helping Your Child: Tips for Parents," National Institute of Diabetes and Digestive and Kidney Diseases (NIDDK), NIH Pub. No. 02-4955, June 2002.

help your child pack a lunch that includes a variety of foods. Get involved in the parent-teacher association (PTA) to support physical education (PE) and after-school sports.

Your child's friends and the media can also affect his or her eating and activity choices. Children may go to fast food places or play video games with their friends instead of playing tag, basketball, or other active games. TV commercials try to persuade kids to choose high-fat snacks and high-sugar drinks and cereals. When parents help their children be aware of peer and media pressures, youngsters are more likely to make healthy choices outside the home.

What should my child eat?

Just like adults, children need to eat a wide variety of foods for good health. Use the Food Guide Pyramid as a starting point for planning family meals and snacks. The Food Guide Pyramid applies to healthy people age 2 years and older. The smaller number of servings in the range is for children age 6 years and under. For 2- to 3-year-old children, the serving size should be smaller, about two-thirds the size of a regular serving (except for milk).

When you help children build healthy eating habits early, they will approach eating with a positive attitude—that food is something to enjoy, help them grow, and give them energy.

Food Guide Pyramid

One Serving Equals

Bread, Cereal, Rice, and Pasta Group

- 1 slice of bread
- 1 ounce of ready-to-eat cereal
- ½ cup of cooked cereal, rice, or pasta

Vegetable Group

- 1 cup of raw or ½ cup of frozen (cooked) leafy vegetables
- ½ cup of other vegetables-cooked or chopped raw
- ¾ cup of vegetable juice

Fruit Group

- 1 medium apple, banana, or orange

- ½ cup of chopped, cooked, or canned fruit
- ¾ cup of fruit juice

Milk, Yogurt, and Cheese Group

- 1 cup of milk or yogurt
- 1½ ounces of natural cheese
- 2 ounces of processed cheese

Meat, Poultry, Fish, Dry Beans and Nuts Group

- 2–3 ounces of cooked lean meat, poultry, or fish
- ½ cup of cooked dry beans or 1 egg counts as 1 ounce of lean meat. Two tablespoons of peanut butter or 1/3 cup of nuts count as 1 ounce of meat.

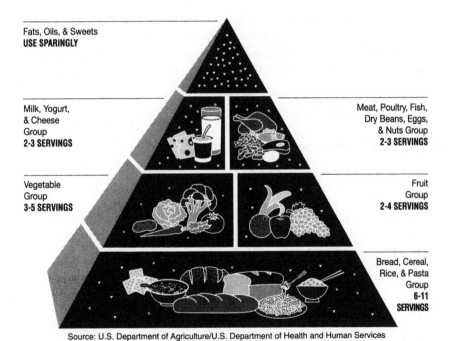

Source: U.S. Department of Agriculture/U.S. Department of Health and Human Services

Figure 37.1. *Food Guide Pyramid: Children 2 to 6 years old need two servings from the milk group per day; children over 6 need three servings. Do not limit fat for children under 2. For older children, aim for a total fat intake of no more than 30 percent of daily calories.*

Sources of Calcium

Calcium helps build strong bones and teeth. Milk and milk products are great sources of calcium. If your child cannot digest milk or if you choose not to serve milk products, there are other ways to make sure he or she gets enough calcium.

- Offer one serving of calcium-fortified fruit juice per day. Fortified juices contain as much calcium per serving as milk.

- Serve calcium-rich vegetables like broccoli, mustard greens, kale, collard greens, and Brussels sprouts.

- Include high-calcium beans like great northern beans, black turtle beans, navy beans, and baked beans in casseroles and salads.

- Try calcium-enriched soy- and rice-based drinks. Serve chilled, use in place of cow's milk in your favorite recipes, or add to hot or cold cereals.

- Serve lactose-reduced or lactose-free dairy products like low-fat or fat-free milk, yogurt, and ice cream. (Lactose is the sugar in milk and foods made with milk. People who cannot digest lactose often have stomach pain and bloating when they drink milk.)

- Try low-fat yogurt or cheese in small amounts—they may be easier to digest than milk.

How can I help my child eat better?

- Give your child a snack or two in addition to his or her three daily meals.

- Offer your child a wide variety of foods, such as grains, vegetables and fruits, low-fat dairy products, and lean meat or beans.

- Serve snacks like dried fruit, low-fat yogurt, and air-popped popcorn.

- Let your child decide whether and how much to eat. Keep serving new foods even if your child does not eat them at first.

- Cook with less fat—bake, roast, or poach foods instead of frying.

- Limit the amount of added sugar in your child's diet. Choose cereals with low or no added sugar. Serve water or low-fat milk more often than sugar-sweetened sodas and fruit-flavored drinks.

- Choose and prepare foods with less salt. Keep the salt shaker off the table. Have fruits and vegetables on hand for snacks instead of salty snack foods.

- Involve your child in planning and preparing meals. Children may be more willing to eat the dishes they help fix.

- Have family meals together and serve everyone the same thing.

- Do not be too strict. In small amounts, sweets or food from fast-food restaurants can still have a place in a healthy diet.

- Make sure your child eats breakfast. Breakfast provides children with the energy they need to listen and learn in school.

*Simple Snack Ideas**

- Dried fruit and nut mix

- Fresh, frozen, or canned vegetables or fruit served plain or with low-fat yogurt

- Rice cakes, whole grain crackers, or whole grain bread served with low-fat cheese, fruit spread, peanut butter, almond butter, or soy nut butter

- Pretzels or air-popped popcorn sprinkled with salt-free seasoning mix

- Homemade fruit smoothie made with low-fat milk or yogurt and frozen or fresh fruit

- Dry cereals served plain or with low-fat or non-fat milk

*Children of preschool age and younger can easily choke on foods that are hard to chew, small and round, or sticky, such as hard vegetables, whole grapes, hard chunks of cheese, raisins, nuts and seeds, and popcorn. Carefully select snacks for children in this age group.

What about physical activity?

Like adults, children should be physically active most, if not all, days of the week. Experts suggest at least 60 minutes of moderate physical activity daily for most children. Walking fast, bicycling, jumping rope, dancing fast, and playing basketball are all good ways for your child to be active.

As children spend more time watching TV and playing computer and video games, they spend less time being active. Parents play a big role in helping kids get up and get moving.

How can I help my child be more active?

- Be a role model for your children. If they see you being physically active and having fun, they are more likely to be active and stay active throughout their lives.

- Involve the whole family in activities like hiking, biking, dancing, basketball, or roller skating.

- Focus on fun. You can do a lot of walking during trips to the zoo, park, or miniature-golf course.

- Include children in household activities like dog-walking, car-washing, or lawn-mowing.

- Limit your children's TV and computer time. Offer them active options, like joining a local recreation center or after-school program, or taking lessons in a sport they enjoy.

- Encourage your child to be physically active every day.

What if my child is overweight?

Children who are overweight are more likely to become overweight adults. They may develop type 2 diabetes, high blood pressure, heart disease, and other illnesses that can follow them into adulthood. Overweight in children can also lead to stress, sadness, and low self-esteem.

Because children grow at different rates at different times, it's not always easy to tell if a child is overweight. For example, it is normal for boys to have a growth spurt in weight and catch up in height later. Your health care provider can measure your child's height and weight and tell you if your child is in a healthy range for his or her gender and age. If your provider finds that your child is overweight, you can help.

How can I help my overweight child?

- Do not put your child on a weight-loss diet unless your health care provider tells you to. Limiting what children eat may interfere with their growth.

- Involve the whole family in building healthy eating and physical activity habits. It benefits everyone and does not single out the child who is overweight.

- Accept and love your child at any weight. It will boost his or her self-esteem.

- Help your child find ways other than food to handle setbacks or successes.

- Talk with your health care provider if you are concerned about your child's eating habits or weight.

Remember, you play the biggest role in your child's life. You can help your children learn healthy eating and physical activity habits that they can follow for the rest of their lives.

Tips for Parents

- Make sure your child eats breakfast. Breakfast provides children with the energy they need to listen and learn in school.

- Offer your child a wide variety of foods, such as grains, vegetables and fruits, low-fat dairy products, and lean meat or beans.

- Talk with your health care provider if you are concerned about your child's eating habits or weight.

- Cook with less fat—bake, roast, or poach foods instead of frying.

- Limit the amount of added sugar in your child's diet. Serve water or low-fat milk more often than sugar-sweetened sodas and fruit-flavored drinks.

- Involve your child in planning and preparing meals. Children may be more willing to eat the dishes they help fix.

- Be a role model for your children. If they see you being physically active and having fun, they are more likely to be active and stay active throughout their lives.

- Encourage your child to be active everyday.

- Involve the whole family in activities like hiking, biking, dancing, basketball, or roller skating.

For More Information

Weight-control Information Network
1 WIN Way
Bethesda, MD 20892-3665
Toll-Free: 877-946-4627
Phone: 202-828-1025
Fax: 202-828-1028
Website: www.niddk.nih.gov/health/nutrit/win.html
E-mail: WIN@info.niddk.nih.gov

Chapter 38

Promoting Fitness in Children

Chapter Contents

Section 38.1

Kids in Action

From "Kids in Action, Fitness for Children," an undated document published by the President's Council on Physical Fitness and Sports, developed in partnership with the Kellogg Company, available online at www.fitness.gov/funfit/action.htm; cited April 2003.

Physical activity is an important part of your child's life; it has a tremendous impact on physical, intellectual, and emotional development. As adults, we have a responsibility to be role models for our children, sharing with them the pleasures and benefits of a physically active lifestyle. Developing a love of sports and a habit of regular physical activity as a child can be the foundation for a long, healthy life.

Good nutrition also is important for your child. As with physical activity, you are a role model. When you choose and prepare healthful foods, your child also will be more likely to follow your example. The first step toward helping your child eat a healthier diet is making a variety of nutritious foods readily available at home. That way your child can choose what he or she likes.

Getting involved in your child's diet and fitness routine will show your support and help foster a great relationship.

The challenge for parents is to find ways to encourage their children to be physically active. This section contains some ideas for activities that you and your children can do together.

Initially, some activities may be more difficult than others. With practice, most activities will become easier. Activity variations are suggested to accommodate children's different abilities.

Each week, try to increase your physical activity using this guide. Here's how to start.

If You Are Inactive
(Haven't thought about activity in years)

Increase daily activities by:

- taking the stairs instead of the elevator

- hiding the TV remote control
- making extra trips around the house or yard
- stretching while standing in line
- walking whenever you can

If You Are Sporadic
(Active some of the time, but not regularly)

Become consistent with activity by increasing activity by:

- finding activities you enjoy
- planning activities in your day
- setting realistic goals

If You Are Consistent
(Active most of the time, or at least four days a week)

Think about the long term as by:

- changing your routine if you start to get bored
- exploring new activities

Activities

Jump the Stick

Parent holds a pole just above the floor and child jumps over. Variations: change pre-height of the pole. Move the pole back and forth. Vary the speed of the pole.

Jump the Brook

Use a towel or mark the sidewalk with the "banks of the brook." Child stands on one side of the brook and attempts to jump the brook without "falling in." Variations: Increase the width of the brook.

Simon Says

Simon says: "Can you touch your toe to your chin?" Select body parts that bend and include stretching. Variations: Touch your ear to your shoulder. Touch your toe to your elbow. Touch your knee to your ankle. Touch tour knee to your elbow. Touch your nose to your knee.

Wall Push-Ups

Stand about arms distance way from a wall with your legs together. Place your hands on the wall just a little wider than your shoulders. Lean forward and touch your nose to the wall and push back to your starting position. Be sure to keep your body in a straight line and your heels on the floor. How many can you do?

Jumping Beans

Hold the child's hands in yours. Child starts bouncing, then jumping up and down. Stop, rest, and start again. Variations: Hop on one foot and then the other. Vary the speed (fast or slow).

Beanbag Balance

Place a beanbag (or soft toy) on the child's head. Ask the child to walk from one place to another without dropping the beanbag. To make it easier, have the child hold the beanbag in place. Variations: Place the beanbag on another body part (for example, back of hand, shoulder, elbow). Use a different toy or more than one toy. Walk around or under things.

Row, Row, Row Your Boat

Parent sits with legs apart, child sits opposite with legs in the middle. Grasp the child's hands. Child leans back as if "rowing a boat" then pulls to upright sit. Repeat. Sing, "Row, row, row your boat."

Wheelbarrow

Child lays face down on the floor. Parent grasps child's ankles and lifts upward. Ask the child to push up with arms until arms are straight. With head up, walk with the hands forward. Child's body should not sag.

Statues

Can you balance on one foot for the count of "4 alligators"? (One alligator, two alligators...) Variations: Count more alligators. Balance in different postures (like statues)

One-Foot Balance Game

Place 5 small objects on an unbreakable dish near another container. Child stands on one foot in front of the dish and container. Ask the child to move the objects one at a time from the dish to the container without losing balance. Variations: Vary the distance between the dish and the container. Time the game.

Inch Worm

Child bends over placing both hands on the floor. The feet are kept stationary while the hands walk forward as far as possible. Then the hands remain stationary while the feet walk forward as close to the hands as possible. Repeat the cycle.

Somersault

Teach your child to roll backwards and forwards. Make sure the child's chin is close to the chest and that weight rests on shoulders and not on head. Be sure to practice on a sofa or cushions.

Up-Up-Down-Down

Repeat the cadence, "up-up-down-down" as parent and child step up (right), step up (left), step down (right), step down (left) on the first step of the stairs.

Clutch Ball

Child sits on floor and holds a ball tightly between legs with hands above head. Parent lifts child in the air by the arms and child tries to keep ball from dropping.

Catch

Parent and child stand 2–3 yards apart. Bounce ball so that each can catch without leaving their place. If child has difficulty with catching a call, use a balloon (Mylar), it travels much slower.

Throw

Can you fly a paper airplane? Child practices throwing paper airplane. Variations: Throw ball made of newspaper or old pantyhose. Throw objects upstairs. (How far up the stairs can you throw ball.)

Section 38.2

Schools Lack Exercise Programs

From "Study Suggests Schools Lacking in Exercise Programs for Children," National Institute of Child Health and Human Development, NIH Press Release, February 10, 2003.

America's young children may not be getting enough vigorous physical exercise through their schools' physical education (PE) programs, suggests the latest analysis by the National Institute of Child Health and Human Development (NICHD) Study of Early Child Care and Youth Development.

Briefly, the third grade children in the study received an average of 25 minutes per week in school of moderate to vigorous activity. Experts in the U.S. have recommended that young people should participate in physical activity of at least moderate intensity for 30 to 60 minutes each day. In addition, *Healthy People 2010*, the Department of Health and Human Services' (HHS) set of health objectives for Americans, seeks to increase the number of schools requiring daily PE for all students.

The current analysis of school PE activities for third graders taking part in the NICHD Study of Early Child Care, appears in the February 2003 *Archives of Pediatrics and Adolescent Medicine*.

The NICHD Study of Early Child Care and Youth Development is not a survey of a representative sample of children in the United States. Rather, the investigators recruited a geographically, economically, and ethnically diverse sample of children from across the United States.

The observations conducted in PE classes provided insight into the amount and types of PE programs offered to 814 third graders at 648 U.S. schools across the country. Observers tracked the activity of a child as he or she participated in school PE classes. The observers used the following categories to describe the activities in each class:

- *Management:* Teachers' activities related to preparing the children for an activity, such as forming a line or moving from one location to another.

- *Knowledge:* Teachers' explanations pertaining to the activity about to take place, such as explaining the rules of a game.

- *Fitness:* Structured physical exercises, such as calisthenics.

- *Skill Practice:* Learning a skill essential to an activity, such as dribbling a basketball.

- *Game Play:* Games or sports, such as softball or basketball.

- *Free Play:* Allowing the children to engage in unstructured activity.

On average, children had 2.1 PE classes per week, totaling 68.7 minutes. Only 5.9 percent of the children had PE five times a week; 2.6 percent, four times a week; 16 percent, three times a week; 45.3 percent, twice a week; and 30.2 percent, once a week. Of the average time children spent in class, 10.4 minutes were spent in game play, 7 minutes on management, 5 minutes on skills practice, 4.8 minutes on fitness, 4.6 minutes on knowledge, and .7 minutes on other activities. For each class, students engaged in only about 4.8 minutes of vigorous physical activity, and 11.9 minutes of moderate to vigorous physical activity.

The authors noted that PE programs vary greatly at the state and local level, with allotted time for classes ranging from 30 minutes per week to 150 minutes per week. Fears that increasing physical activity might have a negative impact on academic performance are unfounded, according to the authors. Earlier studies, published by others, had shown that increasing the length of time in PE classes and the intensity of physical activity in the classes did not have a detrimental effect on academic achievement.

The study also reiterated findings by other researchers that boys spent a greater percentage of class time in moderate to vigorous physical activity (38.3 percent) than did girls (35.6 percent). In addition to calling for more vigorous PE for all children, the authors also called for improvements in the curriculum of PE classes to encourage girls to engage in moderate to vigorous physical activity.

Section 38.3

A Parent's Guide to Fitness for Kids Who Hate Sports

This information was provided by KidsHealth, one of the largest resources online for medically reviewed health information written for parents, kids, and teens. For more articles like this one, visit www.KidsHealth.org, or www.TeensHealth.org. © 2001 The Nemours Center for Children's Health Media, a division of The Nemours Foundation.

Eight-year-old Bradley is a terror on the ice—he lives for hockey practice and spends much of his free time at home slapping a puck around in the driveway. But Bradley's 10-year-old brother, Michael, has no interest in hockey or in any organized sports. He would rather be in his room with a book or riding his bike around the park than playing hockey or basketball with his friends.

The boys' parents worry about Michael's lack of interest in team sports, but do they really have anything to be concerned about? Read this article to find out how you can help to promote fitness in a child who dislikes team sports.

Why Does My Child Hate Sports?

If your child isn't interested in team sports, you should attempt to get to the root of the issue rather than force her to join a team. Kids may not want to participate in sports for many reasons—some of them physical, others emotional.

Children who are physically self-conscious or who feel different from their peers may feel uncomfortable about participating in team activities. Whether this difference is real or imagined, it may lead to self-esteem and body image problems.

Fear of failure or public embarrassment—as well as fear of letting their parents down—can also make some children reluctant to play team sports.

Other children may lack, or believe they lack, the grace or coordination needed to succeed at a particular sport. They may also be afraid of injury or may simply be cautious by nature.

Some children, like many adults, may just not be interested in team sports, but they can still maintain an excellent level of fitness by engaging in other activities that don't emphasize competition. As long as your child does not become sedentary, there's no reason to worry if she resists joining organized sports activities.

Encourage your child to take up lifelong activities like cycling, running, martial arts, or hiking—activities that can promote fitness on an individual, noncompetitive level, suggests Michael Stanwood, PT, ATC, a sports medicine coordinator in Delaware. He also suggests sports such as wrestling or tennis. "Wrestling takes place one on one, but the participants still earn team points."

Ruling out Any Problems

Before beginning any sports or fitness program, your child should have a physical examination by her doctor. Children with undiagnosed medical conditions, vision or hearing problems, or other disorders may have difficulty participating in certain activities. If your child shows uncharacteristic resistance to a particular activity or sudden reluctance to participate in a sport that she previously enjoyed, a visit to her doctor may be in order to rule out any health problems that may be hindering her enjoyment and performance.

Can I Help My Child Learn to Like Sports?

Although you should share your interests with your child, it's never a good idea to force your child into an activity just because you once excelled in it.

In fact, many children may worry that they won't be able to measure up to the success their parents once enjoyed playing a particular sport. Your child needs to know that although you would love to share your love of softball or basketball with her, it would be equally acceptable if she would rather play golf or tennis, or take up gymnastics or karate.

You should also keep your expectations realistic—most children never make it to the city finals or become Olympic medalists no matter how hard they try. The ultimate goal is to help and encourage your child to become fit, healthy, and happy.

Parents should try to remain open-minded about their child's chosen sport. For example, it's possible that your child may enjoy a sports activity that is not offered at her school or that is not offered for girls. If your child wants to try football or ice hockey, help her find a local league or talk to school officials about starting up a new team. Boys may prefer figure skating or ballet. Let your kids know that no matter which sport they choose, they have your support.

You'll also need to be patient with your child if she has difficulty choosing and sticking to an activity. It often takes several tries before a child finds an activity with which she feels comfortable.

Even if your child never belongs to a sports team, there are many other areas of her life where she can learn important skills like teamwork, competition, and cooperation. Clubs, school and volunteer activities, band or music lessons, acting or debating groups, and many other activities teach children to work and get along with others.

Fortunately, there are also many alternative ways to keep fit and active other than organized sports.

What Activities Can My Child Do to Stay Fit?

Many children choose not to join teams, and prefer activities that can be done alone or with friends. Suggested fitness alternatives include:

- cycling
- swimming
- horseback riding
- dancing
- in-line skating
- running
- skateboarding
- hiking
- martial arts

These activities help children build self-esteem, strength, coordination, and general fitness.

How Can I Be a Good Fitness Role Model?

Parents who live sedentary lifestyles may have a hard time motivating their children to stay fit. Try to make exercise a part of your family life by finding fun fitness activities that the whole family can do together, such as swimming, cycling, canoeing, tennis, nature hikes, or walks with the family dog.

Maintain a positive attitude toward exercise and physical activity—be careful not to treat it as a punishment or a chore.

Encourage your child to come up with creative suggestions for family fitness activities; she will be more likely to enjoy an activity if she has a role in planning it.

Parents who attend regular fitness classes or work out at a gym may find it fairly easy to be good fitness role models. Although Stanwood recommends that children under the age of 12 or 13 not get involved in weight training, many gyms offer activities that may interest older children. Some gyms and community centers also offer "Mommy and Me" classes, which introduce fitness to toddlers and preschoolers.

Finally, emphasize the importance of having both a healthy mind and a healthy body, and make it clear to your child that physical activity is an integral part of daily life. By creating a supportive environment, acting as a positive role model, and providing your child with a wide range of fitness choices, you can help your child develop good habits that will last a lifetime.

Chapter 39

The Food Guide Pyramid for Children

The Food Guide Pyramid shows how everybody can make food choices for a healthful diet as described in the Dietary Guidelines for Americans. A special Food Guide Pyramid was developed to help you teach your preschoolers what to eat to help them grow and stay healthy.

The Pyramid divides food into five major food groups: grains, vegetables, fruits, milk, and meat. The foods shown in the Pyramid are those that many children know and enjoy. Each of these food groups provides some, but not all, of the nutrients and energy children need. No one food group is more important than another. For good health and proper growth, children need to eat a variety of different foods every day.

The small tip of the Pyramid shows fats and sweets. These are foods such as salad dressings, cream, butter, margarine, sugars, soft drinks, and candies. Go easy on these foods because they have a lot of calories from fat and sugars, but few vitamins and minerals.

The Food Guide Pyramid adapted for young children focuses on eating a variety of foods. As you increase the variety in your child's diet remember that some fats are necessary for early growth and development. The Dietary Guidelines for Americans suggest that fat in preschoolers' diets be gradually reduced from current levels to the

Excerpted from "Tips for Using the Food Guide Pyramid for Young Children 2 to 6 Years Old," Center for Nutrition Policy and Promotion, United States Department of Agriculture (USDA), March, 1999.

level recommended for most people (no more than 30% of total daily calories) by about 5 years of age.

As parents, you can play a major role in teaching your children how to develop healthful eating habits to last a lifetime. This booklet will help you show your children that food is fun and learning about food is fun, too.

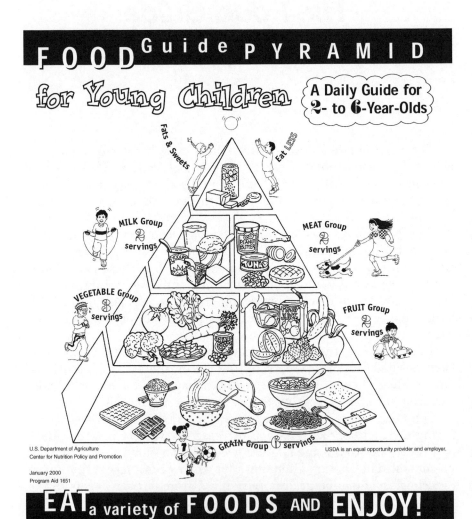

Figure 39.1. *The Food Guide Pyramid for Young Children*

A Guide to Using the Food Guide Pyramid for Young Children

- The small tip shows that it is best to eat less of foods that contain a lot of fat and sugars [See Figure 39.1]. These foods contain calories but few vitamins and minerals.

- The meat group includes protein sources such as eggs, dry beans and peas, and peanut butter, as well as meat, poultry, and fish. These foods are important for protein, iron, and zinc.

- The milk group foods are important for calcium. Two- to 6-year-old children need a total of 2 servings from the milk group each day.

- Your child should eat plenty of foods from the vegetable group and the fruit group for vitamins, minerals, and dietary fiber.

- The grain group forms the base of the Pyramid because the largest number of servings needed each day comes from this food group. Grain products are important for vitamins, minerals, complex carbohydrates, and dietary fiber.

Toddler Tips

Always watch children during meals and snacks. Young children, ages 2 to 3 especially, are at risk of choking on food and remain at risk until they can chew and swallow better by about age 4. Using the Food Guide Pyramid, offer 2- to 3-year-olds the same variety of foods as the rest of the family, but smaller amounts prepared in forms that are easy for them to chew and swallow.

Foods That May Cause Choking Include

- frankfurters
- nuts and seeds
- popcorn
- raw carrots
- chunks of meat
- raisins
- marshmallows
- peanut butter (spoonful)

- chips
- whole grapes
- pretzels
- round or hard candy
- raw celery
- cherries with pits
- large pieces of fruit

Some childhood favorites can be offered if you just change the form:

- Cut frankfurters lengthwise into thin strips.
- Cook carrots or celery until slightly soft, then cut in sticks.
- Cut grapes or cherries in small pieces.
- Spread peanut butter thin.

Healthy Eating Tips: Encouraging Food Choices for a Healthy Diet

Be patient. Young children may not be interested in trying new foods. Offer a new food more than once. Show your child how the rest of the family enjoys it. The food may be accepted when it becomes more familiar to your child.

Be a planner. Most young children need a snack or two in addition to three regular daily meals.

- Offer foods from three or more of the five major food groups for breakfast and lunch.
- Offer foods from four or more of the five major food groups for the "main meal."
- Plan snacks so they are not served too close to mealtime, and offer foods from two or more of the five major food groups.

Be a good role model. What you do can mean more than what you say. Your child learns from you about how and what to eat.

- Eat meals with your children whenever possible.
- Try new foods and new ways of preparing them with your children. Both you and your children can be healthier by eating more dark-green leafy vegetables, deep-yellow vegetables, fruits, and whole grain products.
- Walk, run, and play with your children, don't just sit on the sidelines. A family that is physically active together has lots of fun!

Be adventurous. At the store ask your young child to choose a new vegetable or fruit, from two or three choices, for a weekly "family try-a-new-food" night. At home your child can help you wash and prepare the food.

Be creative. Encourage your child to invent a new snack or sandwich from three or four healthful ingredients you provide. Try a new bread or whole grain cracker. Talk about what food groups the new snack includes and why it tastes good. Is the snack smooth, crunchy, sweet, juicy, chewy, or colorful? When children are offered a balanced diet over time, they will develop good eating habits.

Child-Sized Servings

- Children 2 to 3 years of age need the same variety of foods as 4- to 6-year-olds but may need fewer calories. Offer them smaller amounts. A good estimate of a serving for a 2- to 3-year-old child is about 2/3 of what counts as a regular Food Guide Pyramid serving. Because younger children often eat small portions, offering smaller servings and allowing them to ask for more, satisfies their hunger and does not waste food.

- By the time children are 4 years old, they can eat amounts that count as regular Food Guide Pyramid servings eaten by older family members that is, 1/2 cup fruit or vegetable, 3/4 cup of juice, 1 slice of bread, 2 to 3 ounces of cooked lean meat, poultry, or fish.

- Remember, variety is key for the whole family. Offer a variety of foods from the five major food groups, and let your children decide how much to eat. Offer new foods in small "try me" portions—perhaps 1 or 2 tablespoons. Let your children ask for more.

Young children's appetites can vary widely from day to day, depending on how they are growing and how active they are. As long as they have plenty of energy, are healthy, are growing well, and are eating a variety of foods, they are probably getting enough of the nutrients they need from the foods they eat. If you are concerned about your child eating too much or too little, check with your doctor or other healthcare provider.

What Counts as One Food Guide Pyramid Serving?

Each of the portions listed in the five major food groups below count as one Food Guide Pyramid serving for anyone over 4 years of age. When counting servings, smaller portions count as part of a serving and larger portions count as more than one serving. Two- to 3-year-old children need the variety and the same numbers of servings as older children but may need fewer calories. To get variety but fewer calories, offer 2- to 3-year-olds a smaller portion but count it as one serving. Offer about 2/3 of the portion you would give a 4- to 6-year-old, except for milk. Two- to 6-year-old children need a total of 2 servings from the milk group each day. Foods marked with an "*" may cause choking in 2- to 3-year-old children.

Grain Group Choices (6 Servings Each Day)

Whole grain

- 1/2 cup cooked brown rice
- 2–3 graham cracker squares
- 5–6 whole grain crackers
- 1/2 cup cooked oatmeal
- 1/2 cup cooked bulgur
- *3 cups popped popcorn
- *3 rice or popcorn cakes
- 1 ounce ready-to-eat whole grain cereal
- 1 slice pumpernickel, rye, or whole wheat bread
- *2 taco shells
- 1 7-inch corn tortilla

Enriched

- 1/2 cup cooked rice or pasta
- 1/2 cup cooked spaghetti
- 1/2 English muffin or bagel
- 1 slice white, wheat, French or Italian bread
- 1/2 hamburger or hot dog bun
- 1 small roll
- 6 crackers (saltine size)
- 1 4-inch pita bread
- 1 4-inch pancake
- 1/2 cup cooked grits
- 1/2 cup cooked farina or other cereal
- *9 3-ring pretzels

- 1 ounce ready-to-eat, non-sugar coated, cereal
- 1 7-inch flour tortilla

Offer whole or mixed grain products for at least three of the six grain group choices the Pyramid recommends each day.

Grain products with more fat and sugars

- 1 small biscuit or muffin
- 1 small piece cornbread
- 1/2 medium doughnut
- 9 animal crackers
- 4 small cookies

Vegetable Group Choices (3 Servings Each Day)

Dark-green leafy

- 1/2 cup cooked collard greens
- 1 cup leafy raw vegetables romaine lettuce, spinach, or mixed green salad
- 2 cooked broccoli spears
- 1/2 cup cooked turnip greens, kale, or mustard greens

Deep-yellow

- 1 1/2 whole carrots, cooked
- * 7–8 raw carrot sticks (3" long)
- 1/2 cup winter squash

Starchy

- * 1 medium ear of corn
- 10 French fries, regular size
- 1 baked potato, medium
- 1/2 cup potato salad
- 1/2 cup green peas
- 1/2 cup lima beans
- 1 medium plantain

Dry beans and peas

- 1/2 cup cooked black, kidney, pinto, or garbanzo beans, or black-eyed peas
- 1/2 cup cooked lentils
- 1 cup bean soup
- 1/2 cup cooked split peas

Other

- 1/3 medium cucumber
- 9 raw snow or sugar pea pods
- 1/2 cup cooked green beans
- 4 medium Brussels sprouts
- 6 slices raw summer squash
- 1/2 cup coleslaw
- 1/2 cup cooked cabbage
- *7–8 celery sticks (3" long)
- 1/2 cup tomato or spaghetti sauce
- 3/4 cup vegetable juice
- 1 cup vegetable soup
- 1 medium tomato
- *5 cherry tomatoes

Fruit Group Choices (2 Servings Each Day)

Citrus, melons, berries

- 1/2 cup blueberries or raspberries
- 1/4 medium cantaloupe
- 3/4 cup 100% citrus juice (orange)
- 1/2 grapefruit
- 1/8 medium honeydew
- 1 large kiwi
- 1 medium orange
- 7 medium strawberries
- 1 medium tangerine
- 1/2 cup watermelon pieces

Other

- 1 medium apple, banana, peach, or nectarine
- 2 medium apricots
- *11 cherries
- *1/4 cup dried fruit
- 1/2 cup applesauce
- 2 1/2 canned pineapple slices
- *12 grapes
- 1/2 medium mango
- 1/4 medium papaya
- 1 small pear
- 1/2 cup cut-up fresh, canned, or cooked fruit

Many juice beverages are not 100% juice. Check the ingredient listing to make sure you're getting all juice without added sugars such as corn syrup.

Milk Group Choices (2 Servings Each Day)

One serving of the milk group is based on the amount of calcium in 1 cup of milk. This group is where partial servings are eaten most often. See Table 39.1 for information about the amount of milk servings in a variety of common foods.

Meat Group Choices (2 Servings Each Day)

Two to three ounces of cooked lean meat, poultry, or fish equal one serving from this group. Amounts from this food group should total 5 ounces a day for 4- to 6-year-olds and about 3 1/2 ounces a day for 2- to 3-year-olds. Count 1 egg or 1/2 cup of cooked dry beans as 1 ounce of lean meat. Count 2 tablespoons peanut butter as 1 ounce of meat. Table 39.2 provides information about the amount of meat servings in a variety of common foods.

Counting to see if your child has 5 ounces from the meat group is tricky. Portion sizes vary with the type of food and meal. For example, 5 ounces might come from a combination of: 1 egg for breakfast; 2 ounces of sliced turkey at lunch; and 2 ounces cooked lean hamburger for dinner.

Fat tips: Here are two easy ways to reduce fat. Gradually change from whole milk to lower fat dairy products such as 2% or 1% fat milk or fat-free milk by age 5. Offer lean meats or low-fat luncheon meats instead of higher fat ones. These tips can be used by the whole family.

Table 39.1. Number of milk servings in different foods.

For This Amount of Food	Count This Many Milk Group Servings
1 cup milk	1
1 cup soy milk, calcium fortified	1
1/2 cup milk	1/2
1 cup yogurt (8 ounces)	1
1 1/2 ounces natural cheese	1
2 ounces process cheese	1
1 string cheese (1 ounce)	2/3
1/2 cup cottage cheese	1/4
1/2 cup ice cream	1/3
1/2 cup frozen yogurt	1/2
1/2 cup pudding	1/2

Table 39.2. Number of meat servings in different foods.

For This Amount of Food	Count This Many Ounces
2 ounces cooked lean meat	2 ounces
2 ounces cooked poultry or fish	2 ounces
1 egg (yolk and white)	1 ounce
*2 tablespoons peanut butter	1 ounce
*1 1/2 frankfurters (2 ounces)	1 ounce
2 slices bologna or luncheon meat (2 ounces)	1 ounce
1/4 cup drained canned salmon or tuna	1 ounce
1/2 cup cooked kidney, pinto, or white beans	1 ounce
1/2 cup tofu	1 ounce
1 soy burger patty	1 ounce

Kids in the Kitchen

Children enjoy helping in the kitchen and often are more willing to eat foods they help prepare. Involve your child in planning and preparing some meals and snacks for the family. It is important that you give kitchen tasks appropriate for your child's age. Be patient as your child gains new skills at different ages.

Meal Preparation Activities for Young Children

Children have to be shown and taught how to do these activities. Each child has his or her own pace for learning, so give it time and the skills will come.

2-year-olds:

- Wipe table tops
- Snap green beans
- Scrub vegetables
- Wash salad greens
- Tear lettuce or greens
- Play with utensils
- Break cauliflower
- Bring ingredients from one place to another

3-year-olds can do what 2-year-olds do, plus:

- Wrap potatoes in foil for baking
- Shake liquids in covered container
- Knead and shape yeast dough
- Spread soft spreads
- Pour liquids
- Place things in trash
- Mix ingredients

4-year-olds can do all that 2- and 3-years-olds do, plus:

- Peel oranges or hard cooked eggs
- Mash bananas using fork

- Move hands to form round shape
- Set table
- Cut parsley or green onions with dull scissors

5- to 6-year-olds can do all that 2-, 3-, and 4-years-olds do, plus:

- Measure ingredients
- Use an egg beater
- Cut with blunt knife

When your child is helping you with food preparation, don't forget cleanliness. Wash hands using soap and warm running water before and after handling food or utensils to prepare food. Expect a few spills. It's a small price to pay for helping your children become comfortable around food.

Be Snack-Wise

These snack ideas work at home or "on the go." Snacks marked with an "*" may cause choking in 2- to 3-year-old children.

Snacks from the Grain Group

- Cracker stacks
- Wheat crackers spread with cheese spread
- Ready-to-eat cereals
- Flavored mini rice cakes or popcorn cakes
- Breads of all kinds such as multi-grain, rye, white, wheat
- Ginger snaps or fig bars
- *Popcorn
- *Trail mix...ready-to-eat cereals mixed with raisins or other dried fruit
- Graham crackers

Snacks from the Vegetable Group

- Vegetable sticks such as carrot*, celery*, green pepper, cucumber, or squash
- *Celery stuffed with peanut butter

- Cherry tomatoes cut in small pieces
- Steamed broccoli, green beans, or sugar peas with low-fat dip

Snacks from the Fruit Group

- Apple ring sandwiches, peanut butter on apple rings
- Tangerine sections
- Chunks of banana or pineapple
- Canned fruits packed in juice
- Juice box (100% juice)

Snacks from the Milk Group

- Milk shakes made with fruit and milk
- Cheese slices with thin apple wedges
- String cheese or individually wrapped slices
- Mini yogurt cups

Snacks from the Meat Group

- Hard cooked eggs (wedges or slices)
- Peanut butter spread thin on crackers
- Bean dip spread thin on crackers

For ingredients, stock up on simple foods such as peanut butter; cheese spread or slices; whole grain crackers; little bagels; small pita breads; non-sugar-coated, ready-to-eat cereals; vegetables and fruits.

Plan for Variety

Variety is the key to planning menus using the Pyramid. The foods you offer your child each day should include choices from all five major food groups. Meals and snacks should also include different choices within each food group. For example, offer different breads, whole grain and enriched, different vegetables, especially dark-green leafy and deep-yellow ones, and dry beans and peas.

Most young children need a snack or two in addition to their three regular daily meals.

Chapter 40

Milk Matters for Your Child's Health

Why Do Kids Need Calcium?

Calcium makes bones strong. Bones may seem hard and lifeless, but they are actually growing and alive. Since bones grow most during the childhood and teenage years, these are especially important times to help make them strong and healthy.

By eating and drinking lots of foods with calcium, children and teens can help build their "bone banks" to store calcium for later in life. As adults, this stored calcium can help keep bones strong. It also may help reduce the risk of osteoporosis, a condition where bones become fragile and can break easily later in life. That means it's especially important for children to get enough calcium while they are young.

Bones can also become stronger through weight-bearing exercises. Some examples of weight-bearing exercises are running, dancing, tumbling, and jumping. Swimming is an example of an exercise that is not weight-bearing.

Calcium also keeps teeth and gums healthy throughout life. Even before baby teeth and adult teeth come in, they need calcium to develop properly. And after teeth come in, they remain strong and resist tooth decay by taking in more calcium. Calcium is also important throughout life for preventing gum disease. So be sure to get calcium and drink milk your whole life long.

Excerpted from "Milk Matters for Your Child's Health," National Institute of Child Health and Human Development (NICHD), National Institutes of Health (NIH), http://www.nichd.nih.gov/milk/brochure0105/index.htm, 1999.

Where Can Kids Get Calcium?

Milk and other dairy foods, such as cheese and yogurt, are excellent sources of calcium. One 8-ounce glass of milk has about 300 milligrams (mg) of calcium. Just a few glasses can go a long way toward giving kids the calcium they need each day.

Milk also has other vitamins and minerals that are good for bones and teeth. One especially important nutrient is vitamin D, which helps the body to absorb more calcium.

Other sources of calcium are dark green, leafy vegetables, such as kale, and foods like broccoli, soybeans, tofu made with calcium, orange juice with calcium added, and other calcium-fortified foods.

Breakfast

- pour milk over your breakfast cereal
- have a cup of yogurt
- drink a glass of calcium-fortified orange juice
- add low-fat milk instead of water to oatmeal and hot cereal

Lunch

- add milk instead of water to tomato soup
- add cheese to a sandwich
- have a glass of milk instead of a soda
- make mini-pizzas or macaroni and cheese

Snack

- try flavored milk like chocolate or strawberry
- have a frozen yogurt
- try some pudding made with milk
- make a "smoothie" with fruit, ice, and milk
- dip fruits and vegetables into yogurt

Dinner

- make a salad with dark green, leafy vegetables
- serve broccoli or cooked, dry beans as a side dish

- top salads, soups, and stews with low-fat shredded cheese
- add tofu made with calcium to stir fry and other dishes

Food Nutrition Labels

Reading the food label can be an easy way to find out how much calcium is in one serving of food. For example, one 8-ounce serving of milk has 300 mg of calcium, or 30% of the Daily Value (DV). By looking on the food label, you can see how much calcium a food serving gives toward the total amount needed for the day.

Another way to figure out how much calcium your child is getting is to add a "zero" to the end of the Daily Value number (or multiply by 10). This will show you what the Daily Value equals in milligrams of calcium. For example, a serving of milk that has a Daily Value of 30% has 300 mg of calcium.

The food label can also help you choose between foods if you look to see which ones have the most calcium. A food with a Daily Value of 20% or more is high in calcium. A food with a Daily Value less than 5% is low in calcium. By looking at the labels, you can pick the foods that have the most calcium in them to help your child build strong bones.

What Kind of Milk Is Best?

Fat-free (skim) and low-fat (1%) milk and dairy products have no or little fat so it's easy for kids to get enough calcium without adding extra fat to their diets. However, babies under one year old should drink only breast milk or iron-fortified formula. Children ages one to two should drink whole milk rather than reduced-fat varieties. Between ages two and five, parents should gradually transition children to reduced-fat, low-fat, or fat-free milk.

Whole, low-fat, fat-free, and chocolate milk all have the same amount of calcium, but they have different amounts of fat. 8 ounces of whole milk contains 8 grams of fat; reduced-fat milk has 5 grams of fat; low-fat milk has 2.5 grams of fat; and fat-free milk has 0 grams of fat.

Can Everyone Drink Milk?

Lactose is the sugar found in milk and dairy products and can cause stomach discomfort in some people. A person with lactose intolerance has trouble digesting the sugar in dairy foods. Lactose intolerance is not common among infants and children. Among adults, it tends to be more common in Asian, Hispanic, African-American, and Native American populations.

Many people with lactose intolerance can actually drink 8 ounces of milk each day without getting an upset stomach or abdominal pains. In addition, they can often eat yogurt or cheese without any problems, or have milk combined with other foods, such as cereal with milk. Also, lactose-free milk is available in stores, and there are pills and drops you can buy that make it easier to digest milk and dairy products.

Some people, however, are allergic to milk and dairy products and should avoid eating them. For those people who can't drink milk at all, calcium can come from foods like dark green, leafy vegetables such as kale, calcium supplements, or orange juice, tofu, and soy milk with calcium added. If you have more questions about lactose intolerance or milk allergies, talk to your pediatrician.

Getting Enough Calcium

Getting enough calcium is important for building strong bones and teeth and ensuring future health. Here are three things that parents can do to help kids get enough calcium:

1. Offer your child healthy foods filled with calcium, such as low-fat or fat-free milk and dairy products, and dark green, leafy vegetables.

2. Keep milk and diary products in the house and put milk on the table during meals and snacks.

3. Drink milk yourself and make it part of your whole family's diet. Kids make many food choices by watching their parents so show them milk and calcium are important your whole life long.

Chapter 41

Protect Your Child from Foodborne Illness

Chapter Contents

Section 41.1

How Can Parents Protect Their Children from Foodborne Illness?

This section includes "How Can Parents Protect Their Children from Foodborne Illness?" and "Foodborne Illness in the United States," reprinted with permission from S.T.O.P. — Safe Tables Our Priority, a nonprofit grassroots organization working to prevent suffering, illness, and death from food contaminated by pathogens. © 2002. For additional information, contact S.T.O.P. at P.O. Box 4352, Burlington, VT 05406, 802-863-0555 (voice), 802-863-3733 (fax), 1-800-350-STOP (hotline for victims of foodborne illness), or visit their website at www.SafeTables.org.

Children are exposed to a wide variety of foods prepared a myriad of different ways. To help keep your children safe from foodborne illness, which could prove to be deadly to them, the most important thing a parent can do is be cautious about what children eat. In particular, pay attention to the following:

- Be careful about parties, potlucks, picnics, school lunches, and children sharing lunches, where children may be served or be recipients of foods of unknown origin and preparation standards.

- Ensure that your children eat only thoroughly cooked meat especially ground meat, such as hamburger, sausages, and whole or ground poultry. To ensure your children's safety use a calibrated meat thermometer. Cook ground beef to an internal temperature of 160° F. Chicken dishes and casseroles should reach an internal temperature of 170° F.

- The Food and Drug Administration (FDA) advises that children should not consume uncooked alfalfa because alfalfa sprouts have been linked to outbreaks of Salmonella and *E. coli* O157:H7.

- The Centers for Disease Control and Prevention (CDC) advises that children under the age of 1 should not consume honey to avoid potential infection with infantile botulism.

- S.T.O.P. (Safe Tables Our Priority) advises that children should not drink any unpasteurized juices, unpasteurized milk, or consume unpasteurized milk products including raw milk cheeses. The American Academy of Pediatrics warns against serving children unpasteurized milk due to the potential contamination of cattle-related pathogens. In 1997, the FDA warned specifically that children should not drink unpasteurized apple juice. While bulk liquids are usually pasteurized, retail establishments may not pasteurize their products. Always check if juice is pasteurized before serving it to your children.

- S.T.O.P. advises that children should never eat raw shellfish, due to the risk of *Vibrio*.

- S.T.O.P. advises that children eat only thoroughly cooked shell eggs to avoid *Salmonella*—no tasting cake batter or cookie dough or similar products with raw, unpasteurized eggs. Examples of foods that may contain undercooked eggs are: Hollandaise sauce, Bernaise sauce, timbales, eggs—sunny side up, soft boiled and poached, ice creams, some homemade frostings, eggnog, tartar sauce, mayonnaise, meringue, mousse, soufflés, and fresh Caesar salad dressings. Use pasteurized eggs to reduce the chance of contracting illness if you choose to continue eating raw egg food products. (Note that pasteurization of eggs is ineffective some of the time.) To better understand the potential risk of infection from eggs, you may want to call your state health department and ask how reported infection rates of *Salmonella enteritidis* in your area compare with those of other areas.

- Be aware that restaurants are generally not required to give the same warnings that you may receive on products purchased in stores. For example, while all meat and poultry sold in grocery stores now carries a safe handling label, restaurants do not carry warnings about proper cooking temperatures. Therefore, you might still be asked by a server, "How would you like your hamburger: rare, medium or well done?" The only safe hamburger is one cooked to an internal temperature of 160° F for 1 second throughout (usually well done.) Likewise, in a grocery store, a juice might carry a warning label, while at a juice bar the same juice might be sold as a component of a smoothie without a required warning.

In addition, it is critical to maintain and teach meticulous hygiene. Always thoroughly wash your hands before touching your children and before, during and after a cooking project in which you will be handling foods. Teach your children good bathroom hygiene. Children are prone to touch the toilet seat as they get on and off of it, and they are also likely to let soap run off their hands without working up a good lather. It is critical that children be taught proper hygiene techniques—especially when organisms such as *E. coli* O157:H7 and *Shigella* require only a few organisms to impart life-threatening illness. When teaching children to wash their hands use warm soapy water and briskly rub hands together while washing, singing the "Happy Birthday" song twice through. Then rinse and dry hands on a clean, dry paper towel.

Understanding the Diseases

The list of potential foodborne illnesses is extremely long. S.T.O.P. Here are descriptions of some of the most common:

- *Botulism* and *Infantile Botulism* are two different diseases, associated with *C. botulinum* spores. Botulism can result in paralysis leading to respiratory arrest. Symptoms in adults occur within 12–36 hours and sometimes days, following ingestion of contaminated foods. Infantile botulism occurs specifically in children under 1 year old. The CDC recommends that children under the age of 1 not be fed honey.

- *Campylobacter* is a bacteria particularly common in birds and poultry, including chicken and turkey. Symptoms in adults occur usually within 2–5 days of ingestion with a range of 1 to 10 days.

- *Cryptosporidium* is a parasite.

- *Cyclospora* is another parasite. Infection results in prolonged diarrheal illness measured in weeks. Severe weight loss is a resulting complication.

- *E. coli* O157:H7 is a bacteria found in the intestines of healthy cattle, deer, sheep and possibly other ruminants. Infected children and adults can develop hemolytic uremic syndrome (HUS) in about 10% of cases, resulting in the loss of kidney function, strokes, heart attack, coma, paralysis or death from organ liquefaction. A second complication is thrombotic thrombocytopenic purpura (TTP). Because it takes as few as 1 to 10 organisms to cause life-threatening illness, the organism causes very high rates of infection in group settings. Other pathogenic *E. coli* may cause similar symptoms and complications.

- *Giardia* is a protozoa that is more common to fresh bodies of water. Infected people can be asymptomatic.

- *Hepatitis A* is a virus that causes liver damage, which can be transferred by food handlers.

- *Listeria* is a bacteria particularly dangerous to pregnant women, their fetuses and newborns. Infected people can be asymptomatic or present as mild flu symptoms. The CDC has produced two separate brochures warning of the potential hazards of *Listeria*.

- *Salmonella* is commonly found in poultry but has been associated with the feces of many animals including cattle and pigs. It can be harbored in the ovaries of chickens, thus causing their eggs to carry the bacteria internally. Due to fecal contamination it has become associated as well with raw produce such as alfalfa sprouts. While antibiotic resistant strains of *Salmonella* are on the rise, many cases can be treated. However, salmonellosis can be deadly, particularly to the elderly.

- *Shigella* is a highly infectious bacterium and can cause hemolytic uremic syndrome. Its source is human feces.

- *Vibrio vulnificus* and *perfringens* are unusually deadly bacterium associated with shellfish. When contaminated shellfish, such as oysters, are consumed raw, they can cause a rapid decline in at-risk individuals, including people with liver disease (either from excessive alcohol intake, viral hepatitis, or other causes), hemochromatosis (an iron disorder), diabetes, stomach problems (including previous stomach surgery and low stomach acid—for example, from antacid use), cancer, immune disorders (including HIV infection), and long-term steroid use (as for asthma and arthritis).

Table 41.1. Tips for Packing Fun and Healthy School Lunches

- Make sure the majority of the food in the lunch box is healthy, but compromise and have food items in the lunch box that your child likes.

- Involve your children. Have them go to the grocery store with you and help choose some of the food. Also, include the child in preparing some of the foods and actually packing the lunch.

- Have your children write down a list of healthy foods that they like in categories of sandwiches, fruits, vegetables, snacks or desserts. You can then select one item for each category to pack the lunch.

- Instead of the same old sandwich, you can use different kinds of breads for sandwiches. You could use hamburger rolls, hot dog rolls, tortillas, bagels or pitas. You can also use a cookie cutter to make fun shapes out of bread, meats and cheeses.

- Use your imagination by creating theme lunches. For instance, have the lunch box contain food that is round using a bagel, an orange, and round pieces of carrots. Or have a tea party, complete with finger sandwiches, grapes and mini-muffins served on doll plates.

- Create your own pre-packaged lunches similar to the kinds you can buy in the supermarket. Purchase a plastic, divided container with a lid, and cut out your own shapes of meat, cheese, bread, crackers, vegetables or fruit and pack it all together.

- Create a lunch box pizza by using a piece of unsliced, pita bread. Spread with seasoned tomato sauce, sprinkle it with cheese and heat it in the microwave until the cheese melts. Let it cool, then wrap it up.

- Keep hot foods hot by making sure the food you pack is steaming hot and sent to school in a thermos.

- Keep cold foods cold by using an insulated lunch box with a freezer pack inside. You can also use ice cubes in a leak-proof container or a frozen juice box. The juice will melt for your child to drink at lunch.

- When preparing and packing lunches, keep food, hands and surfaces clean.

- If any perishable food comes home from school in your child's lunch box, be sure to throw it away because it has been out of refrigeration for a long period of time.

Source: From "Tip Sheet, KSU Expert Offers Tips for Packing a Fun and Healthy School Lunch," suggestions from Paula Peters, associate professor of human nutrition at Kansas State University, text prepared by Robyn Horton, © 1999 Kansas State University; reprinted with permission.

Section 41.2

Packing School Lunches

"How to Make School Lunches Safe Lunches," Oregon Department of Agriculture, © 2001, updated 2003; reprinted with permission. Additional information from the Oregon Department of Agriculture is available online at www.oda.state.or.us.

Whether it comes in a Star Wars lunch pail or a brown paper sack, the lunch you send to school with your child needs to be packed with care and consideration in order to ensure good food safety. Now that school is back in session this month, the Oregon Department of Agriculture is offering some helpful hints on how to make that school lunch from home as safe as possible.

Children are more susceptible to food borne illnesses than adults, so it becomes even more important that we protect the lunches they take to school. From the preparation of the food that will go into the lunch to the consumption of the meal at school—and all the steps in between—there are several important factors to keep in mind for the sake of your kids.

It all starts in the kitchen with clean hands, clean surfaces, and the washing of fruits and vegetables before they are put into the school lunch. Avoid cross contamination. Don't use the same surfaces for raw foods that you use for cooked foods. Don't give those bugs a chance to hop into the lunch pail.

Making the lunch the night before is a good idea so that the preparer isn't rushed into doing something improper, such as using dirty surfaces. Putting the lunch in the refrigerator to keep it cold overnight is essential for most foods.

Maintaining a proper temperature for the school lunch is very important. Given the fact that the food is not likely to stay in a refrigerator once the lunch is taken to school, it is critical that steps are taken at home to keep cold foods cold and hot foods hot.

If you are going to send a cold lunch, use a gel-pack, a frozen individual juice box, or a frozen sandwich as a source of cold temperatures so that the entire lunch can stay cold. Depending on the type of container available, there are things you can do to keep food at a safe

397

temperature. An insulated lunch bag is probably best. But even a brown paper bag will work, especially if you double bags to provide a little bit more insulation.

If your child is going to take a hot lunch to school, chances are it will be something like soup, which would probably be inside a thermos. Preheat the thermal container by putting some boiling water in it first, letting it sit for a few minutes, then dump out the hot water. That way, you have a preheated container that will actually keep food safely hot enough to prevent food borne illnesses all the way through the lunch hour."

Chances are the lunch you send to school in the morning will be consumed within a few hours. Still, that's plenty of time for bacteria to grow if the lunch is not stored properly. Once again, maintaining a proper temperature is important. A gel-pack in an insulated lunch bag will probably keep the food safe until lunchtime, but it won't keep the lunch safe all day. Putting the lunch in a locker—someplace quiet and dark—is a good idea. But remember, the lunch should be kept away from direct sunlight or heat sources like a classroom radiator.

Remind the kids that the lunch is to be eaten at lunchtime—or not at all. Leftovers are a no-no in school lunches. Once your child is finished eating, they need to throw the rest of it away. Of course, there may be some exceptions—depending on what foods are packed. Some items are potentially more hazardous than others. It is best to look first at foods that are great for packing into lunches. Crackers, pretzels, raisins, peanut butter sandwiches, and the little individual cans of fruit are all things that are shelf stable and don't require refrigeration. Other foods like whole fruits and vegetables should be washed before they are placed into the lunch bag—then they are safe. Once you begin to cut up the fruits and vegetables, though, they should be kept refrigerated because more surface area has been exposed to potential contamination.

Sandwiches with meat, eggs, or dairy products should be packed directly next to the cold source in the container. The optimum temperature for such a lunch is 41 degrees Fahrenheit. How do you know that's the temperature of the lunch? Put together a "home test" lunch on a Saturday or Sunday. Use a kitchen thermometer and check the reading throughout the day to see how long the cold temperature actually lasts.

Packing leftovers from last night's dinner is okay, as long as that food was chilled within two hours of cooking and kept in the refrigerator overnight.

Another consideration for the school lunch is what your child ultimately does with it. It is common for kids to swap lunch items at school, preferring a classmate's cuisine instead. Remember that your child's friends may have food allergies. It's probably not a good idea for them to share their lunch with other kids unless they are sure those friends are not allergic to what was brought in the lunch.

Finally, remind your children the importance of hand-washing before eating. Many times recess precedes lunch. Even more often, kids will need to go to the bathroom sometime before lunch. Washing hands well and often is a great way to cut down on potential food borne illnesses.

Keeping lunches safe is every bit as important as making them tasty.

Chapter 42

Caffeine, Sugar, Fat, and Your Child

Does your child want to drink a six-pack of soda every day? Is a French fry the only vegetable your kid allows on the plate? If these preferences sound familiar, your child may be consuming the typical American diet—a diet high in sugar, caffeine, and fat. Today's children are much less physically fit than previous generations, and in the United States, the percentage of obese children has more than doubled since 1976.

There are healthy ways that you can reduce the caffeine, sugar, and fat in your child's diet. Keep reading to find out more.

The Truth about Caffeine, Sugar, and Fat

Sometimes it's difficult to determine the truth about food. TV and magazines tantalize consumers with images of tasty, sugary foods. Your child's doctor may tell you that your child's diet is too high in fat, but what's the truth?

Caffeine, totally lacking in nutritional value, does not add taste, texture, or color to a soft drink. Caffeine affects children and adults similarly. A stimulant, caffeine can interfere with sleep and may affect children who are sensitive to it. In addition, because caffeine is a

---

diuretic that causes the body to eliminate water, it can contribute to dehydration. Caffeine is an especially poor choice in hot weather, when children need to replace water lost through perspiration. In addition, children who drink lots of caffeinated beverages may miss getting the calcium they need from milk to build strong bones and teeth.

The U.S. Department of Agriculture (USDA) suggests a maximum of 6 tablespoons of sugar per day for someone consuming 1,600 calories (an amount typical for children 5 years). One 12-ounce soft drink contains about 3 tablespoons of sugar, so in one drink, your child is getting almost half the day's recommended amount of sugar.

Sugar's effects are sometimes misperceived. Sugar does promote tooth decay, but studies show no link between hyperactivity and sugar. When 5-year-olds are running around at a birthday party after eating cake and ice cream, parents joke that they're "high" from the sugar. The reality is they're just being 5-year-olds, explains pediatrician Keith Ayoob, MD.

Sugar does not cause hyperactivity, but it can contribute to excess weight gain. Foods that are high in sugar also tend to be high in calories and fat and low in other valuable nutrients. As a result, a high-sugar diet is often linked with obesity.

There's an important link between calories, sugar, and fat. A calorie is a unit that measures heat, or energy. So, calories describe the amount of energy that different foods supply to people. The amount of heat, measured in calories, is that particular food's caloric content. Before you eat, the energy contained in the food is trapped in the food. The energy is released when your digestive system breaks down the food. Because sugary and fatty foods often are high in calories, it takes the body longer to use up those calories. As a result, excess calories from food equal excess pounds on a person's body.

On the fat front, the American Dietetic Association (ADA) recommends that after age 2, children should consume no more than 30% of daily calories from fat. Infants and toddlers need more fat as they're developing. Excess fat in a child's diet may lead to weight gain. Obese children have a higher incidence of depression and orthopedic problems, reports Jordan Metzl, MD, a pediatrician. Kids who carry excess weight into adulthood have greater risk of heart attacks, high blood pressure, and early death.

Kids who fill up on sugar, fat, and caffeine don't get the nutrients they need from healthy sources, putting them at risk for malnutrition. The average teen consumes about twice as much sugar as the USDA recommends and doesn't get the recommended amounts of fruit and low-fat milk.

Which Foods Contain Caffeine, Sugar, and Fat?

Children get most of their caffeine from cola or other sodas, which also deliver sugar and empty calories (calories that don't provide any nutrients). Caffeine is also in coffee, tea, and chocolate. Some parents may give their children iced tea in place of soda, thinking that it is a better alternative. But iced tea packs as much of a sugar and caffeine punch as cola.

Sugar is found in beverages, juices, pastries, cookies, cake, candy, and frozen desserts. Fruit is a natural source of sugar, but fruit also contains fiber and vitamins that balance out the sugar.

Fat gives food flavor and texture, but it's also high in calories and excess amounts of it cause many health risks. For children and adolescents, desserts (including chocolate, cakes, doughnuts, pastries, and cookies) are a significant source of fat. Kids also get fat from whole milk products and high-fat meats, such as bacon, hot dogs, and non-lean red meat. Butter, cheeses, and oils are major fat foods. Fast-food and take-out meals tend to have more fat than home cooking, and in restaurants, fried dishes are the highest in fat content. Fat is often "hiding" in foods in the form of creamy, cheesy, or buttery sauces or dressings.

Jilting Junk Food

Can you help your kids jilt the junk food habit? Absolutely! Food preferences are learned, so we can relearn, Dr. Ayoob says. One way to cut out sugar and caffeine from your child's diet is to eliminate soda. Offer water, flavored seltzer, or diluted juice as beverages. You can give your child or teen water in squeeze bottles for added convenience.

Try to limit sugary beverages to moderate or occasional use. You may encounter in-school resistance—not from students, but from administrators. Kids drink more soda than ever and purchase much of it in schools, where they fed $750 million into soda and candy vending machines in 1997. Some schools count on revenue from soft drink sales to bolster their budgets.

Parents have to accept the responsibility of becoming good nutritional role models. If your kids see you eating junk food, they will too, Dr. Ayoob says. Keep mainly healthy foods around the house: try having a "healthy" shelf in the refrigerator, with fruit, cut-up vegetables, lean meats, and low-fat cheeses that kids can grab themselves. Buy low-fat or nonfat milk and whole-grain breads. Pack school lunches and meals for family outings, instead of going to fast-food restaurants or relying on your child to make healthy choices in the school cafeteria.

Learn which fruits and vegetables your children enjoy. Your child may hate apples but enjoy grapes, melons, strawberries, oranges, or bananas. Offer slices of mango and papaya, rich in beta-carotene and potassium. A wedge of watermelon, with more water than 8 ounces of juice, helps children re-hydrate in hot weather. Fruits and vegetables provide important vitamins, minerals, and fiber with an added bonus of no caffeine or fat and only natural sugar. If time is scarce, purchase pre-sliced and pre-washed fruit or vegetables at salad bars or the grocery store.

Try planning your child's meal ahead of time to eliminate reliance on fatty and sugary foods. Use the Food Guide Pyramid and plan meals that include lots of grains, fruits, and vegetables, with only small amounts of fats and sweets.

When you dine out, help your children make balanced choices that don't include large amounts of caffeine, sugar, or fat. Make a green salad part of your order and use low-fat dressing on the side. Choose stir-fried or steamed dishes rather than fried. If your children want to skip the burger and just have fries at a fast-food restaurant, suggest they order only a small portion of fries and have it with a salad.

Probably the most effective way to teach your child healthy eating habits is to set a good example. Make healthy food a priority in your life by limiting visits to fast-food restaurants and by teaching your child how to prepare food healthfully.

Exercise Is the Key

It's important to recognize that childhood obesity is a family problem, Dr. Metzl says. Once you've identified your child's sources of sugar, fat, and caffeine, and begun to offer healthier options, the next step is exercise.

Kids today tend to be sedentary. Schools have cut back on physical education programs, and time-starved working parents are glad their children are content in front of the TV or computer screen. But a growing child needs 45 to 60 minutes of physical activity every day. If your children are not used to getting exercise, encourage them to develop active habits. Find out what they like to do and make an effort to support them by doing the activity with them, driving them to the activity, or helping them find peers or teams to play with. Whether you're in a city or a suburb, seek out community sports associations, after school programs, or camps, which offer an array of physical programs all year long. If your child doesn't like team sports, look for programs emphasizing group participation rather than winning. The most important thing is to emphasize an active lifestyle and that exercise can be fun.

Viewing your child's diet and exercise needs as a family issue will help you to think of physical activities to share. Your family can go on walks, short hikes, bike rides, or visits to nature trails together. An active child is burning calories and building muscles—and too busy to be taking in excess sugar, fat, and caffeine.

Chapter 43

Snack Smart for Healthy Teeth

What's Wrong with Sugary Snacks, Anyway?

Sugary snacks taste so good—but they aren't so good for your teeth or your body. The candies, cakes, cookies, and other sugary foods that kids love to eat between meals can cause tooth decay. Some sugary foods have a lot of fat in them too.

Kids who consume sugary snacks eat many different kinds of sugar every day, including table sugar (sucrose) and corn sweeteners (fructose). Starchy snacks can also break down into sugars once they're in your mouth.

Did you know that the average American eats about 147 pounds of sugars a year? That's a big pile of sugar. No wonder the average 17-year-old in this country has more than three decayed teeth.

How Do Sugars Attack Your Teeth?

Invisible germs called bacteria live in your mouth all the time. Some of these bacteria form a sticky material called plaque on the surface of the teeth. When you put sugar in your mouth, the bacteria in the plaque gobble up the sweet stuff and turn it into acids. These acids are powerful enough to dissolve the hard enamel that covers your teeth. That's how cavities get started. If you don't eat much

Excerpted from "Snack Smart for Healthy Teeth!" National Institute for Dental and Craniofacial Research (NIDCR), http://www.nidcr.nih.gov/health/pubs/snaksmrt/main.htm, January 2, 2000.

sugar, the bacteria can't produce as much of the acid that eats away enamel.

How Can I "Snack Smart" to Protect Myself from Tooth Decay?

Before you start munching on a snack, ask yourself what's in the food you've chosen. Is it loaded with sugar? If it is, think again. Another choice would be better for your teeth. And keep in mind that certain kinds of sweets can do more damage than others. Gooey or chewy sweets spend more time sticking to the surface of your teeth. Because sticky snacks stay in your mouth longer than foods that you quickly chew and swallow, they give your teeth a longer sugar bath.

You should also think about when and how often you eat snacks. Do you nibble on sugary snacks many times throughout the day, or do you usually just have dessert after dinner? Damaging acids form in your mouth every time you eat a sugary snack. The acids continue to affect your teeth for at least 20 minutes before they are neutralized and can't do any more harm. So, the more times you eat sugary snacks during the day, the more often you feed bacteria the fuel they need to cause tooth decay.

If you eat sweets, it's best to eat them as dessert after a main meal instead of several times a day between meals. Whenever you eat sweets—in any meal or snack—brush your teeth well with a fluoride toothpaste afterward.

When you're deciding about snacks, think about:

- the number of times a day you eat sugary snacks
- how long the sugary food stays in your mouth
- the texture of the sugary food (chewy? sticky?)

If you snack after school, before bedtime, or other times during the day, choose something without a lot of sugar or fat. There are lots of tasty, filling snacks that are less harmful to your teeth—and the rest of your body—than foods loaded with sugars and low in nutritional value.

Low-fat choices like raw vegetables, fresh fruits, or whole-grain crackers or bread are smart choices. Eating the right foods can help protect you from tooth decay and other diseases. Next time you reach for a snack, pick a food from the list inside or make up your own menu of non-sugary, low-fat snack foods from the basic food groups.

How can you snack smart? Be choosy. Pick a variety of foods from these groups:

Fresh Fruits and Raw Vegetables

- berries
- oranges
- grapefruit
- melons
- pineapple
- pears
- tangerines
- broccoli
- celery
- carrots
- cucumbers
- tomatoes
- unsweetened fruit and vegetable juices
- canned fruits in natural juices

Grains

- bread
- plain bagels
- unsweetened cereals
- unbuttered popcorn
- tortilla chips (baked, not fried)
- pretzels (low-salt)
- pasta
- plain crackers

Milk and Dairy Products

- low or non-fat milk
- low or non-fat yogurt
- low or non-fat cheeses
- low or non-fat cottage cheese

Meat, Nuts, and Seeds

- chicken
- turkey
- sliced meats
- pumpkin seeds
- sunflower seeds
- nuts

Remember

- choose sugary foods less often
- avoid sweets between meals
- eat a variety of low or non-fat foods from the basic groups
- brush your teeth with fluoride toothpaste after snacks and meals

Note to Parents

The foods listed in this chapter have not all been tested for their decay-causing potential. However, knowledge to date indicates that they are less likely to promote tooth decay than are some of the heavily sugared foods children often eat between meals.

Candy bars aren't the only culprits. Foods such as pizza, breads, and hamburger buns may also contain sugars. Check the label. The new food labels identify sugars and fats on the nutrition facts panel on the package. Keep in mind that brown sugar, honey, molasses, and syrups also react with bacteria to produce acids, just as refined table sugar does. These foods also are potentially damaging to teeth.

Your child's meals and snacks should include a variety of foods from the basic food groups, including fruits and vegetables; grains, including breads and cereals; milk and dairy products; and meat, nuts, and seeds. Some snack foods have greater nutritional value than others and will better promote your child's growth and development. However, be aware that even some fresh fruits, if eaten in excess, may promote tooth decay. Children should brush their teeth with fluoride toothpaste after snacks and meals (so should you).

Chapter 44

Disordered Eating

Chapter Contents

Section 44.1

Understanding Eating Disorders

From "Eating Disorders Information Sheet: Parents and Other Care-givers," Girl Power, Office on Women's Health, 2000. The full text of this document including references is available online at www.4woman.gov/BodyImage/bodywise/uf/parents2.pdf.

Parents play a leading role in their children's lives. As a parent or other caregiver, you are in a unique position to educate your children about nutrition and help them maintain a positive body image as they enter their teenage years. This information is designed to provide basic information on eating disorders, how to detect them, and how to dis-courage disordered eating.

Disordered Eating Behaviors

Your child may not have an eating disorder, but she or he could be engaging in disordered eating behaviors. Pre-adolescence and adoles-cence are times of tremendous physical and psychological change. The rate of most rapid weight gain for girls is from age 9 to 14. By the time a girls reaches 18 years, it is likely she will nearly double her weight. This is also a time when young people seek more independence from their parents and approval from their peers. As body image be-comes more important, your child may begin to pay more attention to media images that portray the female body ideal as thin and the male ideal as muscular.

These changes and the pressures they bring can affect how your child relates to food. Instead of eating normally—eating when hun-gry and stopping when satisfied—your child may engage in disordered eating behaviors. For example, she or he may skip meals, binge one day and eat very little on the next day, use diet pill, laxatives, or di-uretics, or try the latest diet fad. If your child is involved in sports or other athletic activities that emphasize low weight and thin body shape, she or he may be particularly likely to restrict food and/or exer-cise in unhealthy ways to lose weight. Stressful situations like moving

412

or losing a family member can also contribute to disordered eating behaviors among children.

Your Child's Developing Body and Mind

Disordered eating behaviors can be very harmful to children's developing bodies and minds. Children who are restricting food can have a hard time concentrating on their school work and often report feeling tired or having headaches. They may fail to get all of the nutrients their bodies need to grow and develop into healthy adults. As a result, their growth can be stunted and menstrual cycles of girls disrupted. Restricting calories can also decrease bone density and increase their risks of experiencing bone fractures and osteoporosis. For some children, disordered eating behaviors can lead to full-blown eating disorders, such as anorexia nervosa or bulimia nervosa, which require intensive treatment.

In a society obsessed with thinness, children may engage in a number of disordered eating behaviors which may not be identified as eating disorders according to established diagnostic criteria. However, these behaviors can have very harmful consequences for children's health. If disordered eating persists, parents should consider consulting with a nutritionist and/or a therapist.

Signs and Symptoms of Possible Eating Disorders

Become familiar with the signs and symptoms of possible eating disorders. The early detection of an eating disorder can increase the likelihood of successful treatment and recovery. In your interactions with your child, you may notice one or more of the physical, behavioral, and emotional signs and symptoms of eating disorders.

Physical

- Weight loss or fluctuation in short period of time.
- Abdominal pain and discomfort.
- Feeling full or "bloated."
- Feeling faint or feeling cold.
- Dry hair or skin, dehydration, blue hands/feet.
- Lanugo hair (fine body hair).
- Headaches, feeling tired and/or cold.

Behavioral

- Dieting or chaotic food intake.
- Pretending to eat, throwing away food.
- Exercising for long periods of time.
- Showing concern with food, weight, or body size.
- Wearing baggy clothes to hide a very thin body.
- Making frequent trips to the bathroom.
- Avoiding food in social situations.

Emotional

- Complaints about appearance, particularly about being or feeling fat.
- Sadness or comments about feeling worthless.
- Perfectionist attitude.
- Always listening to friends' problems; never sharing one's own.

Ethnic and Cultural Groups

Children of all ethnic and cultural groups are vulnerable to developing eating disorders. Although rates of anorexia are higher among Caucasian girls, eating disorders occur among girls of all ethnic and cultural groups. Many immigrant girls, especially those isolated from their own culture, engage in disordered eating behaviors as they become exposed to social norms that value thinness. In addition, hundreds of thousands of boys and men are also experiencing this problem, and they may have difficulty seeking help because it is considered a "girl's" problem.

Family Attitudes

Family attitudes about eating and weight can set the stage for disordered eating behaviors. Although it may not always seem so, your child pays a lot of attention to what you say and do. If you are constantly complaining about your weight or feel pressured to exercise in order to lose weight or change the shape of your body, your child may learn that losing weight is an important concern. If you are always on the lookout for the new miracle diet, your child may learn that restrictive dieting is a good way to lose weight. And if you tell your child she would be much prettier if she lost a few pounds, she will learn that the goal of weight loss is attractiveness and acceptance.

Here are some questions that can help you consider your own attitudes and behaviors:

- Am I unhappy with my body size and shape?
- Am I always on a diet or going on a diet?
- Do I make fun of overweight people?
- Do I tease my child about body shape or weight?
- Do I focus on exercise for body size and shape control or for health?

Parents Do Not Cause Eating Disorders

While parents can contribute to their children's eating disorders, they are not the cause of these disorders. Eating disorders are associated with emotional problems and are closely related to many other health-related issues, such as depression, low self-esteem, physical and sexual abuse, substance abuse, and problems at home or with friends. Many factors, including genetics, can increase the likelihood that a child will develop an eating disorder.

Talk to Your Child

If you are concerned about your child, have a talk with her or him. Pay attention to your child's eating habits. If you notice an intense preoccupation with food, weight, and exercise, especially if it affects different parts of her or his life, it may signal a deeper problem.

Have a talk with your child to gauge what's going on. Ask specific questions about food amounts (too little or too much) and exercise. If she or he becomes angry or defensive, you may consider seeing a professional with expertise in eating disorders. Be sure to validate your child's feelings and encourage discussion.

Things You Can Do

As a parent or other caregiver, you can help your child develop a positive body image and relate to food in a healthy way. Here are some ideas:

- Make sure your child understands that weight gain is a normal part of development, especially during puberty.

- Avoid negative statements about food, weight, and body size and shape.

- Allow your child to make decisions about food, while making sure that plenty of healthy and nutritious meals and snacks are available.

- Compliment your child on her or his efforts, talents, accomplishments, and personal values.

- Restrict television viewing and watch television with your child and discuss the media images presented.

- Encourage your school to enact policies against size and sexual discrimination, harassment, teasing, and name calling; support the elimination of public weigh-ins and fat measurements.

- Keep the communication lines with your child open.

Section 44.2

Boys and Eating Disorders

"Eating Disorders Information Sheet: Boys and Eating Disorders," Girl Power, Office on Women's Health, 2000. The full text of this document including references is available online at www.4woman.gov/BodyImage/bodywise/bp/boys.pdf.

This section provides information on boys and eating disorders. It includes suggestions for creating a school environment that discourages disordered eating and promotes the early detection of eating disorders.

Boys Can and Do Develop Eating Disorders

Eating disorders are often seen as problems affecting only girls. However, 1 in 10 cases of these disorders involve males. This means that hundreds of thousands of boys are affected. Moreover, for one disorder—anorexia—up to one in four children referred to an eating disorders professional is a boy.

Factors Associated with Eating Disorders for Males

Factors associated with eating disorders are similar for males and females. The characteristics of males with eating disorders are similar to those seen in females with eating disorders. These factors include low self-esteem, the need to be accepted, an inability to cope with emotional pressures, and family and relationship problems. Homosexuality and bisexuality also appear to be risk factors for males, especially for those who develop bulimia. Homosexuality can be seen as a risk factor that puts males in a subculture that places the same premium on appearance for men as the larger culture places for women. Both males and females with eating disorders are likely to experience depression, substance abuse, anxiety disorders, and personality disorders.

Students of all ethnic and cultural groups are vulnerable to developing eating disorders. One recent study, for example, reported that Hispanic boys were twice as likely as Caucasian boys to binge eat at least monthly.

Boys May Diet and "Shape" to Achieve the Ideal Body Image

Boys are less likely than girls to consider themselves overweight or in need of dieting. While girls often *feel* fat before they begin dieting, boys are more likely to *be* overweight, usually in the mild to moderate range, when they begin to diet. Males tend to diet as a means to an end. For example, they may diet to avoid being teased about being fat or to improve athletic performance in wrestling, track, swimming, and other sports.

Males often try to achieve a better body image through *shaping*—bodybuilding, weightlifting, and muscle toning—in response to social norms for males, which emphasize strength and athleticism.

Boys Are Less Likely to Be Diagnosed

Boys are less likely to be diagnosed early with an eating disorder. Doctors reportedly are less likely to make a diagnosis of eating disorders in males than females. Other adults who work with young people and parents also may be less likely to suspect an eating disorder in boys, thereby delaying detection and treatment. A study of 135 males hospitalized with an eating disorder noted that the males with bulimia felt ashamed of having a stereotypically "female" disorder, which might explain their delay in seeking treatment.[10] Binge eating disorder may go unrecognized in males because an overeating male is less likely to provoke attention than an overeating female.

Action Figures Are Bulking Up

A recent study noted that some of the most popular male action figures have grown extremely muscular over time. Researchers compared action toys today—including GI Joe and Star Wars' Luke Skywalker and Han Solo—with their original counterparts. They found that many action figures have acquired the physiques of bodybuilders, with particularly impressive gains in the shoulder and chest areas. Some of the action toys have not only grown more muscular but have also developed increasingly sharp muscle definition, such as rippled abdominals. As noted in the study, if the GI Joe Extreme were 70 inches in size, he would sport larger biceps than any bodybuilder in history.

What Can You Do?

Here are some ideas:

- Communicate openly about body image issues, using messages that support acceptance of body diversity, discourage disordered eating, and promote the development of self-esteem.

- Do not tolerate teasing and bullying in school, particularly when focused on a boy's body size or masculinity.

- Conduct media literacy activities that explore the "wedge shape" as the cultural ideal and build skills to resist such messages.

- Develop policies that prohibit student athletes from engaging in harmful weight control or bodybuilding measures.

- Connect young men with positive role models who will encourage personal growth and development.

Section 44.3

Ten Things Parents Can Do to Prevent Eating Disorders

Reprinted with permission from, "10 Things Parents Can Do to Prevent Eating Disorders," by Michael Levine, Ph.D. and Linda Smolak, Ph.D. © 2002 National Eating Disorders Association. All rights reserved. For additional information visit, www.NationalEatingDisorders.org.

1. Consider your thoughts, attitudes, and behaviors toward your own body and the way that these beliefs have been shaped by the forces of weightism and sexism. Then educate your children about:

    • the genetic basis for the natural diversity of human body shapes and sizes, and

    • the nature and ugliness of prejudice.

    Make an effort to maintain positive, healthy attitudes and behaviors. Children learn from the things you say and do.

2. Examine closely your dreams and goals for your children and other loved ones. Are you overemphasizing beauty and body shape?

    • Avoid conveying an attitude which says in effect, "I will like you more if you lose weight, don't eat so much, look more like the slender models in ads, fit into smaller clothes, etc."

    • Decide what you can do and what you can stop doing to reduce the teasing, criticism, blaming, staring, etc. that reinforce the idea that larger or fatter is "bad" and smaller or thinner is "good."

3. Learn about and discuss with your sons and daughters (a) the dangers of trying to alter one's body shape through dieting, (b) the value of moderate exercise for health, and (c) the importance

419

of eating a variety of foods in well-balanced meals consumed at least three times a day.

- Avoid categorizing foods into "good/safe/no-fat or low-fat" vs. "bad/dangerous/ fattening."

- Be a good role model in regard to sensible eating, exercise, and self-acceptance.

4. Make a commitment not to avoid activities (such as swimming, sunbathing, dancing, etc.) simply because they call attention to your weight and shape. Refuse to wear clothes that are uncomfortable or that you don't like but wear simply because they divert attention from your weight or shape.

5. Make a commitment to exercise for the joy of feeling your body move and grow stronger, not to purge fat from your body or to compensate for calories eaten.

6. Practice taking people seriously for what they say, feel, and do, not for how slender or "well put together" they appear.

7. Help children appreciate and resist the ways in which television, magazines, and other media distort the true diversity of human body types and imply that a slender body means power, excitement, popularity, or perfection.

8. Educate boys and girls about various forms of prejudice, including weightism, and help them understand their responsibilities for preventing them.

9. Encourage your children to be active and to enjoy what their bodies can do and feel like. Do not limit their caloric intake unless a physician requests that you do this because of a medical problem.

10. Do whatever you can to promote the self-esteem and self-respect of all of your children in intellectual, athletic, and social endeavors. Give boys and girls the same opportunities and encouragement. Be careful not to suggest that females are less important than males, for example, by exempting males from housework or childcare. A well-rounded sense of self and solid self-esteem are perhaps the best antidotes to dieting and disordered eating.

Part Six

Other Common
Parenting Concerns

Chapter 45

Administering Medications Correctly

Chapter Contents

Section 45.1

How to Give Medicine to Children

by Rebecca D. Williams, *FDA Consumer*, January-February, 1996, revised May 1996, Food and Drug Administration (FDA) Pub. No. 96-3223, http://www. fda.gov/fdac/features/196_kid.html. Despite the age of this document, readers will still find helpful information about giving medications to children.

"Open wide... here comes the choo-choo."

When it comes to giving children medicine, a little imagination never hurts.

But what's more important is vigilance: giving the medicine at the right time at the right dose, avoiding interactions between drugs, watching out for tampering, and asking your child's doctor or the pharmacist about any concerns you may have.

Whether it's a prescription or over-the-counter (OTC) drug, dispensing medicine properly to children is important. Given incorrectly, drugs may be ineffective or harmful.

Read the Label

"The most important thing for parents is to know what the drug is, how to use it, and what reactions to look for," says Paula Botstein, M.D., pediatrician and acting director of the Food and Drug Administration's (FDA) Office of Drug Evaluation. She recommends that a parent should ask the doctor or pharmacist a number of questions before accepting any prescription:

- What is the drug and what is it for?
- Will there be a problem with other drugs my child is taking?
- How often and for how long does my child need to take it?
- What if my child misses a dose?
- What side effects does it have and how soon will it start working?

It's also a good idea to check the prescription after it has been filled. Does it look right? Is it the color and size you were expecting? If not, ask the pharmacist to explain.

Check for signs of tampering in any OTC product. The safety seal should be intact before opening. Also, parents should be extra careful to read the label of over-the-counter medicines.

"Read the label, and read it thoroughly," says Debra Bowen, M.D., an internist and director of FDA's medical review staff in the Office of OTC Drugs. "There are many warnings on there, and they were written for a reason. Don't use the product until you understand what's on the label."

Make sure the drug is safe for children. This information will be on the label. If the label doesn't contain a pediatric dose, don't assume it's safe for anyone under 12 years old. If you still have questions, ask the doctor or pharmacist.

Children are more sensitive than adults to many drugs. Antihistamines and alcohol, for example, two common ingredients in cold medications, can have adverse effects on young patients, causing excitability or excessive drowsiness. Some drugs, like aspirin, can cause serious illness or even death in children with chickenpox or flu symptoms. Both alcohol and aspirin are present in some children's medications and are listed on the labels.

Younger and Trickier

The younger the child, the trickier using medicine is. Children under 2 years shouldn't be given any over-the-counter drug without a doctor's OK. Your pediatrician can tell you how much of a common drug, like acetaminophen (Tylenol), is safe for babies.

Prescription drugs, also, can work differently in children than adults. Some barbiturates, for example, which make adults feel sluggish, will make a child hyperactive. Amphetamines, which stimulate adults, can calm children.

When giving any drug to a child, watch closely for side effects.

"If you're not happy with what's happening with your child, don't assume that everything's OK," says Botstein. "Always be suspicious. It's better to make the extra calls to the doctor or nurse practitioner than to have a bad reaction to a drug."

And before parents dole out OTC drugs, they should consider whether they're truly necessary, Botstein says.

Americans love to medicate—perhaps too much. A study published in the October 1994 issue of the *Journal of the American Medical Association (JAMA)* found that more than half of all mothers surveyed had given their 3-year-olds an OTC medication in the previous month.

Not every cold needs medicine. Common viruses run their course in seven to 10 days with or without medication. While some OTC medications can sometimes make children more comfortable and help them eat and rest better, others may trigger allergic reactions or changes for the worse in sleeping, eating, and behavior. Antibiotics, available by prescription, don't work at all on cold viruses.

"There's not a medicine to cure everything or to make every symptom go away," says Botstein. "Just because your child is miserable and your heart aches to see her that way, doesn't mean she needs drugs."

Dosing Dilemmas

The first rule of safety for any medicine is to give the right dose at the right time interval.

Prescription drugs come with precise instructions from the doctor, and parents should follow them carefully. OTC drugs also have dosing instruction on their labels. Getting the dosage right for an OTC drug is just as important as it is for a prescription drug.

Reactions and overdosing can happen with OTC products, especially if parents don't understand the label or fail to measure the medicine correctly. Similar problems can also occur when parents give children several different kinds of medicine with duplicate ingredients.

"People should exercise some caution about taking a bunch of medicines and loading them onto a kid," Botstein says.

Pediatric liquid medicines can be given with a variety of dosing instruments: plastic medicine cups, hypodermic syringes without needles, oral syringes, oral droppers, and cylindrical dosing spoons.

Whether they measure teaspoons, tablespoons, ounces, or milliliters, these devices are preferable to using regular tableware to give medicines because one type of teaspoon may be twice the size of another. If a product comes with a particular measuring device, it's best to use it instead of a device from another product.

Aspirin and Children

Remember those orange-flavored baby aspirin tablets? They're not usually for kids anymore.

Children and teenagers should never take aspirin or products containing aspirin or other salicylates if they have chickenpox or flu symptoms or are recovering from these or other viral illnesses. Such aspirin use has been associated with Reye syndrome, a rare but serious condition that can cause death.

"The incidence of Reye syndrome has dropped dramatically," says Debbie Lumpkins, an FDA microbiologist in the Office of OTC Drugs, "but that doesn't mean it can't still happen." To reduce fever safely in children, use acetaminophen or ibuprofen products.

—by Rebecca D. Williams

Rebecca D. Williams is a writer in Oak Ridge, Tenn.

Section 45.2

Administering Medication in Various Dosage Forms

Excerpted and reprinted with permission from the following fact sheets in the Kidsmeds, Inc. "Administering Medications" series: "Otic (Ear)," Ophthalmic Eye Drops, Eye Ointment," "Nasal (Nose) Drops, Nasal Spray, Nasal Inhaler," "Oral Inhaler," "Rectal," "Oral Liquids," "Tablets and Capsules," and "Topicals (Skin)," © 1998 Kidsmeds, Inc., updated 2000. For more information from Kidsmeds, Inc. visit their website at www.kids meds.com.

Ear Drops

The following list of instructions will help you to properly administer ear drops to your child:

1. Always wash your hands before giving medication.

2. Warm the medicine to body temperature by holding the bottle between your hands for several minutes. A medicine that is cold and placed in the ear could cause dizziness or nausea.

3. Place child on his side so the affected ear is on top.

4. Straighten the ear canal by:

   - Child younger than 3 years old: Hold ear lobe and pull down and back.

   - Child 3 years and older: Hold upper part of ear and pull up and back.

5. Drop the correct number of drops into the ear. Do not touch the dropper to the ear. Try to place the drops onto the side of the ear canal and not dropped directly down the ear canal.

6. Keep child on his side for 5 minutes.

7. Repeat steps 3 to 6 on other ear if necessary.

Eye Drops and Eye Ointment

Eye Drops

The following list of instructions will help you properly administer eye drops to your child:

1. Always wash your hands before giving medication.

2. Be sure the eye drops are at room temperature before using.

3. Clean your child's eye of all secretions and/or old medication. This can be done by gently wiping the eye with a damp gauze or cotton pad.

4. Have your child stand or sit with his head tilted back.

5. Do not touch the dropper bottle to the eye.

6. Have the child look upward toward the ceiling. Use your index finger and thumb to gently pinch and pull down the lower lid to create a pouch. Drop the prescribed number of drops into the pouch and not directly in the eye.

7. Have child close eyes for 1–2 minutes.

8. If a second type of eye drop is also prescribed, wait at least 5 minutes before giving second drops.

Eye Ointment

The following list of instructions will help you properly administer eye ointment to your child:

1. Always wash your hands before giving the medicine to your child.

2. Be sure the ointment is at room temperature before using.

3. Clean your child's eye of all secretions and/or old medication. This can be done by gently wiping the eye with a damp gauze or cotton pad.

4. Tell the child that the ointment may cause blurred vision. This is normal and will go away rather quickly.

5. Have child lie on his back or sit with his head tilted back.

6. Do not touch the tip of the tube to the eye, eyelashes or eyelids.

7. Pull lower lid down while your child looks up. Squeeze out a line of ointment along the lower lid from the inner to the outer eye. By rotating the tube when you reach the outer eye, you will help detach the ointment from the tube.

8. Keep eyes closed for 1–2 minutes.

9. Gently wipe any excess ointment from the eye while it is closed.

Nasal Drops, Nasal Sprays, and Nasal Inhalers

Nasal Drops

Infant

The following list of instructions will help you properly administer nasal drops to an infant:

1. Wash your hands before giving the medicine.

2. Using a suction bulb, clear the baby's nose. Ask your pharmacist or pediatrician on the proper method for suctioning an infant's nose.

3. Warm the medicine to room temperature if it is cold.

4. Place the infant lying down in your arms with his head tilted back.

5. Draw up enough medicine into the dropper so the correct number of drops can be given.

6. Without touching the dropper to the nose, insert the dropper slightly (about one-third of an inch) into the nostril.

7. Aim dropper toward the back of the nostril and squeeze the prescribed number of drops from the dropper.

8. Repeat on the other side if the other nostril needs medicine.

9. After the drops have been given, tell the child to keep his head tilted back for 5 minutes. Allow the child to spit out any medicine that runs down his throat.

10. If the child coughs, place him upright. Keep him upright and watch for any problems with breathing or excessive coughing. If this occurs, call the pediatrician immediately.

Older Child

The following list of instructions will help you to properly administer nasal drops to an older child:

1. Wash your hands before giving the medicine.

2. Have the child gently blow his nose if he is able.

3. Smaller children (toddler age) should lie on their back with a small pillow between their shoulders. Tilt head back over top of the pillow. Older children can sit in an upright position with their heads tilted back.

4. Warn the child that he may taste the medicine drops.

5. Warm the medicine to room temperature if it is cold.

6. Draw up enough medicine into the dropper so the correct number of drops can be given.

7. Push up gently on the tip of the child's nose.

8. Without touching the dropper to the nose, insert the dropper slightly into the nostril (about one-third of an inch).

9. Instruct the child to breathe through his mouth while the medicine is being placed into the nose.

10. Aim the dropper toward the back of the nostril and squeeze out the prescribed number of drops.

11. Repeat the above steps if the other nostril needs medicine.

12. Tell the child to keep his head tilted back for 5 minutes. Allow him to spit out any medicine that runs down his throat.

13. If the child coughs, place him upright and watch for any problems with breathing or excessive coughing. If either of these should occur, call the pediatrician immediately.

Nasal Spray

The following list of instructions will help you to properly administer nasal spray to your child:

1. Have the child gently blow his nose if able. An infant suction bulb can be used for infants.

2. Have the child sit upright with head tilted back.

3. Plug one nostril with your finger.

4. Place the tip of the sprayer slightly (about one-half inch) into the other nostril.

5. While pointing the sprayer straight back, have the child hold his breath.

6. Squeeze the sprayer quickly and firmly.

7. The child should continue to hold his breath for several seconds.

8. Remove sprayer from nose and allow child to exhale through his mouth.

9. Repeat above steps if more sprays are prescribed, or if the other nostril needs medicine.

10. Have the child keep his head tilted back for at least 2 minutes and avoid blowing nose during this time.

11. Rinse the tip of the sprayer with warm tap water before replacing the cap.

Nasal Inhaler

The following list of instructions will help you to properly utilize a nasal inhaler with your child:

1. Have the child gently blow his nose if able. An infant suction bulb can be used for infants.

2. Shake the inhaler well and remove the protective cap.

431

3. Place the tip of the inhaler inside the child's nostril.

4. While the child holds his breath, firmly press down on the top of the inhaler and then release.

5. Have the child hold his breath for at least 3 more seconds.

6. Remove the inhaler from the child's nose and have him exhale through his mouth.

7. Repeat the above steps if more sprays are prescribed or if the other nostril needs medicine.

8. Instruct child not to blow his nose for at least 2 minutes after the last spray.

Oral Inhalers

Oral Inhaler without Spacer

The following list of instructions will help you properly administer a medication with an oral inhaler:

1. Shake the inhaler well before use.

2. Remove the cap from the inhaler.

3. Ask your child to exhale completely (blow all the air from lungs).

4. Position inhaler about an inch away from the mouth.

5. While child breathes in, press on the top of the inhaler to release a puff of medicine.

6. After child has inhaled completely, have the child hold his breath for 10 seconds or as long as he can hold it.

7. Have the child breathe out slowly.

8. If more than one puff is to be given, wait at least one minute after first puff to give second puff.

9. If several different medicines from different inhalers are to be given, it is best to give the bronchodilator before any other. Examples of bronchodilators include albuterol or metaproterenol. To check if your child is taking a bronchodilator ask your pharmacist or pediatrician.

Oral Inhaler with Spacers

There are three different types of popular spacers. They are the Aerochamber with mask, the Aerochamber with mouthpiece, and the Inspirease spacer. The following list of instructions for each type will allow you to properly help your child use a spacer.

Aerochamber with Mask

The following list of instructions will allow you to help your child properly use an Aerochamber with mask:

1. Shake the inhaler well before use.

2. Place the whole inhaler unit onto the end of the spacer.

3. Place the masked end of the spacer up to the child's face.

4. Be sure the mask fits tightly over both the child's mouth and nose. If it isn't a snug fit, you may have the wrong size. The masks come in several different sizes. Check with your pediatrician or pharmacist if you think you need a different size mask.

5. Press on top of the inhaler to release medicine into the spacer.

6. Instruct the child to breathe in and out slowly several times, taking deep breaths and holding for several seconds.

7. If the spacer squeaks or whistles while the child is inhaling or exhaling, then the child is breathing too fast. Instruct the child to take slower breaths.

8. If more than 1 puff is necessary, wait at least one minute after first puff.

9. If several different medicines from different inhalers are to be given, it is best to give the bronchodilator before any other. Examples of bronchodilators include albuterol or metaproterenol. To check if your child is taking a bronchodilator ask your pharmacist or pediatrician.

Aerochamber with Mouthpiece

The following list of instructions will allow you to help your child properly use an Aerochamber with mouthpiece:

1. Shake the inhaler well before use.

2. Place the whole inhaler unit onto the end of the spacer.

3. Place the other end of the spacer (mouthpiece) in the child's mouth.

4. Press on top of the inhaler to release medicine into the spacer.

5. Instruct the child to breathe in and out slowly several times, taking deep breaths and holding for several seconds.

6. If the spacer squeaks or whistles while the child is inhaling or exhaling, then the child is breathing too fast. Instruct the child to take slower breaths.

7. If more than 1 puff is necessary, wait at least one minute after first puff.

8. If several different medicines from different inhalers are to be given, it is best to give the bronchodilator before any other. Examples of bronchodilators include albuterol or metaproterenol. To check if your child is taking a bronchodilator ask your pharmacist or pediatrician.

Inspirease Spacer

The following list of instructions will allow you to help your child properly use an Inspirease spacer:

1. Shake the inhaler well before use.

2. Take the medicine chamber out of the inhaler and place it on the top of the mouthpiece on the Inspirease spacer.

3. Place the mouthpiece of the spacer in the child's mouth.

4. Press on top of the medicine chamber to release medicine into the spacer.

5. Instruct the child to breathe in and out slowly several times, taking deep breaths and holding for several seconds.

6. If the spacer squeaks or whistles while the child is inhaling or exhaling, then the child is breathing too fast. Instruct the child to take slower breaths.

7. If more than 1 puff is necessary, wait at least one minute after first puff.

8. If several different medicines from different inhalers are to be given, it is best to give the bronchodilator before any other. Examples of bronchodilators include albuterol or metaproterenol. To check if your child is taking a bronchodilator ask your pharmacist or pediatrician.

Capsule Inhaler

There is one type of capsule inhaler currently on the market: the Rotahaler®. This is only used with Ventolin Rotacaps®. The following list of instructions will allow you to help your child properly use a Rotahaler®:

1. Twist the back of the inhaler all the way to the right.

2. Place the small end of the capsule into the opening on the back of the inhaler.

3. To release the medicine from the capsule, twist the back of the inhaler all the way to the left.

4. Tell the child to breathe out completely (exhale).

5. Tilt the child's head back slightly.

6. Have the child place his/her lips around the top of the inhaler.

7. Tell the child to inhale quickly and hold his/her breath for 10 seconds or as long as he/she can.

8. Remove the inhaler from mouth and tell the child to exhale.

9. Repeat the above steps until no medicine is left in the inhaler.

10. Clean the Rotahaler® by rinsing with water after each use and allow to air dry.

Nebulizer

The following list of instructions will allow you to help your child properly use a nebulizer.

1. Place the prescribed volume of medicine and diluting liquid into the reservoir (usually a plastic cup at the end of the mouthpiece).

2. Turn the nebulizer on.

3. Be sure a mist is coming out of the mouthpiece before placing it into your child's mouth.

4. Place the end of the mouthpiece into the child's mouth and have the child breathe normally.

5. The child is usually finished when there is no more liquid in the cup.

6. Clean the nebulizer after each use by rinsing the mouthpiece and reservoir with water. Once a week the mouthpiece and reservoir should be soaked in soapy water, then rinsed and allowed to air dry.

Oral Liquids

When giving your child liquid medicine always use either an oral syringe, a medicine dropper, a medicine spoon, or a medicine cup which sometimes accompanies children's medications. You can also buy any of these items at your local pharmacy. Do not use a kitchen utensil such as a teaspoon or tablespoon. These do not deliver the correct amount of liquid.

Sometimes children refuse to take liquid medicine because it tastes bad. One method used to overcome this problem is to mix the medicine in a small amount of water or fruit juice. Not all medications, however, can be mixed with water or fruit juice. Contact the child's pharmacist and/or pediatrician for more information.

If your child spits out the medicine, vomits shortly after taking it, or drools some of the dose down his/her face, do not give another dose. Consider this a partial dose and call your pharmacist and/or pediatrician for further instructions.

The following guidelines should help make it easier to administer a liquid medication by each method.

Oral Syringe

The easiest method for getting the liquid into the syringe is to pour a small amount into a paper cup, or any small cup. Place the tip of the syringe into the liquid in the cup and pull back on the plunger. This should pull the liquid into the syringe. To avoid air bubbles from entering, keep the tip below the level of the liquid. Draw up enough liquid to equal the dosage amount, and place the remaining liquid back into the medicine bottle.

Sometimes a syringe adapter can be used to get the liquid into the syringe. This is a plastic device that fits between the medicine bottle and the oral syringe. This way the whole bottle of medicine can be turned upside down and the correct amount of liquid drawn out. These adapters can also be found at your local pharmacy.

When giving the medicine, slowly squirt into the side of the child's mouth so the child will swallow the liquid naturally. Do not squirt onto the back of the throat as this will cause gagging. The oral syringe should be rinsed in warm water after each use.

Medicine Dropper

Droppers are usually part of the medicine bottle you receive at the pharmacy. Withdraw the correct dose (volume) into the dropper. Squeeze the rubber end of the dropper and drop the liquid into the side of the child's mouth to avoid gagging. The dropper should be rinsed with warm water after each use.

Medicine Spoon

Hold the medicine spoon upright. Pour the correct volume of medicine into the spoon. Use the markings on the side of the spoon as a guide. Put the spoon up to the child's lips and tilt it slowly. The liquid should flow into the mouth slowly enough so the child can swallow normally. Rinse the medicine spoon with warm water after each use.

Medicine Cup

Some over-the-counter medications come with a medicine cup included in the package. You should only use the cup with that particular medicine. There are slight differences in the cups from different manufacturers. Pour the correct volume of medicine into the cup. Use the markings on the side of the cup as a guide. Usually this method is only used when measuring volumes for older children (usually teaspoonsful). Do not try to measure something for an infant or small toddler with a medicine cup. The result will not be accurate.

Rectal

Suppository

The following list of instructions will help you to properly administer a rectal suppository to your child:

1. Wash your hands before administering the medicine.

2. Have the child lie on his left side. The left leg should be straight and the right leg should be bent up towards his chest.

3. Before unwrapping the suppository, run it under cold water to make sure it is firm.

4. Put on a pair of medical gloves and remove the suppository from its wrapper.

5. With one hand, gently separate the child's buttocks so you can see the anal opening.

6. With the other hand, dip the suppository into some cold water or place a small amount of Vaseline or KY Jelly on the tip. Gently insert the smooth, rounded end of the suppository into the anal opening.

7. With one finger (child under 3 years old, use pinky finger; child over 3 years old, use index finger) gently push the suppository into the rectum until there is no resistance (maximum distance = 2–3 inches). Check with your pediatrician on the proper distance for your child.

8. Remove your finger and check to make sure the suppository is still in the rectum. If it is inserted far enough, the suppository should stay in place. If it comes out, reinsert it again slightly farther than before.

9. After the suppository has been inserted, hold the child's buttocks together until the immediate urge to go to the bathroom passes.

10. Have the child remain in the same position for about 20 minutes. If this becomes impossible, the child should at least sit or lie down for about 20 minutes without going to the bathroom.

Ointment

The following list of instructions will help you to properly administer a rectal ointment to your child:

1. Wash your hands and put on a pair of medical gloves.

2. Have the child lie on his left side. The left leg should be straight and the right leg bent up toward his chest.

438

3. Place the applicator that comes with the ointment onto the end of the tube. Place a small amount of Vaseline or KY Jelly onto the tip of the applicator.

4. With one hand, gently separate the child's buttocks so you can see the anal opening.

5. With the other hand, gently insert the applicator into the anal opening.

6. Once the applicator is inside, squeeze the tube to insert the prescribed amount of ointment.

7. Remove the applicator from the rectum. Detach the applicator from the tube and clean applicator with soap and warm water.

8. Have the child remain in the same position for about 20 minutes. If this becomes a problem, the child should at least sit or lie down for this amount of time without going to the bathroom.

Tablets and Capsules

Older Children

Tablets and capsules are usually swallowed whole and taken with water. Some tablets and capsules have a protective coating which prevents the stomach from getting upset. This coating may also keep the medicine from being destroyed by the acid in the stomach. Other tablets and capsules may be extended-release or have long-acting properties. If these tablets and capsules are cut open, crushed, or chewed, these properties may be destroyed. The medicine could then possibly harm your child. Do not crush, chew, or cut open these tablets or capsules unless advised to do so by a physician or pharmacist. This will ensure that the proper amount of medicine is delivered to your child.

Younger Children

Taking a tablet or capsule represents a problem when they are unable to swallow it. Certain medications are not available in liquid form. In this case, certain tablets can be crushed and certain capsules opened and mixed into ice cream or applesauce. Not all tablets and capsules may be crushed or opened—you must first check with your child's pharmacist or pediatrician.

439

Certain tablets and capsules can be converted into a liquid form at some pharmacies. Check with your local pharmacist to see if your pharmacy will prepare a liquid form for you.

Topical Medications for Skin

The following list of instructions will help you apply topical medications to your child:

1. Always wash your hands before applying a topical medication.

2. Wash the affected area of the skin and pat dry with a towel. Do not wash the skin if a physician has directed you otherwise.

3. If no specific directions have been given, follow these general guidelines:

    *   Creams, ointment, gels, solutions, lotions: Use only a thin layer of medicine and rub well into skin.

    *   Aerosol: Shake well; hold can 6 inches away from skin and spray for several seconds.

4. Be careful not to get any topical medication into your child's eyes, ears, or mouth.

5. Wash your hands after the topical medicine has been applied.

Section 45.3

Liquid Medication and Dosing Devices

Excerpted from "Avoiding Problems Liquid Medication and Dosing Devices," by *FDA Consumer*, by Paula Kurtzweil, October 1994, Food and Drug Administration (FDA) Pub. No. 94-3209, http://www.fda.gov/fdac/reprints/drugdose.html. Reviewed January 2001 by Dr. David A. Cooke, MD, Diplomate, American Board of Internal Medicine. Tips listed for common dosing instruments are excerpted from "How to Give Medicine to Children," by Rebecca D. Williams, *FDA Consumer*, January-February, 1996, e-text revised May 1996, Food and Drug Administration (FDA) Pub. No. 96-3223, http://www.fda.gov/fdac/features/196_kid.html.

In the Walt Disney movie, Mary Poppins suggests a "spoonful" as the correct dose of sugar to ease the not-so-pleasant things in life, like taking bad-tasting medicine. But when giving or taking medicine, the Food and Drug Administration (FDA) warns consumers to put away their spoons and use a more exact measure—the proper dosing device.

Dosing Made Accurate

Consumers can get various types of dosing instruments for liquid medicines: hypodermic and oral syringes, oral droppers, cylindrical dosing spoons, and plastic medicine cups. They measure in one or more units of ounces, teaspoons, tablespoons, cubic centimeters, or milliliters. These devices are more accurate than tableware teaspoons, dessertspoons (a spoon between a teaspoon and tablespoon in size), and tablespoons commonly used to measure doses.

Common tableware teaspoons come in many sizes. They may be as small as 2.5 milliliters (mL) or larger than 9.5 mL, according to *U.S. Pharmacist*. The measuring teaspoon holds 5 mL, so on oral syringes and droppers, the teaspoon mark is at the same place as the 5-mL mark. Syringes offer additional benefits: They're easy to use, especially with infants, young children, and ailing older adults; relatively inexpensive; and available in various sizes. There are two types: an oral syringe designed especially for administering liquid medicines and the standard hypodermic syringe without the needle.

Health professionals frequently give patients hypodermic syringes rather than oral syringes because they cost less. In some cases, the health-care professional draws the medicine into the syringe for the customer to demonstrate how it is done.

Potential Problems

Both types of syringes often come with caps. According to the American Pharmaceutical Association, manufacturers "cap" their syringes to protect the syringe's nozzle. The cap also may keep medicine from leaking out of the syringe. This is useful in health-care facilities, so the syringe can be capped between the time the nurse or pharmacist measures the medicine and it is given to a patient. Parents whose children are in day care may also fill syringes and recap them for later administration by a day-care worker. The caps are supposed to be removed before the medicine is drawn up into any syringe and administered. But because the caps sometimes are not distinct from the rest of the syringe, the care giver may be unaware that a cap is there. And, with hypodermic syringes, the medicine can be drawn up and given with the cap in place. This creates a potentially life-threatening situation if the cap gets into the child's windpipe or esophagus.

Also, if the caps are not properly thrown away, infants and toddlers may pick them up and put them in their mouths. If they swallow, they are likely to choke.

Inappropriately marked plastic dosing cups also have posed some problems. In 1992, FDA received a report of a child who had been given three times the safe dose of a liquid acetaminophen product, 2 teaspoons. The dosing cup packaged with the drug gave measurements in tablespoons rather than teaspoons. The parents measured to the 2-tablespoon level marked on the cup, and the child got triple the recommended dose.

How to Use Dosing Instruments

- Remove caps from hypodermic and oral syringes before drawing medicine and giving it to yourself or another person. Keep the caps out of reach of infants and toddlers.

- For oral dosing syringes, unless the syringe is filled with medicine for later use, do not recap. Throw out caps immediately.

- For hypodermic syringes, do not recap; throw out caps immediately.

- Follow label directions for dosage amounts and time intervals. If you have any questions, call your pharmacist.

- Use the plastic dosing cup that comes with the medicine; don't substitute a cup from another drug product.

- Verify that dosing instrument measurements are compatible with product label.

- Use a standard measuring spoon or proper dosing device to measure medicines—not tableware spoons.

- Follow package directions for the proper cleaning and handling of dosing devices.

Safety Tips

- Use child-resistant caps, and do not leave medicine uncapped.

- Store medicine as directed and in a safe place out of reach of children.

- Don't give medicine to children unless it is recommended for them on the label or by a doctor.

- Don't take drugs prescribed for someone else or give yours to someone else.

- Don't use medicine for purposes not mentioned on the container or in package directions, unless so directed by a doctor.

- Don't try to remember the dose used during previous illnesses; read the label each time.

- Keep liquid medicines in their original bottles; don't transfer them to other containers.

- Use a prescribed medicine for as long as the doctor recommends to ensure complete recovery.

- Check with your doctor or pharmacist if you have any problems with or questions about your medicine.

The following are some tips for using common dosing instruments:

Syringes. Syringes are convenient for infants who can't drink from a cup. A parent can squirt the medicine in the back of the child's mouth where it's less likely to spill out. Syringes are also convenient for storing a dose. The parent can measure it out for a baby-sitter to use later.

443

Some syringes come with caps to prevent medicine from leaking out. **These caps are usually small and are choking hazards.** Parents who provide a syringe with a cap to a baby-sitter for later use should caution the sitter to remove the cap before giving the medicine to the child. The cap should be discarded or placed where the child can't get at it. There are two kinds of syringes: oral syringes made specifically for administering medicine by mouth, and hypodermic syringes (for injections), which can be used for oral medication if the needles are removed. For safety, parents should remove the needle from a hypodermic syringe. Always remove the cap before administering the medication into the child's mouth.

Droppers. These are safe and easy to use with infants and children too young to drink from a cup. Be sure to measure at eye level and administer quickly, because droppers tend to drip.

Cylindrical dosing spoons. These are convenient for children who can drink from a cup but are likely to spill. The spoon looks like

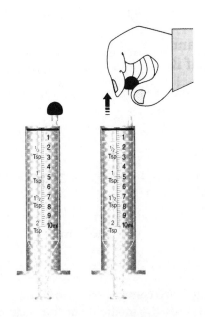

Figure 45.1. Always remove the cap before giving medication to the child. Throw it away or place it out of reach of children.

a test tube with a spoon formed at the top end. Small children can hold the long handle easily, and the small spoon fits easily in their mouths.

Dosage cups. These are convenient for children who can drink from a cup without spilling. Be sure to check the numbers carefully on the side, and measure out liquid medicine with the cup at eye level on a flat surface.

—by Paula Kurtzweil

Paula Kurtzweil is a member of FDA's public affairs staff.

Section 45.4

Use Antibiotics Appropriately

From "Miracle Drugs vs. Superbugs," by Tamar Nordenberg, *FDA Consumer*, November-December 1998, http://www.fda.gov/fdac/features/1998/698_bugs.html.

The historical scourge known as the bubonic plague killed up to one-third of Europe's population in the 1300s. But in modern times, it has been controlled handily with the help of antibiotic drugs such as streptomycin, gentamicin, and chloramphenicol.

That is, until 1995, when a plague infection in a 16-year-old boy from Madagascar failed to respond to the usual antibiotic treatments. This first documented case of an antibiotic-resistant plague, reported in the September 1997 *New England Journal of Medicine*, eventually succumbed to another antibiotic.

In the United States and globally, many other infectious germs, including those that cause pneumonia, ear infections, acne, gonorrhea, urinary tract infections, meningitis, and tuberculosis, can now outwit some of the most commonly used antibiotics and their synthetic counterparts, antimicrobials.

Antibiotic resistance isn't a new problem; resistant disease strains began emerging not long after the discovery of antibiotics more than

50 years ago. Penicillin and other antibiotics, which were initially viewed as miracle drugs for their ability to cure such serious and often life-threatening diseases as bacterial meningitis, typhoid fever, and rheumatic fever, soon were challenged by some defiant strains.

"What's different now," explains David Bell, MD, an expert on antimicrobial resistance with the national Centers for Disease Control and Prevention (CDC), "is that we've reached a situation where it's no longer an isolated problem of this bug or that bug; virtually all important human pathogens treatable with antibiotics have developed some resistance."

Too Much of a Good Thing

Experts say that doctors are sometimes quick to prescribe antibiotics for all sorts of symptoms, even though antibiotics work only against bacterial infections, not viruses such as the flu or the common cold. More than 50 million of the 150 million antibiotic prescriptions written each year for patients outside of hospitals are unnecessary, according to a recent CDC study.

Sometimes, doctors lack knowledge about the symptoms and natural course of respiratory illnesses, which contributes to overuse. Also, many doctors have told CDC they sometimes write prescriptions simply to meet patient demands.

Patients therefore must take some of the responsibility for the overprescribing problem, according to Stuart Levy, MD, director of Tufts University's Center for Adaptation Genetics and Drug Resistance. "Patients have been left out of the formula. Overuse of antibiotics was felt to be a physicians' problem when it is really as much a patient problem."

Patients can do their part to help curb resistance:

- Don't demand an antibiotic when the health-care provider determines one isn't appropriate.

- Finish each prescription. Even when the symptoms of an illness have disappeared, some bacteria may still survive and reproduce if the patient doesn't complete the course of treatment.

- Don't take leftover antibiotics or antibiotics prescribed for someone else. These antibiotics may not be appropriate for the current symptoms, and taking the wrong medicine could delay getting appropriate treatment and allow bacteria to multiply.

Preventing infection in the first place may therefore be the best defense against an antibiotic-resistant infection.

Frequent and thorough hand washing is one key to preventing the spread of infection. Good kitchen habits, such as storing foods at the proper temperature, washing fruits and vegetables thoroughly, and cooking foods completely, can also reduce the chance of getting a food-borne illness.

"Take your basic precautions," Bell advises. "That means practicing common hygiene, as well as food safety in your kitchen."

Additional information about antibiotic use and drug resistance is available from the CDC online at www.cdc.gov/drugresistance/.

—by Tamar Nordenberg

Tamar Nordenberg is a staff writer for *FDA Consumer*.

Chapter 46

Alternative Medicine and Your Child

As you wander the aisles of your local health food store, you stumble on one that is full of bottles that look like they belong in the drug store. Looking up, you notice that the name of the aisle is Alternative Medicine.

Seeing the phrase "alternative medicine" might conjure up images of pungent herbal teas, poultices, chanting, or meditation. In fact, both herbal remedies and meditation, as well as dozens of other treatments, fall under the heading of complementary and alternative medicine (CAM). Although there is no strict definition of alternative medicine, it generally includes any healing practices that are not part of mainstream medicine—that means any practice that is not widely taught in medical schools or frequently used by doctors or in hospitals.

But the boundaries of alternative medicine in the United States are constantly changing as different types of care become more accepted by doctors and more requested by patients. A few practices (such as hypnosis) that were dismissed as nonsense 20 years ago are now considered helpful therapies in addition to traditional medicine. Can alternative medicine help your child?

449

Types of Alternative Care

The National Center for Complementary and Alternative Medicine (NCCAM) at the National Institutes of Health recognizes seven general areas of alternative care (some of which have been put through rigorous scientific testing, but many have not).

Alternative medical systems generally fall outside the conventional medical system of doctors and hospitals. They include acupuncture, the practice of stimulating points on the body (usually with a needle) to promote healing; traditional Oriental medicine, which focuses on diagnosing disturbances of energy in the body; homeopathy, treating health problems with very diluted substances; and community-based healers like midwives, herbalists, and practitioners of Native American medicine.

Herbal remedies include a wide range of plants used for medicine or nutrition. They are available in grocery stores, in health food stores, or through herbalists and are often in the form of teas, capsules, and extracts. The U.S. Food and Drug Administration (FDA) does not regulate these substances. About one third of American adults regularly take some sort of herb, anything from a cup of chamomile tea to soothe nerves to Echinacea to fight a cold.

Manual healing treats medical problems by manipulating and realigning body parts. Perhaps the most widely known method is chiropractic care, which focuses on the nervous system and adjusting the vertebra of the spine. Other forms of manual healing include massage therapy; osteopathic medicine, which uses manipulation in addition to traditional medicine and surgical treatment; and healing touch, where practitioners place their hands on or near the patient's body to direct energy.

Making a change in diet or lifestyle is an area of alternative medicine that almost everyone has practiced at some time. Many people take supplements if their regular diet does not have enough vitamins or minerals. And people with chronic conditions such as heart disease or diabetes often change their diet (more whole grains and vegetables and less salt or processed sugar) or habits (regular exercise) to keep the problem in check. This is one of the most useful forms of alternative care because altering your diet and habits not only helps treat numerous diseases but can help prevent them as well. This area of alternative medicine is widely accepted in the traditional medicine model.

Mind-body control focuses on the mind's role in conditions that affect the body. Hypnosis, a sort of conscious sleep or trance, can help some people deal with addictions, pain, or anxiety, whereas treatments like psychotherapy, meditation, and yoga are used for relaxation. Many people also turn to support groups and prayer to cope with an illness or feel more connected to others.

Drugs and vaccines that have not yet been accepted by mainstream medicine are also considered alternative. Eventually, after extensive testing and approval by the FDA, some of these medications or vaccines may become regularly prescribed treatments.

Lastly, an emerging area of study looks at how changes in the body's electromagnetic fields can affect health. Bioelectromagnetics is based on the idea that electrical currents in all living organisms produce magnetic fields that extend beyond the body.

How Does It Differ from Traditional Medicine?

Alternative therapy is frequently distinguished by its holistic methods, which means that the doctor or practitioner treats the "whole" person and not just the disease or condition. In alternative medicine, many practitioners address patients' emotional and spiritual needs as well. This "high touch" approach differs from the "high tech" practice of traditional medicine, which tends to concentrate on the physical side of illness.

Most alternative practices have not found their way into mainstream hospitals or doctors' offices, so you or your child's doctor may not be aware of them. However, new centers for integrative medicine offer a mix of traditional and alternative treatments. There, you might receive a prescription for pain medication (as you might get from a traditional health care provider) and massage therapy to treat a chronic back problem. Such centers usually employ both medical doctors and certified or licensed specialists in the various alternative therapies.

Despite the growth in the field, the majority of alternative therapies are not covered by medical insurance. This is largely because few scientific studies have been done to prove whether the treatments are effective (unlike traditional medicine, which relies heavily on studies). Rather, most alternative therapies are based on long-standing practice and word-of-mouth stories of success.

What Are the Risks?

The lack of scientific study means that some potential problems associated with alternative therapies may be difficult to identify.

451

What's more, the studies that have been done used adults as test subjects; there is little research on the effects of alternative medicine on children. Although approaches such as prayer, massage, and lifestyle changes are generally considered safe complements to regular medical treatment, some therapies—particularly herbal remedies—might harbor risks.

Unlike prescription and over-the-counter medicines, herbal remedies are not rigorously regulated by the U.S. Food and Drug Administration (FDA). They face no extensive tests before they are marketed, and they do not have to adhere to a standard of quality. That means when you buy a bottle of ginseng capsules, you might not know what you're getting; the amount of herb can vary from pill to pill, with some capsules containing much less of the active herb than stated on the label. Depending on where the herb originated, there might also be other plants, even drugs like steroids, mixed in the capsules. Herbs that come from developing countries are sometimes contaminated with pesticides and heavy metals.

"Natural" does not equal "good" and many parents don't consider that herbal remedies can actually cause health problems for their children. Medicating a child without consulting the child's doctor could result in harm. For example, certain herbal remedies can cause high blood pressure, liver damage, or severe allergic reactions. Consider these examples:

- Ephedra (often sold as the Chinese herb ma huang) was on the market for years until it was linked to several deaths in people with heart problems.

- Alone and in combination with prescription drugs, several dietary supplements—such as chaparral, comfrey, germander, and ephedrine—have been linked to severe illness, liver damage, and even death.

Parents might also give their children much more of an herb than recommended, thinking that because it's natural, higher doses won't hurt. But many plants contain potent chemicals; in fact, approximately 25% of all prescription drugs are derived from plants.

Choosing a practitioner can pose another problem. Although many states have licensing boards for specialists in acupuncture or massage, for instance, there is no organization in the United States that monitors alternative care providers or establishes standards of treatment. Basically, almost anyone can claim to be a practitioner, whether he or she has any training.

Perhaps the greatest risk, however, is the potential for people to delay or stop traditional medical treatment in favor of an alternative therapy. Illnesses such as diabetes and cancer require the care of a doctor. Relying entirely on alternative therapies for any serious chronic or acute conditions will only jeopardize the health of your child.

Can Alternative Care Help Your Child?

Many parents turn to a cup of chamomile tea or ginger as a first line of treatment against the flu or nausea. Anxious children can learn to relax with the help of meditation or yoga. Such alternative therapies complement traditional care and can give you and your child a greater sense of control over his health.

If you want to try alternative medicine for your child, you should first discuss the proposed treatment with your child's doctor or talk to your pharmacist to make sure it is not dangerous or will not conflict with any traditional care your child receives. Your child's doctor can also give you information about treatment options and perhaps recommend a reputable specialist. By coordinating alternative and traditional care, you don't have to choose between them. Instead, you can get the best of both.

Chapter 47

Toileting Concerns

Chapter Contents

Section 47.1

Toilet Teaching Your Child

Toileting (or using the potty) is one of the most basic physical needs of young children. It is also one of the most difficult topics of communication among parents, child care providers, and health care professionals when asked to determine the "right" age a child should be able to successfully and consistently use the toilet.

Most agree that the methods used to potty train can have major emotional effects on children. The entire process—from diapering infants to teaching toddlers and preschoolers about using the toilet—should be a positive one. Often, and for many reasons, toilet learning becomes an unnecessary struggle for control between adults and children. Many families feel pressured to potty train children by age two because of strict child care program policies, the overall inconvenience of diapering, or urging from their pediatricians, early childhood columnists, researchers, other family members, friends, etc.

The fact is that the ability to control bladder and bowel functions is as individual as each child. Some two-year-olds are fully potty trained, and some are not. But those that aren't should not be made to feel bad about it. There are also many cultural differences in handling potty training, therefore it is important that families and program staff sensitively and effectively communicate regarding these issues.

The purpose of toilet learning is to help children gain control of their body functions. If a child is ready, the process can provide a sense of success and achievement. Here are some helpful hints on determining when young children are ready to begin the potty training process and suggestions on how to positively achieve that task.

Ready, Set, Go!

Children are most likely ready to begin toilet learning when they:

456

- show a preference for clean diapers—a preference adults can encourage by frequent diaper changing and by praising children when they come to you for a change.

- understand when they have eliminated and know the meaning of terms for body functions. For example, "wet," "pee," "poop," and "b.m." are words commonly used by children to describe bladder and bowel functions.

- indicate that they need to use the potty by squatting, pacing, holding their private parts, or passing gas.

- show that they have some ability to hold it for a short period of time by going off by themselves for privacy when filling the diaper or staying dry during naps.

Become a Cheerleader

- There may be times during the learning process when children accidentally go in their diapers or training pants. This can be very distressing and may cause them to feel sad—especially if they have been successfully using the chair for some period of time. When this happens, change the diaper without admonition—a caring adult can then try to pick up the child's spirits with encouragement that she is doing well and will get better with practice.

- The most common cause of resistance to potty training occurs when children have been scolded, punished, or lectured too often about using the potty, or have been forced to sit on it for too long. This learning process usually is not fast or consistent. Children need your patience and support.

Have a Plan

- Parents and child care providers should decide together when a child is ready and then negotiate a plan that will be consistent and manageable in both settings. Some questions may include the following:
  - Is special equipment needed—step stool, toilet seat deflector, potty chair?
  - Are extra clothing items needed?
  - Are good hygiene practices in place, for example, hand washing for children and staff, a system for handling soiled clothing, and a routine for disinfecting equipment?

457

• It's a good idea for families and child care professionals to exchange information on the words for body functions most preferred by each child in order to avoid confusion and provide a consistent message for everyone engaged in the process.

Successfully learning to use the potty is a major accomplishment for young children, and patience and praise from the adults who care for them is an extremely important component to their healthy emotional and physical development. Each child will individually provide signals as to when he or she is ready to make that leap. Good communication, appropriate expectations, and a consistent plan on the part of parents and caregivers make it easier to support this process and is the surest route to success.

Section 47.2

Urinary Incontinence in Children

"Urinary Incontinence in Children," National Kidney and Urologic Diseases Information Clearinghouse, National Institute of Diabetes and Digestive and Kidney Diseases (NIDDK), NIH Pub. No. 02-4095, May 2002.

Urination, or voiding, is a complex activity. The bladder stores urine, then releases it through the urethra, the canal that carries urine to the outside of the body. Controlling this activity involves nerves, muscles, the spinal cord, and the brain. Failures in this control mechanism result in incontinence. Reasons for this failure range from the simple to the complex.

Occasional incontinence is a normal part of growing up and treatment is available for most children who have difficulty controlling their bladders. Incontinence happens less often after age 5: About 10 percent of 5-year-olds, 5 percent of 10-year-olds, and 1 percent of 18-year-olds experience episodes of incontinence. It is twice as common in boys as in girls.

What Causes Nighttime Incontinence?

After age 5, wetting at night—often called bedwetting or sleep-wetting—is more common than daytime wetting in boys. Experts do not know what causes nighttime incontinence. Young people who experience nighttime wetting tend to be physically and emotionally normal. Most cases probably result from a mix of factors including slower physical development, an overproduction of urine at night, a lack of ability to recognize bladder filling when asleep, and, in some cases, anxiety. For many, there is a strong family history of bedwetting, suggesting an inherited factor.

Slower Physical Development

Between the ages of 5 and 10, incontinence may be the result of a small bladder capacity, long sleeping periods, and underdevelopment of the body's alarms that signal a full or emptying bladder. This form of incontinence will fade away as the bladder grows and the natural alarms become operational.

Excessive Output of Urine During Sleep

Normally, the body produces a hormone that can slow the making of urine. This hormone is called antidiuretic hormone, or ADH. The body normally produces more ADH at night so that the need to urinate is lower. If the body doesn't produce enough ADH at night, the making of urine may not be slowed down, leading to bladder overfilling. If a child does not sense the bladder filling and awaken to urinate, then wetting will occur.

Anxiety

Experts suggest that anxiety-causing events occurring in the lives of children ages 2 to 4 might lead to incontinence before the child achieves total bladder control. Anxiety experienced after age 4 might lead to wetting after the child has been dry for a period of 6 months or more. Such events include angry parents, unfamiliar social situations, and overwhelming family events such as the birth of a brother or sister.

Incontinence itself is an anxiety-causing event. Strong bladder contractions leading to leakage in the daytime can cause embarrassment and anxiety that lead to wetting at night.

Genetics

Certain inherited genes appear to contribute to incontinence. In 1995, Danish researchers announced they had found a site on human chromosome 13 that is responsible, at least in part, for nighttime wetting. If both parents were bedwetters, a child has an 80 percent chance of being a bedwetter also. Experts believe that other, undetermined genes also may be involved in incontinence.

Obstructive Sleep Apnea

Nighttime incontinence may be one sign of another condition called obstructive sleep apnea, in which the child's breathing is interrupted during sleep, often because of inflamed or enlarged tonsils or adenoids. Other symptoms of this condition include snoring, mouth breathing, frequent ear and sinus infections, sore throat, choking, and daytime drowsiness. In some cases, successful treatment of this breathing disorder may also resolve the associated nighttime incontinence.

Structural Problems

Finally, a small number of cases of incontinence are caused by physical problems in the urinary system in children. Rarely, a blocked bladder or urethra may cause the bladder to overfill and leak. Nerve damage associated with the birth defect spina bifida can cause incontinence. In these cases, the incontinence can appear as a constant dribbling of urine.

What Causes Daytime Incontinence?

Daytime incontinence that is not associated with urinary infection or anatomic abnormalities is less common than nighttime incontinence and tends to disappear much earlier than the nighttime versions. One possible cause of daytime incontinence is an overactive bladder. Many children with daytime incontinence have abnormal voiding habits, the most common being infrequent voiding.

An Overactive Bladder

Muscles surrounding the urethra (the tube that takes urine away from the bladder) have the job of keeping the passage closed, preventing urine from passing out of the body. If the bladder contracts strongly and without warning, the muscles surrounding the urethra may not be able to keep urine from passing. This often happens as a consequence of urinary tract infection and is more common in girls.

Infrequent Voiding

Infrequent voiding refers to a child's voluntarily holding urine for prolonged intervals. For example, a child may not want to use the toilets at school or may not want to interrupt enjoyable activities, so he or she ignores the body's signal of a full bladder. In these cases, the bladder can overfill and leak urine. Additionally, these children often develop urinary tract infections (UTIs), leading to an irritable or overactive bladder.

Other Causes

Some of the same factors that contribute to nighttime incontinence may act together with infrequent voiding to produce daytime incontinence. These factors include

- a small bladder capacity
- structural problems
- anxiety-causing events
- pressure from a hard bowel movement (constipation)
- drinks or foods that contain caffeine, which increases urine output and may also cause spasms of the bladder muscle, or other ingredients to which the child may have an allergic reaction, such as chocolate or artificial coloring

Sometimes overly strenuous toilet training may make the child unable to relax the sphincter and the pelvic floor to completely empty the bladder. Retaining urine (incomplete emptying) sets the stage for urinary tract infections.

What Treats or Cures Incontinence?

Growth and Development

Most urinary incontinence fades away naturally. Here are examples of what can happen over time:

- Bladder capacity increases.
- Natural body alarms become activated.

- An overactive bladder settles down.

- Production of ADH becomes normal.

- The child learns to respond to the body's signal that it is time to void.

- Stressful events or periods pass.

Many children overcome incontinence naturally (without treatment) as they grow older. The number of cases of incontinence goes down by 15 percent for each year after the age of 5.

Medications

Nighttime incontinence may be treated by increasing ADH levels. The hormone can be boosted by a synthetic version known as desmopressin, or DDAVP, which recently became available in pill form. Patients can also spray a mist containing desmopressin into their nostrils. Desmopressin is approved for use by children.

Another medication, called imipramine, is also used to treat sleep-wetting. It acts on both the brain and the urinary bladder. Unfortunately, total dryness with either of the medications available is achieved in only about 20 percent of patients.

If a young person experiences incontinence resulting from an overactive bladder, a doctor might prescribe a medicine that helps to calm the bladder muscle. This medicine controls muscle spasms and belongs to a class of medications called anticholinergics.

Bladder Training and Related Strategies

Bladder training consists of exercises for strengthening and coordinating muscles of the bladder and urethra, and may help the control of urination. These techniques teach the child to anticipate the need to urinate and prevent urination when away from a toilet. Techniques that may help nighttime incontinence include:

- determining bladder capacity

- stretching the bladder (delaying urinating)

- drinking less fluid before sleeping

- developing routines for waking up

Unfortunately, none of the above has demonstrated proven success.

Techniques that may help daytime incontinence include:

- urinating on a schedule, such as every 2 hours (this is called timed voiding)

- avoiding caffeine or other foods or drinks that you suspect may contribute to your child's incontinence

- following suggestions for healthy urination, such as relaxing muscles and taking your time

Moisture Alarms

At night, moisture alarms can awaken a person when he or she begins to urinate. These devices include a water-sensitive pad worn in pajamas, a wire connecting to a battery-driven control, and an alarm that sounds when moisture is first detected. For the alarm to be effective, the child must awaken or be awakened as soon as the alarm goes off. This may require having another person sleep in the same room to awaken the bedwetter.

Incontinence Is Also Called Enuresis

- Primary enuresis refers to wetting in a person who has never been dry for at least 6 months.

- Secondary enuresis refers to wetting that begins after at least 6 months of dryness.

- Nocturnal enuresis refers to wetting that usually occurs during sleep (nighttime incontinence).

- Diurnal enuresis refers to wetting when awake (daytime incontinence).

Additional Resources

American Foundation for Urologic Disease
1128 North Charles Street
Baltimore, MD 21201
Toll-Free: 800-242-2383
Phone: 410-468-9235
Website: http://www.afud.org
E-mail: admin@afud.org

National Association for Continence
P.O. Box 8310
Spartanburg, SC 29305
Toll-Free: 800-BLADDER
Phone: 864-579-7900
Website: http://www.nafc.org
E-mail: memberservices@nafc.org

National Kidney and Urologic Diseases Information Clearinghouse
3 Information Way
Bethesda, MD 20892-3580
Website: http://www.niddk.nih.gov/health/kidney/nkudic.htm

National Kidney Foundation, Inc.
30 East 33rd Street
New York, NY 10016
Toll-Free: 800-622-9010
Phone: 212-889-2210
Website: http://www.kidney.org
E-mail: info@kidney.org

The Simon Foundation for Continence
P.O. Box 835
Wilmette, IL 60091
Toll-Free: 800-23-SIMON
Phone: 847-864-3913
Website: http://www.simonfoundation.org
E-mail: simoninfo@simonfoundation.org

Society of Urologic Nurses and Associates
P.O. Box 56
East Holly Avenue
Pitman, NJ 08071
Toll-Free: 888-TAP-SUNA
Phone: 856-256-2335
Website: http://www.suna.org
E-mail: suna@ajj.com

Section 47.3

What Parents Need to Know about Bedwetting

"Childhood Bed-Wetting: Cause for Concern," by Dixie Farley, originally in *FDA Consumer*, currently available at http://www.fda.gov/bbs/topics/CONSUMER/CON00083.html; reviewed and revised by David A. Cooke May 2002.

Fourteen percent of 5- to 13-year-olds wet the bed, according to a recent population study. For many such children, the consequences are humiliation and damaged self-esteem. Fortunately, this common childhood affliction, known medically as "primary enuresis," usually disappears on its own, and proper treatment can often hurry it on its way.

Bedwetting is considered normal up to age 5. When the problem persists, however, a visit to the doctor is in order. Bedwetting rarely signals a health problem, but daytime wetting—which often occurs with bedwetting yet may be overlooked if it's only a dribble—can represent serious illness. Indeed, if the wetting disorders known as dysfunctional voiding go untreated, kidney failure—even death—can result.

Delayed Development and Other Causes

The precise cause of bedwetting is unknown. Most cases appear to be due to delayed physical development. Bladder capacity may be less than half what is considered normal for the child's age. Bedwetting is up to three times more common in boys than girls—linked, perhaps, to boys' slower rate of maturation. Some researchers, in fact, have argued that boys aren't normally dry at night until age 8.

Several studies point to a genetic link in enuresis. When both parents had the problem as youngsters, 77 percent of the children in these studies developed it. But the figure dropped to 44 percent when only one parent had wet the bed in childhood. By contrast, when neither parent had enuresis, only 15 percent of the children did.

A frequent cause of bedwetting is constipation. In fact, treatment of constipation in enuretic children often resolves the wetting. Attempts to hurry toilet training may backfire and actually contribute to bedwetting; experts advise letting a child develop bladder control at his or her own pace.

Other contributing factors include hospitalization (especially between ages 2 and 4), arrival of a baby, loss of a parent, and entering school. In rare cases, emotionally disturbed children may respond to their illness with loss of bladder and bowel control. Urinary tract infection also can result in bedwetting. These infections often cause additional symptoms, such as painful urination, foul-smelling urine, and daytime wetting.

To Treat, or Not

The choice of therapy and effectiveness of individual treatments depend on the severity of the problem, the child's age and emotional maturity, and the level of commitment of the child and parents. Certainly, scolding and punishment are ineffective and inappropriate.

Behavior Modification

For behavior modification to be effective, child and parents must be highly motivated to follow the physician's instructions exactly and to persist long enough, which may mean several months. It's very easy to become lax or give up. Rewards alone—no punishments—are used. Among the techniques:

Responsibility reinforcement training. The child takes charge of making one last trip to the bathroom, changing and laundering soiled bed linens, and charting progress (dry nights earn rewards). These responsibilities should help improve the child's feelings of self-worth and prevent parental anger over a wet bed. Hints from the Mayo Clinic: Use a plastic mattress pad and pillowcases, and buy lots of inexpensive sheets and blankets for storage in a tightly sealed plastic bag for weekly washing.

Urinary alarm. Many experts believe this is the best form of treatment for enuresis. Wetting sets off the battery-powered alarm; the child wakens, turns off the switch, and finishes urinating in the bathroom. Eventually, the child is supposed to learn to wake before wetting. Lightweight pajamas are best because thick ones slow down the time between the first drops of urine and the sounding of the alarm. It's a good idea to replace batteries at set intervals because weakened ones may not trigger the alarm and may damage the device. The success rate with the alarm is as high as 92 percent, but the relapse rate can be as high as 30 percent. Maizels says that, by combining the alarm with other therapies, he and his colleagues can correct about 80 percent of wetting within the first month or two, with a relapse rate of only around 13 percent.

Bladder capacity. Another treatment often reported involves retaining urine to enlarge bladder capacity. But Terry Allen, M.D., urology professor at Southwestern Medical School in Dallas, says "this is bad policy because it puts undue pressure on the urinary tract."

Drugs Have Drawbacks

The Food and Drug Administration has approved imipramine (Tofranil), an antidepressant, as safe and effective for bedwetting. It can immediately produce dry nights, but there are drawbacks. It can cause a number of side effects, including blood pressure changes, irregular heartbeat, anxiety, insomnia, dry mouth, blurred vision, nausea, vomiting, diarrhea, dizziness, drowsiness, and headache. Bedwetting often resumes when treatment stops. And, while the drug is safe at recommended dosages, an overdose can cause convulsions, coma and death.

A newer drug called oxybutynin chloride (Ditropan) is also used to treat enuresis. It inhibits contraction of the bladder. It is less hazardous than imipramine, but can have many of the same side effects.

A third drug which has become popular for treatment of enuresis is desmopressin, also known as DDAVP or Stimate. This is a synthetic form of a natural hormone produced in the brain which reduces urinary output. It is usually administered as a nasal spray, and may be modestly effective in children with enuresis in the absence of a correctable cause.

The difficulty with all drug therapies for enuresis is that relapses tend to occur when the drugs are stopped. Still, they may be appropriate in some children. They may also be helpful for specific events, such as overnight trips, when enuresis might cause embarrassment.

Dysfunctional Voiding

Sometime between ages 1 and 2, a toddler first senses bladder fullness and, so, starts to hold back urine by contracting the sphincter muscle of the urethra, the urinary tract opening out of the body. As the bladder gradually stretches to hold more urine, increased inner pressure causes the bladder's powerful detrusor muscle to contract to expel its contents. By age 4 or 5, most children learn to suppress detrusor contractions so they can retain urine and to relax the urethral sphincter during detrusor contractions so they can pass urine.

Certain children, however, get stuck in this transition with a condition known as dysfunctional voiding. Some don't learn to coordinate the urinary muscles; others learn coordination, but so persist in holding back urine that the bladder greatly overstretches. In both abnormal patterns, the contained urine becomes stagnant and infected. Dysfunctional voiding reflects neither disease nor physical defect but, rather, a hitch in the child's beginning efforts at bladder control. Such children make up about 40 percent of the outpatient practice of pediatric urologists.

With early detection and muscle retraining, dysfunctional voiding is often cured. Allowed to progress, this abnormal wetting can lead to permanent damage to the urinary tract—even kidney failure and death.

To ward off this dangerous situation, proper diagnosis and treatment are vital. If the problem is detected before damage requires surgical correction, the child begins a simple retraining program that centers on urinating frequently, completely, and in a relaxed manner. This may require months or even years. The child goes to the bathroom at two-hour intervals, tries to maintain a continuous stream by remaining completely relaxed, and then tries to urinate again and again until unable to pass any more urine. Some investigators suggest intermittent catheterization (a catheter is threaded through the urethra into the bladder for complete emptying) and the use of any of a number of drugs: the tranquilizer diazepam (Valium) to relax the sphincter, the antidepressant imipramine (Tofranil) to help control wetting, and the antispasmodic oxybutynin chloride (Ditropan) to decrease bladder pressure.

Section 47.4

Stool Soiling in Children

What are the causes of stool soiling?

Stool soiling (messing the underwear with stool) affects about 2%
of children. Most often, the soiling occurs because of constipation.
In a few children, stool soiling is caused by a disease or a birth defect.

When stool soiling is caused by constipation, it's called encopresis. In children with encopresis, formed, soft or liquid stools that often have a very bad smell leak from the anus (the outside opening to
the rectum) around a mass of stool that is stuck in the lower bowel.
Most often, the amount of soiling in children with constipation is small
and just stains the underwear.

Stool soiling is involuntary—your child does not mean to soil his
or her pants. Soiling can occur just sometimes, or it can occur once a
day or many times a day. The consistency of the stools found in the
underwear is usually loose and sort of runny or like clay.

How are stool soiling and constipation related?

Children who have problems with constipation may have stool soiling. They also may have painful bowel movements, or they may have
incomplete emptying of stool. Sometimes they may have only 3 bowel
movements a week. Some constipated children have daily bowel movements, but they pass only small amounts of stool. Once in a while, they
have a very large bowel movement, sometimes large enough to clog
the toilet. In children who have incomplete emptying of stool, the
amount of stool left in the rectum becomes so large that stool leaks
out of the anus and produces stool soiling. Other symptoms of constipation are extreme straining during a bowel movement, abdominal
pain and bloating, crankiness, tiredness, loss of appetite between

bowel movements, wetting during the day or night, and extreme reluctance to use the toilet.

What causes constipation in a child?

Constipation may occur if your child is not eating enough high-fiber foods or drinking enough fluids. But in many children, no cause for the constipation can be found. Sometimes a child may have gotten a cut or crack in the skin around the anus from passing a large stool. Having a bowel movement may have been so painful that the child began resisting the urge to have a bowel movement. Not having a bowel movement when the urge occurs can lead to constipation.

A tendency toward constipation runs in some families. An illness that leads to poor food intake, physical inactivity, or fever can also result in constipation and stool soiling that remain a problem after the illness goes away.

What is the treatment for stool soiling due to constipation?

The first step in treating your child is to remove the stool that has collected in the lower bowel. Your doctor will probably do this in the office by giving your child an enema or a suppository. It is also possible that your doctor may have you give your child high doses of laxatives to remove the stool.

After the stool has been removed, it is important to be sure that your child can have bowel movements easily. Easy bowel movements will help prevent another large collection of stool. Treatment includes changing your child's diet to include more fluids and fiber-rich foods, having your child sit on the toilet several times a day, and giving your child laxatives every day to help soften the stools.

Why does my child need to sit on the toilet several times a day?

Having your child sit on the toilet several times a day is a way to train your child how to have a bowel movement in the toilet. Your child should sit on the toilet at least 3 times a day, for 5 minutes each time, to try to have a bowel movement. A good time to have your child sit on the toilet is after each meal. Be certain that while your child is sitting on the toilet, his or her feet can touch the floor or a footstool. Having his or her feet on the floor or a footstool will help your child pass a stool if your child needs to strain to have a bowel movement.

Give praise and rewards for sitting on the toilet and, later, for having bowel movements into the toilet or for having clean underwear.

What laxatives should my child take?

Your doctor can tell you which laxatives to use and how much to give your child. The most commonly used laxatives are milk of magnesia, mineral oil, and sorbitol. During the retraining period, a laxative must be given every day to get your child's body into a routine. If your child's stools are too loose, you can reduce the amount of laxative, but keep giving your child the laxative every day. Some laxatives taste better if they are mixed with orange juice, chocolate milk, or other drinks.

How do I know if the treatment is working?

Every day, keep a written record of your child's bowel movements, soiling episodes, and the use of medicines. This record will help you and your doctor figure out if the treatment is working.

While your child is receiving laxatives, he or she should have daily bowel movements and less soiling or no soiling at all. Large, hard bowel movements, soiling, or abdominal bloating and pain usually are signs that changes need to made in the treatment program.

Stool soiling is a problem that requires patience and effort on your part. Talk with your doctor regularly so he or she is aware of how the treatment is progressing. Your doctor can help you make any changes in the treatment plan or can give you advice about other types of treatment.

Chapter 48

Children and Sleep

Chapter Contents

Section 48.1

Healthy Sleep Is Important

From "Healthy Sleep," "Why Sleep Is Important," "Sleep Disorders,"
and, "Sleep Tips for Your Children," National Institutes of Health,
National Heart, Lung, and Blood Institute (NHLBI), 2001.

Healthy Sleep

Children ages 7 to 11 require at least nine hours of sleep each night on a consistent basis to be well-rested, but getting them to sleep at night can be a challenge. Here are some resources to help put your child to sleep for a good night's rest, so that they can be healthy and rested.

Why Sleep Is Important

Sleep Is a Basic Human Need

Sleep is a natural part of everybody's life, but many people know very little about how important it is, and some even try to get by with little sleep. Sleep is something our bodies need to do; it is not an option. Even though the exact reasons for sleep remain a mystery, we do know that during sleep many of the body's major organ and regulatory systems continue to work actively. Some parts of the brain actually increase their activity dramatically, and the body produces more of certain hormones.

Sleep, like diet and exercise, is important for our minds and bodies to function normally. In fact, sleep appears to be required for survival. Rats deprived of sleep die within two to three weeks, a time frame similar to death due to starvation.

An internal biological clock regulates the timing for sleep. It programs each person to feel sleepy during the nighttime hours and to be active during the daylight hours. Light is the cue that synchronizes the biological clock to the 24-hour cycle of day and night.

Problem Sleepiness Has Serious Consequences

Sleepiness due to chronic lack of adequate sleep is a big problem in the United States and affects many children as well as adults.

Children and even adolescents need at least 9 hours of sleep each night to do their best. Most adults need approximately 8 hours of sleep each night.

When we get less sleep (even one hour less) than we need each night, we develop a "sleep debt." If the sleep debt becomes too great, it can lead to problem sleepiness—sleepiness that occurs when you should be awake and alert, that interferes with daily routine and activities, and reduces your ability to function. Even if you do not feel sleepy, the sleep debt can have a powerful negative effect on your daytime performance, thinking, and mood, and cause you to fall asleep at inappropriate and even dangerous times.

Problem sleepiness has serious consequences—it puts adolescents and adults at risk for drowsy driving or workplace accidents. In children, it increases the risk of accidents and injuries. In addition, lack of sleep can have a negative effect on children's performance in school, on the playground, in extracurricular activities, and in social relationships.

Inadequate sleep can cause decreases in:

- Performance
- Concentration
- Reaction times
- Consolidation of information learning

Inadequate sleep can cause increases in:

- Memory lapses
- Accidents and injuries
- Behavior problems
- Mood problems

Signs of Sleep Disorders

A child who has not obtained adequate nighttime sleep is at high risk for symptoms of physical and/or mental impairment. The child may fall asleep in school, have difficulty concentrating in school and other activities, and/or exhibit behavioral problems. Some children who are sleepy become agitated rather than lethargic and may be misdiagnosed as hyperactive. Not getting enough sleep is one cause of problem sleepiness. Undiagnosed/untreated sleep disorders can also cause problem sleepiness.

Sleep Disorders

Sleep disorders affect more than 70 million Americans, including children. The most common sleep disorders are obstructive sleep apnea, insomnia, restless legs syndrome, and narcolepsy. If your child is having trouble with sleeping, or with daytime alertness, talk to your pediatrician. Note especially if your child:

- Snores loudly frequently or always

- Stops breathing for brief intervals during sleep

- Has trouble staying awake during the day

Sleep deprivation can cause daytime hyperactivity and decrease in focused attention. This can be mistaken for attention deficit hyperactivity disorder (ADHD) or other behavior disorders.

Sleep Tips for Your Children

Here are some important things you can do to ensure that your child gets enough sleep:

- Set a regular time for bed each night and stick to it.

- Establish a relaxing bedtime routine, such as giving your child a warm bath or reading him or her a story.

- Make after-dinner playtime a relaxing time. Too much activity close to bedtime can keep children awake.

- Avoid feeding children big meals close to bedtime.

- Avoid giving children anything with caffeine less than six hours before bedtime.

- Set the bedroom temperature so that it's comfortable—not too warm and not too cold.

- Make sure the bedroom is dark. If necessary, use a small nightlight.

- Keep the noise level low.

Section 48.2

Sleepwalking in Children

What is sleepwalking?

Sleepwalking is a disorder in which a child partly, but not completely, awakens during the night. The child may walk or do other things without any memory of doing so.

What are the symptoms of sleepwalking?

The child may sit up in bed and repeat certain movements, such as rubbing his or her eyes or fumbling with clothes. The child may get out of bed and walk around the room. The child may look dazed, and his or her movements may be clumsy. When you talk to your child, he or she usually will not answer you.

What should I do if my child sleepwalks?

The most important thing you can do is prevent injury by removing dangerous objects from areas that your child might reach. You should keep doors and windows closed and locked. This is especially important if you live in an apartment. If necessary, your child may have to sleep on the ground floor of your home.

When you find your child sleepwalking, you should gently guide your child back to bed. You shouldn't yell or make a loud noise to wake your child up. You shouldn't shake your child. Finally, you should never make your child feel ashamed about sleepwalking.

Should I worry if my child sleepwalks?

No. Most children who sleepwalk don't have emotional problems.

What happens to children who sleepwalk?

Most children outgrow sleepwalking. If your child sleepwalks for a long time, talk to your doctor. Your doctor may want to look at the problem more closely. Some medicines can be used to treat sleepwalking.

Section 48.3

Nightmares and Night Terrors in Children

Reprinted with permission from http://familydoctor.org/handouts/ 566.html. Copyright © 2000 American Academy of Family Physicians, updated July 2002. All Rights Reserved.

What are nightmares?

Nightmares are scary dreams. Most children have them from time to time. One out of every 4 children has nightmares more than once a week. Most nightmares happen very late in the sleep period (usually between 4 a.m. and 6 a.m.). Your child may wake up and come to you for comfort. Usually, he or she will be able to tell you what happened in the dream and why it was scary. Your child may have trouble going back to sleep. Your child might have the same dream again on other nights.

What are night terrors?

Some children have a different kind of scary dream called a "night terror." Night terrors happen during deep sleep (usually between 1 a.m. and 3 a.m.). A child having a night terror will often wake up screaming. He or she may be sweating and breathing fast. Your child's pupils (the black center of the eye) may look larger than normal. At this point, your child may still be asleep, with open eyes. He or she will be confused and might not answer when you ask what's wrong. Your child may be difficult to wake. When your child wakes, he or she usually won't remember what happened.

478

Will my child keep having nightmares or night terrors?

Nightmares and night terrors don't happen as much as children get older. Often, nightmares and night terrors stop completely when your child is a teenager. Some people, especially people who are imaginative and creative, may keep having nightmares when they are adults.

When should I worry about nightmares or night terrors?

Nightmares and night terrors in children are usually not caused by mental or physical illness. Often nightmares happen after a stressful physical or emotional event. In the first 6 months after the event, a child might have nightmares while he or she gets used to what happened in the event. If nightmares keep happening and disturb your child's sleep, they can affect your child's ability to function during the day. Talk with your doctor about whether treatment will help your child.

What should I do?

Night terrors and sleepwalking require that you protect your child during sleep. Be sure your home is safe (use toddler gates on staircases and don't use bunk beds for children who have nightmares or night terrors often). Talk with your doctor if your child ever gets hurt while sleeping. Your doctor may want to study your child during sleep.

Chapter 49

Child Care Choices

Chapter Contents

Section 49.1

Choosing Child Care

From "Choosing Child Care," Michigan Department of Consumer and Industry Affairs, Copyright © 2003 State of Michigan; reprinted with permission.

What to Look for in a Family Child Care Home

Quality family child care is the friendly and warm environment provided by a family child care parent. Good child care provides the necessary ingredients for a child's healthy growth and development: intellectually, physically, socially, and emotionally.

Family Day Care Home Checklist

Does the family child care parent:

- Appear to be warm and friendly?

- Seem calm and gentle?

- Treat each child as an individual with a different personality?

- Accept and respect your family and cultural values?

- Read and talk to the children?

- Encourage the children to express themselves?

- Have previous experience working with children?

- Have specialized training in child development?

- Have attitudes and methods of guiding and controlling behavior which you agree with?

- Serve nutritious meals and snacks?

- Take time to discuss your children with you regularly?

- Seem to have a sense of pride in the important job of caring for children?

Are there opportunities for children to:

- Be a part of a family?
- Make friends with other children?
- Receive individual attention?
- Visit nearby places of interest like the park, library, museum, or fire house?
- Use books, creative materials, games, and toys regularly?
- Study and do homework?
- Play actively and quietly both in and out-of-doors?

Does the child care home have:

- A license?
- A clean and comfortable look?
- A "children are welcome" look?
- Space for all the day care children?
- Adequate space for each child to take a nap?
- Safety caps on electrical outlets?
- A locked cabinet for the storage of medicine, household cleaners, and poisons?
- An alternate exit in case of fire?
- Adequate heat, light, and ventilation?
- A safe outdoor play area?

Do you feel that:

- Being in this day care home will be a fun and happy experience for your children?
- You can develop a relaxed, sharing relationship with this family day care parent?

Be sure to discuss:

- Total fees to be paid.
- Name, address, and phone number of parent at home/at work.

- A plan for an emergency or a child's illness.

- Who will provide food for meals and snacks, and the number of meals to be served.

- Arrangements for children to be taken to and picked up from the child care home and by whom.

- Any special arrangements for holidays or vacations.

- The time that children will arrive and leave the child care home, and any arrangement if this changes.

- Any special characteristic of your child such as food likes, habits, allergies, special medical needs.

How to Choose a Good School-Age Child Care Program

The parent's responsibilities:

- Assess the appropriateness of the program for your child.

- Communicate with your child and the care provider.

- Help the child make a smooth transition from home to school and school to home.

- Understand the operating policies of the program.

- Provide emergency information.

The child's responsibilities:

- Talk with your parents and your care provider.

- Provide information about what you are interested in doing and complete the activities you have chosen.

- Understand the rules for the activities and for getting along with others. Know the consequences of inappropriate behavior.

- Be responsible for your own behavior and your own belongings.

- Respect and take care of the provided materials and equipment.

The program's responsibilities:

- Provide written policies and procedures including emergency procedures and financial policies.

- Provide opportunities for communication among the care providers, the child, the parent, the teacher, and school personnel.

- Provide a comfortable, fun, relaxing environment that is purposefully different from academically oriented activities but promotes the child's development in all areas and supports the academic work of the school day.

- Provide for leisure time as defined by the child.

- Provide time for diverse activities such as homework, recreation, physical development, socialization and the development of friendship, leisure, and outdoor play.

- Respect and promote the spontaneity and serendipity of childhood.

- Provide equipment and learning/play materials that are age-appropriate and encourage diverse choices.

- Provide a well-organized program with a predictable daily routine.

- Provide a place for each child's individual belongings.

- Provide an accessible drop-off and pick-up arrangement including a place for parents to wait while the child completes an activity.

- Provide nutritious snacks.

Get answers to these questions:

- Is this program licensed?

- What are the hours and days the program is open? Holidays?

- What are the fees? When must they be paid?

- How are parents involved? Are parents welcome at any time?

- Who makes major policy decisions?

- What is the discipline policy?

- Is transportation provided?

- Are the children grouped by age, interest area, or ability?

- Who is the main person responsible?

- How many children is each care provider responsible for (adult/child ratio)?

Child Care Is a Service: You Are the Consumer

Warning signals:

- The caregiver/center does not permit or encourage parents to observe or visit while children are in care.
- Children are left in care without the immediate and direct supervision of an adult.
- The caregiver spends much of the time scolding, ordering, and belittling children:
  - screaming, yelling, or swearing at the children.
  - making fun of the children, or a specific child.
  - ridiculing or threatening a child.
  - criticizing a child.
- Caregiver(s) are physically rough and abusive with the children.
- The home or center is filthy and/or unsafe.
- Complaints from your child about the care, or your child starts to act nervous or distressed about the child care program. Investigate immediately.
- A child repeatedly gets bruises or injuries; the presence of a bruise or injury is unexplainable.

After Child Care Begins

- Talk with your children about the day care home or center.
- Ask very specific questions about your child's day and the events of that day.
- Listen to what your child is saying.
- Visit your child's day care at unexpected times of the day.
- Speak with your provider about any concerns or questions you have.

Section 49.2

Four Steps to Selecting a Child Care Provider

Excerpted and adapted from "Four Steps to Selecting a Child Care Provider," Administration for Children and Families, U.S. Department of Health and Human Services, http://www.acf.dhhs.gov/programs/ccb/faq1/4steps.htm, June 2001.

Four Steps to Selecting a Child Care Provider

One: Interview Caregivers

Call prospective caregivers and ask questions such as: Is there an opening for my child? What hours and days are you open? Where are you located? How much does care cost? Is financial assistance available? How many children are in your care? What age groups do you serve? Do you provide transportation? Do you provide meals (breakfast, lunch, dinner, snacks)? Do you have a license, accreditation, or other certification? When can I come to visit?

Next, visit—visit more than once, and stay as long as you can. Be sure to ask about policies regarding discipline, sickness, emergencies, training of staff and substitutes, immunization requirements, licensing or certification, use of back-up caregivers, naps, and toileting. Also ask for references.

Two: Check References

Ask other parents questions such as: Is the caregiver reliable on a daily basis? How does the caregiver discipline your child? Does your child enjoy the child care experience? How does the caregiver respond to you as a parent? Is the caregiver respectful of your values and culture? Would you recommend the caregiver without reservation? If your child is no longer with the caregiver, why did you leave?

Ask your local child care resource and referral program or licensing office what regulations child care providers should meet. Also ask about how you can check to see if there is a record of complaints about the child care provider you are considering.

Three: Make the Decision for Quality Care

From what you heard and saw, ask yourself which available caregiver will provide affordable care with an atmosphere where your child will be happy and have his or her special needs met. Also consider which caregiver's values are most compatible with your family's values.

Four: Stay Involved

Talk to your child's caregiver every day, and talk to your child every day about how the day went. Visit and observe your child in care at different times of the day. Be involved in your child's activities.

Work with your caregiver to resolve issues and concerns that may arise. Stay informed about your child's growth and development while in care. Promote good working conditions for your child care provider, and network with other parents.

Section 49.3

Be Sure Your Child Care Setting Is as Safe as It Can Be

Excerpted from "Be Sure Your Child Care Setting Is as Safe as It Can Be," an undated document produced by the U.S. Consumer Product Safety Commission (CPSC), CPSC Doc. No. 242, available online at http://www.cpsc.gov/cpscpub/pubs/chldcare.html.

In a recent national study, Consumer Product Safety Commission (CPSC) staff visited a number of child care settings and found that two-thirds of them had one or more potentially serious hazards. Use the safety tips in this checklist to help keep young children safe.

* *Cribs.* Make sure cribs meet current national safety standards and are in good condition. Look for a certification safety seal. Older cribs may not meet current standards. Crib slats should be no more than 2 3/8" apart, and mattresses should fit snugly.

- *Soft bedding.* Be sure that no pillows, soft bedding, or comforters are used when you put babies to sleep. Babies should be put to sleep on their backs in a crib with a firm, flat mattress.

- *Playground surfacing.* Look for safe surfacing on outdoor playgrounds—at least 12 inches of wood chips, mulch, sand or pea gravel, or mats made of safety-tested rubber or rubber-like materials.

- *Playground maintenance.* Check playground surfacing and equipment regularly to make sure they are maintained in good condition.

- *Safety gates.* Be sure that safety gates are used to keep children away from potentially dangerous areas, especially stairs.

- *Window blind and curtain cords.* Be sure mini-blinds and Venetian blinds do not have looped cords. Check that vertical blinds, continuous looped blinds, and drapery cords have tension or tie-down devices to hold the cords tight. These safety devices can prevent strangulation in the loops of window blind and curtain cords.

- *Clothing drawstrings.* Be sure there are no drawstrings around the hood and neck of children's outerwear clothing. Other types of clothing fasteners, like snaps, zippers, or hook and loop fasteners (such as Velcro), should be used. Drawstrings can catch on playground and other equipment and can strangle young children.

- *Recalled products.* Check that no recalled products are being used and that a current list of recalled children's products is readily visible. Recalled products pose a threat of injury or death. Displaying a list of recalled products will remind caretakers and parents to remove or repair potentially dangerous children's toys and products.

Section 49.4

Choosing a Babysitter

Commonly Asked Questions

How do I choose a babysitter?

- Ask friends, neighbors, and coworkers to suggest a reliable sitter.

- Ask your child's doctor, your local recreation center, or an American Red Cross chapter for suggestions.

- You may want to interview the person before you hire him. Find out if he has experience with children, if he knows infant and child CPR, and if he has other qualifications that are important to you (able to provide transportation, cook, etc.).

- Invite the sitter to your home so you and your children can get to know him. Watch how he talks and plays with your children. How do your children respond to him?

What should my babysitter know?

- Give the sitter a brief tour of your house.

- Explain your family's full emergency plan for fire, weather, and first aid emergencies.

- Show the sitter where he can find first aid and other emergency supplies (fire extinguishers, candles, first aid, etc.).

- Let the sitter know of any special problems that your child has, such as allergies or wetting the bed.

- Tell the sitter any special rules you have for the children (TV time, bed times, snacks, having friends over, etc.).

- What should your sitter do if your child breaks a rule? (Time out, to bed early, etc.).

- Where and when can you be reached? By what name?

- Should the sitter answer your phone? How? Should he take messages?

- Make your expectations clear. If you do not want the sitter to have friends over, tell him. Can the sitter leave the house with the children? Drive the children? Use the phone to call friends?

What are some general rules to follow?

Make sure the sitter knows a few general safety rules:

- Do not give your child any medicine without your permission.

- Do not leave your child, alone, even for a minute.

- Be alert when your child is near water or taking a bath. Children can drown in only a few inches of water if they are not watched carefully.

- Do not feed your child under 4 years old large pieces of solid food. Cut food like grapes and hotdogs into small pieces. Do not give your child nuts, popcorn, hard candy, raw carrots, or other hard, smooth foods.

- Do not let your child play with plastic bags, latex balloons, coins, or other small objects. These are all choking hazards.

- Keep your child away from electrical outlets, stairs, and stoves.

What information should I leave?

- Where you will be at all times and phone numbers where you can be reached.

- Leave an emergency phone list by the phone, including numbers for: poison control, police, fire, ambulance, doctor, and hospital.

- Leave a phone list of neighbors, friends, and family members who can be contacted in case of emergency.

- Write down your home phone number, address, and general directions to your house.

- If your child needs to be given medication, write down specific instructions for the sitter.

- Leave a medical release for emergency care.

- Use the checklist to make sure you covered everything.

How did things go?

- When you return home, ask the sitter how things went. Were there any problems? Any questions? How did the children behave?

- After the sitter leaves, ask your children the same questions. Did they enjoy the sitter?

Chapter 50

Help Your Child Use the Internet Responsibly

A Note to Parents

The same advances in computer and telecommunication technology that allow our children to reach out to new sources of knowledge and cultural experiences are unfortunately also leaving them vulnerable to exploitation and harm by computer-sex offenders. The information in this chapter is intended to help you to begin to understand the complexities of online child exploitation. For further information, please contact your local FBI office or the National Center for Missing and Exploited Children at 800-843-5678.

Introduction

While online computer exploration opens a world of possibilities for children, expanding their horizons and exposing them to different cultures and ways of life, they can be exposed to dangers as they hit the road exploring the information highway. There are individuals who attempt to sexually exploit children through the use of online services and the internet. Some of these individuals gradually seduce

This chapter includes text excerpted from "A Parent's Guide to Internet Safety," Federal Bureau of Investigation (FBI), U.S. Department of Justice, and "Rules in Cyberspace," U.S. Department of Justice, updated May 31, 2002. Additional glossary terms were excerpted from [1] "Parents Guide to the Internet," U.S. Department of Education, November 1997; and [2] "Glossary of Terms," Chapter 3, *Guide to Web Browsing*, U.S. Department of the Interior, revised December 2002.

their targets through the use of attention, affection, kindness, and even gifts. These individuals are often willing to devote considerable amounts of time, money, and energy in this process. They listen to and empathize with the problems of children. They will be aware of the latest music, hobbies, and interests of children. These individuals attempt to gradually lower children's inhibitions by slowly introducing sexual context and content into their conversations.

There are other individuals, however, who immediately engage in sexually explicit conversation with children. Some offenders primarily collect and trade child-pornographic images, while others seek face-to-face meetings with children via online contacts. It is important for parents to understand that children can be indirectly victimized through conversation (that is, "chat") as well as the transfer of sexually explicit information and material. Computer-sex offenders may also be evaluating children they come in contact with online for future face-to-face contact and direct victimization. Parents and children should remember that a computer-sex offender can be any age or sex—the person does not have to fit the caricature of a dirty, unkempt, older man wearing a raincoat to be someone who could harm a child.

Children, especially adolescents, are sometimes interested in and curious about sexuality and sexually explicit material. They may be moving away from the total control of parents and seeking to establish new relationships outside their family. Because they may be curious, children/adolescents sometimes use their online access to actively seek out such materials and individuals. Sex offenders targeting children will use and exploit these characteristics and needs. Some adolescent children may also be attracted to and lured by online offenders closer to their age who, although not technically child molesters, may be dangerous. Nevertheless, they have been seduced and manipulated by a clever offender and do not fully understand or recognize the potential danger of these contacts.

What Are Signs That Your Child Might Be at Risk Online?

- Your child spends large amounts of time online, especially at night.

- You find pornography on your child's computer.

- Your child receives phone calls from men you don't know or is making calls, sometimes long distance, to numbers you don't recognize.

- Your child receives mail, gifts, or packages from someone you don't know.

- Your child turns the computer monitor off or quickly changes the screen on the monitor when you come into the room.

- Your child becomes withdrawn from the family.

- Your child is using an online account belonging to someone else.

What You Should Do If You Suspect Your Child Is Communicating with a Sexual Predator Online

- Consider talking openly with your child about your suspicions. Tell them about the dangers of computer-sex offenders.

- Review what is on your child's computer. If you don't know how, ask a friend, coworker, relative, or other knowledgeable person. Pornography or any kind of sexual communication can be a warning sign.

- Use the Caller ID service to determine who is calling your child. Most telephone companies that offer Caller ID also offer a service that allows you to block your number from appearing on someone else's Caller ID. Telephone companies also offer an additional service feature that rejects incoming calls that you block. This rejection feature prevents computer-sex offenders or anyone else from calling your home anonymously.

- Devices can be purchased that show telephone numbers that have been dialed from your home phone. Additionally, the last number called from your home phone can be retrieved provided that the telephone is equipped with a redial feature. You will also need a telephone pager to complete this retrieval.

- This is done using a numeric-display pager and another phone that is on the same line as the first phone with the redial feature. Using the two phones and the pager, a call is placed from the second phone to the pager. When the paging terminal beeps for you to enter a telephone number, you press the redial button on the first (or suspect) phone. The last number called from that phone will then be displayed on the pager.

- Monitor your child's access to all types of live electronic communications (such as chat rooms, instant messages, internet relay chat, etc.), and monitor your child's e-mail. Computer-sex offenders

495

almost always meet potential victims via chat rooms. After meeting a child online, they will continue to communicate electronically, often via e-mail.

Should any of the following situations arise in your household, via the internet or online service, you should immediately contact your local or state law enforcement agency, the FBI, and the National Center for Missing and Exploited Children:

1. Your child or anyone in the household has received child pornography;

2. Your child has been sexually solicited by someone who knows that your child is under 18 years of age;

3. Your child has received sexually explicit images from someone that knows your child is under the age of 18.

If one of these scenarios occurs, keep the computer turned off in order to preserve any evidence for future law enforcement use. Unless directed to do so by the law enforcement agency, you should not attempt to copy any of the images and/or text found on the computer.

What You Can Do to Minimize the Chances of an Online Exploiter Victimizing Your Child

*   Communicate, and talk to your child about sexual victimization and potential online danger.

*   Spend time with your children online. Have them teach you about their favorite online destinations.

*   Keep the computer in a common room in the house, not in your child's bedroom. It is much more difficult for a computer-sex offender to communicate with a child when the computer screen is visible to a parent or another member of the household.

*   Utilize parental controls provided by your service provider and/or blocking software. While electronic chat can be a great place for children to make new friends and discuss various topics of interest, it is also prowled by computer-sex offenders. Use of chat rooms, in particular, should be heavily monitored. While parents should utilize these mechanisms, they should not totally rely on them.

*   Always maintain access to your child's online account and randomly check his/her e-mail. Be aware that your child could be

contacted through the U.S. mail. Be up front with your child about your access and reasons why.

- Teach your child the responsible use of the resources online. There is much more to the online experience than chat rooms.

- Find out what computer safeguards are utilized by your child's school, the public library, and at the homes of your child's friends. These are all places, outside your normal supervision, where your child could encounter an online predator.

- Understand, even if your child was a willing participant in any form of sexual exploitation, that he/she is not at fault and is the victim. The offender always bears the complete responsibility for his or her actions.

- Instruct your children:
  - to never arrange a face-to-face meeting with someone they met online;
  - to never upload (post) pictures of themselves onto the internet or online service to people they do not personally know;
  - to never give out identifying information such as their name, home address, school name, or telephone number;
  - to never download pictures from an unknown source, as there is a good chance there could be sexually explicit images;
  - to never respond to messages or bulletin board postings that are suggestive, obscene, belligerent, or harassing;
  - that whatever they are told online may or may not be true.

Rules for Kids In Cyberspace

DO

1. DO use the internet to help with schoolwork. The internet is a source of great volumes of information. It's like having the world's largest library at your fingertips.

2. DO use the internet to "visit" museums in far away places.

3. DO use the internet to meet children in other countries or to keep in touch with pen pals who live far away in this country or other countries. Some online services host chat rooms especially for children, and monitor them periodically for safety.

497

4. DO be careful about talking to "strangers" on a computer network. Who are these people anyway? Some people say and do things which are NOT NICE.

5. DO use the internet to learn more about universities and colleges that you may be interested in attending.

6. DO respect the privacy of other users on the internet, just as you expect your privacy to be respected.

7. DO be careful when you "download" (copy) programs from the internet. Use a virus scan program before loading it on your computer.

DON'T

1. DON'T give your password to anyone. Passwords are intended to protect your computer and your files. It's like giving the key to your house away.

2. DON'T answer messages that make you feel uncomfortable because they seem improper, indecent, or threatening. TELL A GROWN-UP RIGHT AWAY.

3. DON'T give any personal information, such as your family's address, phone number, credit card or calling card numbers, your school's name, or your picture to anyone on a computer network that you don't personally know.

4. DON'T arrange to meet anyone you've met on the internet without telling your parents. Some people on the internet lie about who they are, how old they are, and why they want to meet you.

5. DON'T try to break into computers. It's not a game. It's a crime and it's an invasion of privacy.

6. DON'T steal copyrighted computer programs ("software") by copying it from the internet. This is the same as stealing it from a store.

7. DON'T make copies of any copyrighted material, like books, magazines, or music without the permission of the author, publisher or artist.

8. DON'T copy material that you find on the internet and pretend that it's your own work. It's the same as copying a book or magazine article and pretending that you wrote it.

Frequently Asked Questions

My child has received an e-mail advertising for a pornographic website, what should I do?

Generally, advertising for an adult, pornographic website that is sent to an e-mail address does not violate federal law or the current laws of most states. In some states it may be a violation of law if the sender knows the recipient is under the age of 18. Such advertising can be reported to your service provider and, if known, the service provider of the originator. It can also be reported to your state and federal legislators, so they can be made aware of the extent of the problem.

Is any service safer than the others?

Sex offenders have contacted children via most of the major online services and the internet. The most important factors in keeping your child safe online are the utilization of appropriate blocking software and/or parental controls, along with open, honest discussions with your child, monitoring his/her online activity, and following the tips in this chapter.

Should I just forbid my child from going online?

There are dangers in every part of our society. By educating your children to these dangers and taking appropriate steps to protect them, they can benefit from the wealth of information now available online.

Helpful Definitions

address: The unique location of an information site on the internet, a specific file (for example, a web page), or an e-mail user. [1]

applets: Small Java programs that are embedded in an HTML page. See also HTML, Java. [2]

bookmark: A saved link to a website that has been added to a list of saved links so that you can simply click on it rather than having to retype the address when visiting the site again. [1]

browser: Application software that creates an interactive graphical interface for searching, finding, viewing and managing information over the internet. [2]

CD-ROM (Compact Disk Read Only Memory): A computer disk that can store large amounts of information and is generally used on computers with CD-ROM drives. [1]

chat: Real-time text conversation between users in a chat room with no expectation of privacy. All chat conversation is accessible by all individuals in the chat room while the conversation is taking place.

.com: This refers to commercial, and is the designation at the end of a web address that means the site is a commercial site. See also .gov, .org [2]

domain name: The unique name of each internet site. A domain name consists of two or more name separated by a dot. [2]

download: To copy a file from one computer system to another. From the internet user's point of view, to download a file is to request it from another computer (or from a web page on another computer) and to receive it. [1]

electronic mail (e-mail): A function that provides for the transmission of messages and files between computers over a communications network similar to mailing a letter via the postal service. E-mail is stored on a server, where it will remain until the addressee retrieves it. Anonymity can be maintained by the sender by predetermining what the receiver will see as the "from" address. Another way to conceal one's identity is to use an "anonymous re-mailer," which is a service that allows the user to send an e-mail message repackaged under the re-mailer's own header, stripping off the originator's name completely.

file server: A computer whose principal purpose is to store files and provide network access to those files. [2]

freenet: A community network that provides free online access, usually to local residents, and often includes its own forums and news. [1]

FTP (file transfer protocol): The language that is used to transfer a program or file over the internet. [2]

GIF (graphic interchange format): The standard format for image files on the Web. [2]

hardware: A term for the nuts, bolts, and wires of computer equipment and the actual computer and related machines. [1]

.gov: This refers to government, and is the designation at the end of a web address that means the site is a government site. See also .com, .org [2]

home page: The site that is the starting point on the World Wide Web for a particular group or organization. [1]

HTML (hyper text markup language): This is the code that is used to program all web pages. [2]

hypertext link: An easy method for retrieving information by choosing highlighted words or icons on the screen. The link will take you to related documents or sites. [1]

hypertext transfer protocol (http): A standard used by World Wide Web servers to provide rules for moving text, images, sound, video, and other multimedia files across the internet. [1]

icon: A small picture on a Web page that represents the topic or information category of another Web page. Frequently, the icon is a hypertext link to that page. [1]

instant messages: Private, real-time text conversation between two users in a chat room.

internet: An immense, global network that connects computers via telephone lines and/or fiber networks to storehouses of electronic information. With only a computer, a modem, a telephone line, and a service provider, people from all over the world can communicate and share information with little more than a few keystrokes.

internet service provider (ISP): These services offer direct, full access to the internet at a flat, monthly rate and often provide electronic-mail service for their customers. ISPs often provide space on their servers for their customers to maintain World Wide Web (WWW) sites. Not all ISPs are commercial enterprises. Educational, governmental, and non-profit organizations also provide internet access to their members.

IP address: The internet protocol address which is a 32-bit address assigned to a host.

JPEG (Joint Photographic Experts Group): A popular method used to compress and display images on the Web. [2]

modem: A device that allows computers to communicate with each other over telephone lines or other delivery systems by changing digital signals to telephone signals for transmission and then back to digital signals. Modems come in different speeds: the higher the speed, the faster the data is transmitted. [1]

netiquette: Rules or manners for interacting courteously with others online (such as not typing a message in all capital letters, which is equivalent to shouting). [1]

online service: A company such as America Online (AOL) that provides its members access to the internet through its own special user interface as well as additional services such as chat rooms, children's areas, travel planning, and financial management. [1]

.org: This refers to organization, and is the designation at the end of a web address that means the site is an organizational site. See also .com, .gov [2]

real time: When you and another user are linked at the same time, as with the "chat" function. On the other hand, e-mail communication is delayed. [2]

search engine: A program that performs keyword searches for information on the internet. [1]

server: A host computer in a network that provides information to other computers in the form of HTTP and FTP. [2]

software: A computer program or set of instructions. System software operates on the machine itself and is invisible to you. Application software allows you to carry out certain activities, such as word processing, games, and spreadsheets. [1]

URL (uniform resource locator): The World Wide Web address of a site on the internet. For example, the URL for the White House is http://www.whitehouse.gov. [1]

virus: A piece of programming code inserted into other programming to cause some unexpected and usually undesirable event, such as lost or damaged files. Viruses can be transmitted by downloading programming from other sites or be present on a diskette. The source of the file you're downloading or of a diskette you've received is often unaware of the virus. The virus lies dormant until circumstances cause its code to be executed by the computer. [1]

website: This is a location on the internet. It can be accessed by typing in a specific URL (address). [2]

World Wide Web (WWW): A hypertext-based system that allows you to browse through a variety of linked internet resources organized by colorful, graphics-oriented home pages. [1]

Chapter 51

Your Child and Media-Related Concerns

Chapter Contents

Section 51.1

Teaching Your Child Good TV Habits

"Children and TV Viewing," by Dr. Russell Robertson. © 1999 Medical College of Wisconsin; reprinted with permission of the Medical College of Wisconsin/MCW HealthLink (http://healthlink.mcw.edu). Dr. Russell Robertson is an Associate Dean for Faculty Affairs and an Associate Professor of Family and Community Medicine at the Medical College of Wisconsin.

Two sets of information came my way about the unhealthy effects of too much television on children.

The first showed a clear association between the amount of time spent in front of the TV and scores on standardized testing. The kids who watched the most TV (up to six hours per day) scored the lowest, while those who watched the least scored the highest.

The second demonstrated a link between time spent watching TV and obesity in children. It comes as no surprise that those children who watched more TV were less physically active and more likely to be overweight. Although the study did not mention computer games or prolonged time on the internet it would be reasonable to come to the same conclusions.

I recommend the following to limit the time spent watching TV or at the computer:

- Ask your kids to tell you what their favorite shows are and together predetermine which ones they are going to watch.

- Set limits to time spent on the computer when not engaged in schoolwork. More than one to two hours per day is excessive, in my opinion.

- Help them to structure the rest of their time by looking for opportunities in the community such as after-school sports, school-based clubs, scouting, and school or community artistic endeavors (band, orchestra, etc.). Do not ask them if they wish to participate but rather which one or two activities they will choose, with your guidance.

- Make frequent trips to the library and bring home age-appropriate books for your kids to read.

- Play games or sports with them.

- Last but not least, set a good example.

Section 51.2

Who's Watching What They're Watching?

"Who's Watching What They're Watching?" by Russell Robertson. © 2001 Medical College of Wisconsin; reprinted with permission of the Medical College of Wisconsin/MCW HealthLink (http://healthlink.mcw.edu). Dr. Russell Robertson is an Associate Dean for Faculty Affairs and an Associate Professor of Family and Community Medicine at the Medical College of Wisconsin.

How many parents would consciously serve their children polluted water to drink? How many of us would make a meal consisting of rancid or decaying food for our families? These things would temporarily sicken them at the least and would most likely pass through the digestive system with most likely no long-term ill effects. Yet many of us are content to allow our children sit for countless hours basking in the cold blue light of the television as it spews forth a multiplicity of images that often indelibly imprint themselves in the minds of our children.

There are unmistakable connections between poor school performance and the number of hours of television children watch.

Two landmark studies in Canada and South Africa demonstrated a clear correlation linking televised violence to increased violence in the community. A recent study confirmed again the fact that daytime television dramas depict irresponsible sexual behavior with little or no mention of contraception or measures to prevent the spread of sexually transmitted diseases. The so called "V" chip and the generous commitment of the major networks to produce three hours per week of children's programming are hollow promises that look far better on paper and in political campaigns that they will in reality.

As parents, it is unmistakably clear that we cannot trust network executives to program material that is safe for consumption by children. It is also clear that we must and can do a better job of monitoring their media consumption habits.

The American Academy of Pediatrics and the American Medical Association have recently published new guidelines for parents that if implemented would greatly benefit all Americans. I've listed the majority here for your review.

1. Be alert to the shows that your children see.

2. Avoid using television, videos, or video games as a babysitter.

3. Limit the use of all media. TV should be watched for no more than two hours per day. Set situation limits as well: no TV or video games before school, during daytime hours, during meals, or before homework is done.

4. Keep TVs and video players out of your child's bedrooms.

5. Turn the TV off during meals.

6. Plan the shows you watch and avoid "seeing what's on."

7. Don't make the TV the focal point of the house.

8. Watch what your children are watching.

9. Be careful of viewing TV just before bedtimes as emotion-invoking images may intrude into sleep.

10. Learn about the movies that are playing and the videos available for rental or purchase. (Several movie guides are printed by family friendly organizations)

11. Become media literate in order to learn how and why the media does what it does.

12. Set a good example by limiting your own TV viewing.

13. Let your voice be heard by insisting on better programming for our children.

Section 51.3

How to Talk to Your Child about the News

Excerpted from "Discussing the News with 3- to 7-Year-Olds: What to
Do?" by Sydney Gurewitz Clemens. © 1998 by the National Association
for the Education of Young Children; reprinted with permission.

It is hard for most of us to move toward talking about an awful
subject like war, or death, or divorce, or earthquake, or flood or ... the
list is endless. But children need someone to help them unpack their
thinking and their fears, and to help them know what the emergency
plan is for them.

After any important event occurs, the TV repetition makes sure
the children will know something is going on. It is important that
teachers and parents of young children allow them the time to express
what is on their minds. The following recommendations are based on
children aged 3 and up.

- In a circle or with small groups ask a provocative question. Be
  willing to leave a long silence. (Start counting and don't say
  anything before 75.) Probably one child or more will have a
  great deal to say.

- Let each of the children speak at length.

- Resist the temptation to correct errors as the children explain what they think is going on. Validate what they are
  feeling.

- Keep notes, and take a turn for yourself—at the end or at a
  later time that day.

- When it's your turn, tell them what you think is going on. Don't
  turn attention to their errors, but tell the version you think is
  accurate. Do pay attention to their emotions.

- You can help a child write a letter about what they feel and
  send it to the proper recipient.

- You can suggest that the child make a picture.

Your job is to reassure the child he or she is safe and will be cared for. If the children are in danger, you can point out that adults (including you) are responsible not only for taking care of the danger, but also for taking care of the children.

Section 51.4

Talking to Your Children about War

Excerpted and reprinted with permission from *Parents' Guide for Talking to Their Children about War*, © 2003 National Center for Children Exposed to Violence. For additional information, visit www.nccev.org.

Why Should I Talk about This with My Children?

With increasing news about war and with talk about the threats of terrorism, children, their parents, and caregivers may feel uncertain and robbed of a basic sense of safety and security. We all share concerns about the horrors and dangers of war and terrorism. However, as adults and parents, it is our job to help our children and each other cope as best as we can with concerns that will confront us as individuals, families, communities, and as a nation.

Your clam ability to listen to your children's concerns is one of the most powerful ways of helping them to learn, understand, and feel safe and secure in the most important part of their world—their families.

When Using These Guidelines What Should I Keep in Mind?

- Children whose family members or friends are directly involved in war or are in the military will be more directly impacted.

- Ongoing threats of terrorism may add to children's distress related to war and war may heighten concerns about terrorism.

- Children who have experienced trauma and loss or have long-standing emotional problems are most vulnerable during periods of new threats.

- Reactions will vary from child to child depending upon a variety of factors including their personality, age, developmental level, and personal history.

- Not all children will appear to be affected by news of war. For some children, especially younger ones, it is not helpful to "force the issue" if it does not appear to have an impact.

- When thinking about how to talk to your children, take your lead from them in terms of what they need and what they are thinking and feeling.

- Helping children deal with a difficult event is hard work—parents should seek help and support from other adults when needed.

What Reactions May I Notice in My Child?

There is no one way in which children express worries and fears at times of greater stress. Here are some examples of how children communicate their upset feelings:

- Irritability or difficulty in being calmed and soothed

- Tearfulness, sadness, or talking about scary ideas or scary feelings

- Anger directed towards specific communities or ethnic groups

- Fighting with peers, parents, or other adults or not being able to get along

- Changes in sleep patterns, nightmares, or waking in the night

- Wanting to stay close to their parents or refusing to go to school

- Physical complaints such as stomachaches, headaches, or changes in toileting habits

How Can I Help My Children?

For some children, talking about their concerns with the adults they trust can help them feel less alone. Giving them time to ask questions can be very helpful. For some children, talking might be very hard. Recognizing your children's many different reactions can be the most important beginning to helping your children.

General Guidelines

- *Television and Information:* Watching too much television coverage of war, violence, and terrorism, especially graphic images, can be harmful to children of all ages. Monitor and limit the amount of news coverage they watch. Pre-school and younger school-age children will be especially worried the more war news they see and hear. If your school-age and older child is interested in watching news, watch with them when you can so that you can talk about what you have seen and heard.

- *Talking about the Daily Events:* Do not assume that you know what your children are thinking and feeling. Create a safe and comfortable environment to talk to them. Take cues from them in terms of how much they want to discuss what is going on in the world. It is important that routine and structure are maintained in children's lives and that they continue to enjoy life, with their friends and family.

What Questions Are Children Likely to Have?

Are we safe and can we be attacked?

When children ask questions about safety, often they are really looking for reassurance that their immediate world of family, friends, and other important figures in their lives are safe now. The amount of details about safety and security in the broader world that children will find useful will depend on their age.

Whose fault is it?

Many adults have very strong feelings about our country going to war. Parents should respond honestly to questions about their views of war that their children may ask.

What does this mean to me? How is this going to change my life?

During stressful times, children may become even more concerned about what affects them personally than usual. Expect your children to think more about themselves, at least at first. Once they feel that their needs are being met, they are more likely to think about helping others.

How can I help?

Some children may want to express personal opinions about war or to find ways of helping the country at a time of crisis. They can start by taking care of themselves—telling you what's on their minds, about their views, their fears, and their hopes. They can also offer help by listening to the views and feelings of other members of their community—their friends and classmates, their teacher, and other adults. Over time, they can think about how they, along with other members of their community, might be able to do something helpful for our armed forces and their families as well as for other children and families who also suffer the effects of war.

What If My Children Don't Seem Upset by Events around War?

Many children may appear disinterested and even irritated by the continued attention focused on war. The size and scope of a child's world is smaller than that of an adult—the situation may simply not have affected them directly and they appropriately may be far more concerned about their own life. Young children may not understand, or even know, much about what has happened or what it means. Other children may be concerned, but afraid to ask questions or to share their feelings. Children may visit their concerns briefly, but then turn to play or involve themselves in schoolwork rather then letting themselves feel overwhelmed. Paying attention to changes in behavior and mood as well as asking about children's ideas are the first steps to recognizing whether and when they may have concerns about war.

What If I Have More Questions? Where Can I Turn for Answers?

You may have many more questions or concerns. If you are concerned about your children, please contact a trusted professional in your community. If you would like further information, you may also contact the National Center for Children Exposed to Violence through our website at www.nccev.org or by calling 877-49-NCCEV (62238).

511

Chapter 52

It's Not Too Early to Talk about Alcohol, Tobacco, and Other Drugs

Chapter Contents

Section 52.1

Parents Can Make a Difference

Excerpted from *Keeping Youth Drug Free*. Center for Substance Abuse Prevention, Substance Abuse and Mental Health Services Administration, DHHS Publication No. (SMA)-3772. Rockville, MD, 2002.

Note: In this chapter, a child is referred to as "him" in some places and "her" in others. This is done for easier reading. Every point is the same for girls and boys, unless otherwise specified.

If You Love a Child, You Need to Know This

By the time they enter preschool, most children have seen adults smoking cigarettes or drinking alcohol either in real life or in the media, or both. Children today are exposed to illegal drugs as early as elementary school, so it's never too early to talk with your child about drugs.

You may wonder how useful the information is to you and your child. Some parents aren't aware of how common alcohol, tobacco, and illegal drugs are in their child's life. The facts may surprise you. However, they shouldn't discourage you. Parents have an incredible influence on their child's decision whether or not to use drugs. Research shows that parental influence is a primary reason that youth don't use drugs. Most teens who do not use alcohol, tobacco, or illegal drugs credit their parents as a major factor in that decision.

Differences Boys and Girls

There's no denying that boys and girls are different. Differences between the sexes become more obvious with the onset of puberty, as do boys' and girls' needs when it comes to resisting alcohol, tobacco, and illegal drug use. Boys and girls experience adolescence differently because of various social, cultural, physiological, and psychological challenges. For example, among boys, puberty tends to increase aggressive behavior, while among girls puberty tends to bring a higher incidence of depression. Studies show that girls may lose self-confidence and self-worth during this pivotal time, become less physically active, perform less well in school, and neglect their own interests and aspirations. During these years, girls are more vulnerable to negative outside influences and to mixed messages about risky behaviors. Girls are also at higher risk than boys for sexual abuse, which has been associated with substance abuse.

Puberty generally occurs a year or two later in boys than it does in girls. The physical changes boys go through can cause a lack of coordination that may lead to injury. Boys tend to experience mood swings and can have feelings of anxiety during puberty. During these years, boys crave exploration of things associated with being grown up, including sexual behavior or experimentation with alcohol, tobacco, or illegal drugs.

But boys and girls also have a lot in common. They need the same kinds of guidance, information, and nurturing from their parents to help them grow into healthy, well-informed adolescents and adults. Both boys and girls are less likely to smoke, drink, or use illegal drugs if they have:

- A positive attitude, an ability to adapt to changing circumstances, and a belief in their ability to "handle things."

- A warm close-knit family and parental supervision with consistent discipline.

- Close friends, an extended family that provides support, community resources, and

- Family and community attitudes that do not tolerate substance abuse.

Establish and Maintain Good Communication with Your Child

Get into the habit of talking with your child every day. Your child is an individual with hopes, fears, likes, dislikes, and special talents. The more you know about your child, the easier it will be to guide her toward more positive activities and friendships. As a result, your child will be less likely to experiment with alcohol, tobacco, or illegal drugs. Establishing a close relationship with your child now will make it easier for her to come to you when she has a problem.

It's important not to be critical. Positive reinforcement and constructive support are more effective in influencing children's behavior than criticism.

Action Steps to Good Communication

1. Know your child. How well do you know your child? Can you answer the following questions:

    *   What is your child's favorite color?

    *   Who is your child's best friend?

    *   What are the names of your child's teachers? Who is your child's favorite teacher? Do you know why?

    *   Who are some of your child's role models? What does he admire about those individuals?

    *   What would your child wish for if she saw a falling star?

    *   What is your child's favorite food?

    *   What is your child's favorite movie or TV show?

    *   What three words would your child use to describe himself? To describe you?

    *   What are your child's hobbies?

    *   What are your child's future goals?

    Ask your child what the answers are and let him lead you into a longer conversation. You can talk about one question a day or one a week. Think of other questions you can ask one another. Consider making the questions and conversations part of your daily routine.

2. Set aside a few minutes a day to talk about problems or challenges that might have come up during the day and discuss how you handled them.

3. Validate your child's feelings.

4. Practice active listening.

5. Ask questions. Children have a lot to share when they think their opinions matter.

Communication Is Important Because Some Kids Use Drugs to Satisfy Curiosity

Children are very curious about alcohol, tobacco, and illegal drugs. They are exposed to drug messages on TV, in the movies and videos, in newspapers and magazines, at school, on the internet, and in conversations with friends and family. Even if we have done an outstanding job of educating and nurturing the children in our care, some children will remain curious about alcohol, tobacco, and illegal drugs. Their sources of drug information may not always be accurate or have their best interests at heart. But you do. That's why it's important for you to know about the drugs your child may be exposed to and for you to communicate the consequences associated with them.

Decision Making Skills Are Important

Children learn how to make decisions. You can guide them with a key set of questions to ask when faced with a choice:

- What am I trying to decide and what do I know about it?
- How do I know my information is accurate? Who gave me the information?
- What more do I need to know before going ahead?
- Who has the added information I need?

And once the decision is made, ask these questions:

- What are the good effects of this decision?
- What are the bad effects?

After this, you can ask your child to reconsider a decision and take responsibility for the consequences.

Get Involved in Your Child's Life

Young people are much less likely to use drugs when they have positive activities to do and when caring adults are involved in their lives. Get involved in your child's life by participating in his activities (for example, bring a snack for the soccer team, volunteer in your child's classroom, attend his recital or play, help with his science project) and praise his accomplishments. Your participation and encouragement tell your child that these activities are worthwhile and may help him identify and pursue other positive activities as he gets older.

Action Steps to Get Involved

1. Spend at least 15 minutes a day in a "child-directed" activity (doing something your child wants to do).

517

2. Identify at least one opportunity each week for you and your child to do something special together.

3. Support your child's activities.

4. Recognize good behavior consistently and immediately.

5. Use meal times as opportunities to share news of the day or to discuss current affairs.

Being Involved Helps You to Become Aware when Your Child Is under Stress

Being young doesn't necessarily mean you are never unhappy or anxious. Young people often cite stress as a reason they use alcohol, tobacco, and illegal drugs. Let's face it; young people today have to deal with issues such as:

*   Changing family structures.

*   Easy access to alcohol, tobacco, and illegal drugs.

*   Lack of adult supervision.

*   Lack of safe places to learn, play, and socialize.

*   Lack of good role models.

*   Peer pressure.

*   Pressure to be sexually active.

*   Violence and gangs.

Some young people think that alcohol or illegal drugs will cheer them up, make them forget about problems they have, or make them feel part of the group. Adults and children sometimes develop unhealthy ways of dealing with stress. How many times have we heard people say, "Boy, I could use a drink," as an antidote to stress? How many of us smoke tobacco to reduce stress? How many of us truly know how to deal with stress in healthy ways? Just like some adults, children need to learn how to deal with stress, how to make healthy decisions, and how to relax.

Children also need someone to help them through difficult times—someone to whom they can express their concerns and apprehensions without fear of rejection or recrimination. One of the most important things that can help children choose not to use alcohol and drugs is the love and support of at least one caring adult who helps guide them through the many phases of childhood.

Reducing Stress

There are many ways to help reduce stress in a child's life:

- Allow your child to express her feelings and concerns.

- Promote healthy eating, sleep, and exercise patterns during the early years so they become habits for a lifetime.

- Let your child know that you also experience pain, fear, anger, and upset.

- Look at your own coping skills. Are you setting a good example?

- Teach your child relaxation exercises, such as deep breathing and sitting quietly for 10 to 20 minutes as a way to calm down or reduce stress.

- Set goals based on the child's abilities—not on your expectations.

- Teach your child that it's okay to be angry, but it's also important to let the anger go.

- Help your child express anger positively, without resorting to verbal or physical violence.

- Give your child a big hug before or after a stressful situation.

- Establish a special time each day for just the two of you.

- Show confidence in your child's ability to handle problems and tackle new challenges.

- Get your child's input on how a stressful situation can be improved. Discuss his ideas. They may not always be realistic, but this exercise will help him develop problem-solving skills.

- Help your child learn from mistakes.

If you are or your child is experiencing symptoms of stress and you're not sure how to handle the situation, your doctor or a counselor could help. Or call the Substance Abuse and Mental Health Services Administration (SAMHSA)'s National Mental Health Information Center at 800-789-2647 for resources and referrals near you.

Make Clear Rules and Enforce Them with Consistency and Appropriate Consequences

Would it surprise you to learn that parents' permissiveness is a bigger factor in teenage drug use than is peer pressure? If you let your child know up front that you don't approve of using tobacco or illegal drugs, or underage drinking, your child is less likely to use those substances.

Making rules, explaining the need for them, and enforcing them consistently are important. Parents need to establish regularly enforced rules to guide their children in developing daily habits of self-discipline. Research shows that parents who have either very harsh rules or no rules at all are more likely to have children who are at greater risk for drug-taking behavior. Parents who have a warm relationship with their children, while maintaining rules for behavior, can teach children self-discipline.

Action Steps to Make Clear Rules and Enforce Them

1. Discuss your rules and expectations in advance.

2. Follow through with the consequences you have established.

3. Acknowledge when they follow the rules.

4. Discuss why using tobacco and illegal drugs, and underage drinking are not acceptable.

What Is an "Appropriate Consequence"?

Appropriate consequences will vary based on the age of your child, the seriousness of the situation, and your child's personality. Here are a few examples that may help you establish your own guidelines.

- Less time on the computer
- Phone privileges taken away
- No later bedtime/earlier bedtime
- No friends over during the week
- No friends over during the weekend
- Tickets to a concert or sports event taken away
- Less time to watch television

When possible, try to relate the consequence you impose to the behavior they exhibit.

Rules and Consequences Are Important Because Some Kids Use Drugs to Take Risks and Rebel

Taking risks is part of growing up. Children may take an emotional risk by letting someone know that they don't like what they are doing. They may take a physical risk by testing their balance climbing up a tree. They may take a social risk by introducing themselves to someone they don't know.

To grow, a child must learn skills that, as adults, we may take for granted. For example, we may forget how hard it was to go to our first dance. We had to risk that no one would ask us to dance, that we would not be able to dance very well, or that someone would make fun of us. For a child, these are big risks.

As children approach the teen years, almost everything holds some risk because everything feels so new and unexplored. As risks are overcome, most young people continue to look for other new, challenging opportunities.

Parents can help children take healthy risks. These risks may include trying out for a play, joining a community youth group, or going on a survival skills training course. It's important to do so because youth who don't grow and learn with positive challenging opportunities may look for other risks to take. However, they will be unclear about boundaries and unsure of rules and expectations. So, if they are not clearly guided into making smart and healthy decisions about these risks, they may think it's okay to include using alcohol, tobacco, or illegal drugs as part of that risk taking they are trying on.

Some youth may think that using these substances will help them prove that "I'm cool. I can handle anything." This desire to feel grownup, combined with media images of people drinking, smoking, and taking drugs, send a message to some young people that it's ok to take this risk.

By stating and enforcing clear rules and expectations about the use of alcohol, tobacco, and illegal drugs, you can help ensure that your child is less likely to view using drugs or alcohol as an acceptable risk.

Be a Positive Role Model

Children like to imitate adults. How many times have children imitated the way we speak, tried on our clothes or makeup, had a make-believe tea party or cocktail party, or pretended to "go to work"?

Every child wants to be a grownup. Being "grown up" means freedom. Being grown up means making your own decisions. Being grown up means being able to eat and drink anything you want, wherever you want.

Young people like to "try on" our behaviors along with our adult clothes. Lots of things fit into the grownup category: driving a car, working, drinking alcohol, getting married, smoking cigarettes, having babies, and so forth.

If we ask young people about the messages we send them about drinking alcohol, smoking, or using drugs, what might they say? We might be surprised to find out that we influence their attitudes toward alcohol, tobacco, or any substance when we involve them in our own substance use by asking them to get us a beer from the refrigerator or an ashtray from the cupboard.

A child can understand and accept the differences between what adults may do legally and what is appropriate and legal for children. We should continue to reinforce this understanding by not abusing legal substances like alcohol, or by using illegal drugs. Children are exposed to media messages and images that glamorize the use of substances. We must help them understand these messages are neither glamorous nor healthy.

A parent or caregiver using alcohol, tobacco, or illegal drugs may increase a child's chances of using and becoming dependent on a substance.

Action Steps to Being a Positive Role Model

1. Do not engage in illegal, unhealthy, or dangerous drug use.

2. Don't involve your child in your use of alcohol, tobacco, or illegal drugs.

3. When possible, point out examples of bad behavior linked to substance use or abuse and the consequences.

Being a Positive Role Model Is Important Because Some Kids Use Drugs to Feel Grown Up

We must keep in mind that our children grow up. Some of the ways children behave are part of a natural and healthy separation, which generally starts in the early teen years between ages 11 and 14. While we need to set limits, we also must allow room for growth.

But that doesn't mean you should "check out." Know your children, their friends, where they hang out, and what they are doing. If adults have set the example of responsible behavior, children are much more likely to make positive decisions and choices. Parents are a child's first and best teachers.

Teach Your Child to Choose Friends Wisely

As parents, we often worry about how much influence peers have on our child. We've all heard the phrase "peer pressure." However, recent research suggests that most youth don't feel overt pressure from their peers to use alcohol, tobacco, or illegal drugs. Youth say that the pressure to do drugs, smoke, or drink comes more from wanting to be accepted, wanting to belong, and wanting to be noticed. In other words, youth drug use often has more to do with the need for peer acceptance than an inability to "just say no" to their peers.

Action Steps to Help Your Children Cope with Peer Pressure

1. Establish the clear message that you, as a caring adult, do not want them to use alcohol, tobacco, and illegal drugs.

2. Help your child practice resisting peer pressure.

3. Help your child feel comfortable in social situations.

4. Teach your child to analyze media messages.

Teaching Your Child to Choose Friends Wisely Is Important Because Some Kids Use Drugs to Fit in

Wanting to fit in, to belong, is one of *the* most natural parts of growing up. In fact, if we really listen, we may find that, for some, it is the most important part of growing up. By teaching your child to choose friends wisely, you are giving her skills she needs to feel confident in her own judgment. This can help her resist peer influences to use alcohol, tobacco, or illegal drugs or engage in other dangerous behavior.

Monitor Your Child's Activities

Monitoring your child's activities is an important deterrent to alcohol, tobacco, and illegal drug use. One study found that latchkey youth who were home alone 2 or more days per week were four times more likely to have gotten drunk in the past month than those youth who had parental supervision five or more times a week. Another study found that children who had the least monitoring initiated drug use at earlier ages. And the earlier a child starts using drugs, the greater the likelihood that a serious problem will develop as a result.

Action Steps to Monitor Your Child's Activities

1. Establish relationships with your child's friends.

2. Get to know other parents.

3. When your child goes out, make sure you know where he's going, who he'll be with, and what he'll be doing.

4. Have your child check in at regular times and make it easy for her to contact you.

5. Make sure your child has access to enjoyable, drug-free, structured activities.

Monitoring Your Child's Activities Is Important Because Some Kids Use Drugs When They Think They Have Nothing Better to Do

Many youth say they started smoking marijuana or using illegal drugs out of "boredom." In fact, having significant amounts of unsupervised time is a risk factor for youth substance abuse. Unfortunately, changes over the years in family structures and neighborhood networks have increased the amount of time that many young people spend unsupervised. Even if you aren't able to be with your child during the after-school hours, you can seek out activities your child can participate in. Involvement in supervised activities not only occupies free time that could otherwise permit involvement in harmful or dangerous activities, but it helps young people develop skills, establish friendships, identify their talents, and develop a strong sense of self-esteem. They learn self-confidence and skills that last a lifetime, and studies show they are much less likely to use drugs or alcohol.

Section 52.2

Drug Facts You Need to Know

Excerpted from *Keeping Youth Drug Free*. Center for Substance Abuse Prevention, Substance Abuse and Mental Health Services Administration, DHHS Publication No. (SMA)-3772. Rockville, MD, 2002.

When you talk with your child about alcohol, tobacco, and illegal drugs, it's best to know as much background information as you can. The following descriptions are by no means comprehensive, but they give you a broad overview of the substances your child may be exposed to or ask you about.

Alcohol

- *Product names:* Beer, gin, vodka, bourbon, whiskey, tequila, liqueurs, wine, brandy, champagne, rum, sherry, port, coolers.

- *Street names:* Booze, Sauce, Brews, Brewskis, Hard Stuff, Juice.

- *Symptoms of use:* Slurred speech, impaired judgment and motor skills, incoordination, confusion, tremors, drowsiness, agitation, nausea and vomiting, respiratory ailments, depression.

- *Potential consequences:* Impaired judgment can result in inappropriate sexual behavior, sexually transmitted diseases (including HIV/AIDS), injuries, and auto crashes. Habitual use can lead to an inability to control drinking, high tolerance level, blackouts and memory loss, interference with personal relationships, cirrhosis of the liver, vitamin deficiencies, damage to heart and central nervous system, sexual impotence, weight gain.

- *Route of administration:* Ingested.

- *Medical uses:* For appetite stimulation and mild sedation.

- *Legal status:* Illegal under 21.

Cannabis (Marijuana)

- *Product names:* Delta-9-tetrahydrocannabinol (THC), Cannabis sativa, marijuana, hashish, hashish oil.

- *Street names:* Weed, Pot, Grass, Reefer, Mary Jane, Joint, Roach, Nail, Blunt. (Blunt refers to a cigar into which marijuana is rolled.)

- *Symptoms of use:* Mood swings, euphoria, slow thinking and reflexes, dilated pupils, increased appetite, dryness of mouth, increased pulse rate, delusions, hallucinations.

- *Potential consequences:* Amotivational syndrome, memory impairment, weight gain, increased risk for cancer, lower sperm counts and lower testosterone levels for men, increased risk of infertility for women, psychological dependence requiring more of the drug to get the same effect. Marijuana serves as a barrier against self-awareness, and users may not be able to learn key developmental skills.

- *Routes of administration:* Ingested and smoked.

- *Medical use:* The use of THC as an appetite stimulant in people with severe wasting disease is controversial.

- *Legal status:* Illegal.

Cocaine/Crack Cocaine

- *Product names:* Cocaine, crack cocaine.

- *Street names:* Cocaine—Coke, Snow, Blow, Toot, Nose Candy, Flake, Dust, Sneeze. Crack Cocaine—Crack, Rock, Base, Sugar Block, Rox/Roxanne.

- *Symptoms of use:* Excitability, euphoria, talkativeness, anxiety, increased pulse rate, dilated pupils, paranoia, agitation, hallucinations.

- *Potential consequences:* High risk for addiction, violent or erratic behavior, hallucinations, cocaine psychosis, eating or sleeping disorders, impaired sexual performance, ongoing respiratory problems, ulceration of the mucous membrane of the nose, collapse of the nasal septum, death from cardiac arrest or respiratory arrest.

- *Routes of administration:* Sniffed and smoked.

- *Medical use:* None.

- *Legal status:* Illegal.

Depressants

- *Product names:* Sleeping pills and tranquilizers (Seconal, Nembutal, Quaalude, Miltown, Norcet, Placidyl, Valium, Librium, Ativan, Xanax, Serax).

- *Street names:* Downers, Ludes, Vs, Blues, Goofball, Red Devil, Blue Devil, Yellow Jackets, Yellow Bullets, Pink Ladies, Christmas Trees, Phennies, Peanuts.

- *Symptoms of use:* Drowsiness, confusion, incoordination, tremors, slurred speech, depressed pulse rate, shallow respiration, dilated pupils.

- *Potential consequences:* Anxiety, depression, restlessness, psychotic episodes, chronic fatigue, insomnia, changes in eyesight, irregular menstruation, stopped breathing, suicide, dependence requiring more of the drug to get the same effect, severe withdrawal symptoms.

- *Route of administration:* Ingested.

- *Medical uses:* For tranquilization, sedation, and sleep.

- *Legal status:* Prescription only.

Hallucinogens

- *Product names:* LSD (lysergic acid diethylamide), PCP (phencyclidine), DMT (dimethyltryptamine), Mescaline, MDA (methylenedioxyamphetamine), STP (dimethoxymethamphetamine), psilocybin, Rohypnol, GHB (gamma-hydroxybutyric acid), MDMA (methylenedioxymethamphetamine).

- *Street names:* LSD—A, Acid, Blotter, Microdots, Windowpane. PCP—Angel Dust, Angel Mist, Animal Tranquilizer. Psilocybin—Mushrooms, Magic Mushrooms, Shrooms. MDMA—Ecstasy, E, X, XTC. Rohypnol—R-2, Roofies, Roaches, "The Date Rape Drug." GHB—Liquid Ecstasy, Liquid X, Georgia Home Brew, Georgia Home Boyz.

- *Symptoms of use:* Trance-like state, excitation, euphoria, increased pulse rate, insomnia, hallucinations.

- *Potential consequences:* Impaired judgment and coordination can result in greater risk for injury, self-inflicted injury, violent behavior, paranoia, depression or anxiety, unpredictable flash-backs.

- *Route of administration:* Ingested.
- *Medical use:* None, except OxyContin.
- *Legal status:* Illegal.

Inhalants

- *Product names:* Organic solvents, nitrous oxide, nitrites, aerosols, airplane glue, nail polish remover, lighter fluid, gasoline, paints, hair spray.
- *Street names:* Glue, Kick, Bang, Sniff, Huff, Poppers, Whippets, Texas Shoeshine.
- *Symptoms of use:* Slurred speech, incoordination, nausea, vomiting, slowed breathing.
- *Potential consequences:* Brain damage; pains in chest, muscles, and joints; heart trouble; severe depression; toxic psychosis; nerve damage; fatigue; loss of appetite; bronchial tube spasm; sores on nose or mouth; nosebleeds; diarrhea; nausea; bizarre or reckless behavior; sudden death; suffocation.
- *Route of administration:* Sniffed.
- *Medical use:* Nitrous oxide only, for anesthesia.
- *Legal status:* Most products available in retail stores.

Narcotics

- *Product names:* Heroin, morphine, codeine, Dilaudid, Demerol, Percodan, Methadone, Talwin.
- *Street names:* Heroin—Smack, Junk, Horse, H, Tar. Morphine—Mojo, Mud, Mary, Murphy, M, Miss Emma, Mister Black. Codeine—Schoolboy, Cody, Captain Cody. Methadone—Dollies, Fizzies.
- *Symptoms of use:* Lethargy, drowsiness, euphoria, nausea, constipation, constricted pupils, slowed breathing.
- *Potential consequences:* HIV infection, heart or respiratory problems, mood swings, chronic constipation, tremors, toxic psychosis, high potential for addiction.

- *Routes of administration:* Injected and ingested.

- *Medical use:* For pain relief (except heroin and methadone).

- *Legal status:* Illegal except by prescription.

Stimulants

- *Product names:* Amphetamine, Methamphetamine, Biphetamine, Dexedrine, Desoxyn, Tenuate, Ionamin, Tepanil, Methcathinone.

- *Street names:* Methamphetamine—Speed, Crystal, Meth, Ice, Glass, Crank, Go. Methcathinone—Cat, Jeff, Goob, Stat, Star. Amphetamine—Bennies, Benz, Uppers. Dexedrine—Dexies, Brownies.

- *Symptoms of use:* Excitability, tremors, insomnia, sweating, dry mouth and lips, bad breath, dilated pupils, weight loss, paranoia, hallucinations.

- *Potential consequences:* Weight loss, nutritional deficiency, chronic sleep problems, high blood pressure, paranoia, anxiety or nervousness, decreased emotional control, severe depression, violent behavior, death from heart failure or suicide.

- *Route of administration:* Ingested.

- *Medical uses:* For narcolepsy, obesity, hyperkinesis.

- *Legal status:* Prescription only.

Tobacco

- *Product names:* Cigarettes, cigars, chewing tobacco.

- *Street names:* Cancer Sticks, Sticks, Bidis (flavored, hand-rolled cigarettes), Cloves (60% tobacco/40% cloves), Chew, Smoke, Bone, Butt, Coffin Nail.

- *Symptoms of use:* Smelly hair, clothes, and breath; yellowing of teeth; coughs; increased asthma attacks; shortness of breath and poorer athletic performance. After only a few weeks, users of spit tobacco can develop cracked lips, white spots, sores, and bleeding in the mouth.

- *Potential consequences:* Addiction; respiratory problems such as emphysema and chronic bronchitis; heart and cardiovascular disease; cancer of the lung, larynx, esophagus, bladder, pancreas, kidney, and mouth.

- *Routes of administration:* Smoked or ingested orally (chew or spit tobacco).

- *Medical use:* None.

- *Legal status:* Illegal for youth under 19 in Alabama, Alaska, and Utah. Illegal for youth under 18 in all remaining states.

Section 52.3

Help Your Kids Overcome Peer Influence on Smoking

Excerpted from "Got a Minute? Give It to Your Kids," reviewed July 2002, and "You(th) and Tobacco," reviewed March 2003, National Center for Chronic Disease Prevention and Health Promotion, Centers for Disease Control and Prevention; along with text from "Parents' Involvement Helps Kids Overcome Peer Influence on Smoking," National Institute of Child Health and Human Development, NIH Press Release, December 23, 2002.

Every day, 6,000 youth try cigarettes for the first time—and one out of three smokers will die from the addiction. Preteens who report they regularly eat meals, follow a family calendar, and discuss free-time activities with their parents are less likely to smoke. And more likely to live longer, healthier lives.

Most parents don't expect their child to smoke. But youth are exposed to millions of misleading images glamorizing tobacco. That's one reason one out of eight middle school students use tobacco.

Parents Can Help Keep Kids Tobacco-Free

Despite the impact of movies, music, and TV, parents can be the greatest influence in their kids' lives. Talk directly to children about the risks of tobacco use; if friends or relatives died from tobacco-related illnesses, let your kids know. If you use tobacco, you can still make a difference. Your best move, of course, is to try to quit. Meanwhile, don't use tobacco in your children's presence, don't offer it to them, and don't leave it where they can easily get it.

Start the dialog about tobacco use at age 5 or 6 and continue through their high school years. Many kids start using tobacco by age 11, and many are addicted by age 14.

Know if your kids' friends use tobacco. Talk about ways to refuse tobacco. Discuss with kids the false glamorization of tobacco on billboards, and other media, such as movies, TV, and magazines.

Having involved parents—those who know a lot about their children's friends, activities, and how they're doing in school—can help children overcome peer influence to start smoking, according to a study by a researcher at the National Institute of Child Health and Human Development (NICHD).

The study also confirmed earlier findings that the more widespread children think smoking is, the more likely they are to start. Moreover, children who are socially competent—who have the ability to exercise self control and good judgment—and have parents who monitor their behavior tend not to start smoking.

While researchers have known that both peers and parents play an important role in whether young teens and preteens start smoking, they've known less about whether the effects of peer influence on starting smoking is affected by other factors, such as parents' involvement, children's adjustment to school, and their degree of social competence.

"Many children start to experiment with smoking in early adolescence, " said Duane Alexander, M.D., Director of the NICHD. "Many then go on to develop a life-long addiction that can cause them serious health problems later in life. This study shows that by staying involved in their children's lives, parents can help them to avoid the smoking habit."

Section 52.4

Talk to Your Child about Alcohol

Excerpted from "Make a Difference: Talk to Your Child About Alcohol,"
National Institute on Alcohol Abuse and Alcoholism (NIAAA),
NIH Pub. No. 00-4314, revised 2002.

You Should Know

Your child looks to you for guidance and support in making life decisions—including the decision not to use alcohol.

"But my child isn't drinking yet," you may think. "Isn't it a little early to be concerned about drinking?" Not at all. This is the age at which some children begin experimenting with alcohol. Even if your child is not yet drinking, he or she may be receiving pressure to drink. Act now. Keeping quiet about how you feel about your child's alcohol use may give him or her the impression that alcohol use is OK for kids.

It's not easy. As children approach adolescence, friends exert a lot of influence. Fitting in is a chief priority for teens, and parents often feel shoved aside. Kids will listen, however. Study after study shows that even during the teen years, parents have enormous influence on their children's behavior.

The bottom line is that most young teens don't yet drink. And parents' disapproval of youthful alcohol use is the key reason children choose not to drink. So make no mistake: You can make a difference.

Talking with Your Child about Alcohol

For many parents, bringing up the subject of alcohol is no easy matter. To boost your chances for a productive conversation, take some time to think through the issues you want to discuss before you talk with your child. Also, think about how your child might react and ways you might respond to your youngster's questions and feelings. Then choose a time to talk when both you and your child have some "down time" and are feeling relaxed.

Keep in mind, too, that you don't need to cover everything at once. In fact, you're likely to have a greater impact on your child's drinking by having a number of talks about alcohol use throughout his or her adolescence. Think of this discussion with your child as the first part of an ongoing conversation.

And remember, do make it a conversation, not a lecture. Following are some topics for discussion:

- *Your Child's Views about Alcohol.* Ask your young teen what he or she knows about alcohol and what he or she thinks about teen drinking. Ask your child why he or she thinks kids drink. Listen carefully without interrupting. Not only will this approach help your child to feel heard and respected, but it can serve as a natural "lead-in" to discussing alcohol topics.

- *Important Facts about Alcohol.* Although many kids believe they already know everything about alcohol, myths and misinformation abound. Here are some important facts to share:

  - Alcohol is a powerful drug that slows down the body and mind. It impairs coordination; slows reaction time; and impairs vision, clear thinking, and judgment.

  - Beer and wine are not "safer" than hard liquor. A 12-ounce can of beer, a 5-ounce glass of wine, and 1.5 ounces of hard liquor all contain the same amount of alcohol and have the same effects on the body and mind.

  - On average, it takes 2 to 3 hours for a single drink to leave the body's system. Nothing can speed up this process, including drinking coffee, taking a cold shower, or "walking it off."

  - People tend to be very bad at judging how seriously alcohol has affected them. That means many individuals who drive after drinking think they can control a car—but actually cannot.

  - Anyone can develop a serious alcohol problem, including a teenager.

- *The "Magic Potion" Myth.* The media's glamorous portrayal of alcohol encourages many teens to believe that drinking will make them popular, attractive, happy, and "cool." Research shows that teens who expect such positive effects are more likely to drink at early ages. However, you can help to combat these dangerous myths by watching TV shows and movie videos with your child and discussing how alcohol is portrayed in them.

- *Good Reasons Not to Drink.* In talking with your child about reasons to avoid alcohol, stay away from scare tactics. Most young teens are aware that many people drink without problems, so it is important to discuss the consequences of alcohol use without overstating the case. For example, you can talk about the dangers of riding in a car with a driver who has been drinking without insisting that "all kids who ride with drinkers get into crashes." Some reasons not to drink include:

  - You want your child to avoid alcohol. Your values and attitudes count with your child, even though he or she may not always show it.

  - To maintain self-respect.

  - Drinking is illegal.

  - Drinking can be dangerous.

  - You have a family history of alcoholism.

- *How to Handle Peer Pressure.* It's not enough to tell your young teen that he or she should avoid alcohol—you also need to help your child figure out how. Brainstorm with your teen for ways that he or she might handle difficult situations, and make clear how you are willing to support your child. An example: "If you find yourself at a home where kids are drinking, call me and I'll pick you up—and there will be no scolding or punishment." The more prepared your child is, the better able he or she will be to handle high-pressure situations that involve drinking.

Six Ways to Say No to a Drink

At some point, your child will be offered alcohol. To resist such pressure, teens say they prefer quick "one-liners" that allow them to dodge a drink without making a big scene. It will probably work best for your teen to take the lead in thinking up comebacks to drink offers so that he or she will feel comfortable saying them. But to get the brainstorming started, here are some simple pressure-busters—from the mildest to the most assertive.

1. No thanks.

2. I don't feel like it—do you have any soda?

3. Alcohol's NOT my thing.

4. Are you talking to me? FORGET it.

5. Why do you keep pressuring me when I've said NO?

6. Back off!

Taking Action: Prevention Strategies for Parents

While parent-child conversations about drinking are essential, talking isn't enough—you also need to take concrete action to help your child resist alcohol. Research strongly shows that active, supportive involvement by parents and guardians can help teens avoid underage drinking and prevent later alcohol misuse.

- Monitor alcohol use in your home
- Connect with other parents
- Keep track of your child's activities
- Develop family rules about teen drinking
- Set a good example
- Don't support teen drinking (or imply support through the telling of "funny" alcohol-related stories)
- Help your child build healthy friendships
- Encourage healthy alternatives to alcohol

Warning Signs of a Drinking Problem

While the following behaviors may indicate an alcohol or other drug problem, some also reflect normal teenage growing pains. Experts believe that a drinking problem is more likely if you notice several of these signs at the same time, if they occur suddenly, and if some of them are extreme in nature.

- Mood changes: flare-ups of temper, irritability, and defensiveness.
- School problems: poor attendance, low grades, and/or recent disciplinary action.
- Rebelling against family rules.
- Switching friends, along with a reluctance to have you get to know the new friends.

- A "nothing matters" attitude: sloppy appearance, a lack of involvement in former interests, and general low energy.

- Finding alcohol in your child's room or backpack, or smelling alcohol on his or her breath.

- Physical or mental problems: memory lapses, poor concentration, bloodshot eyes, lack of coordination, or slurred speech.

Section 52.5

A Parents' Guide to Preventing Inhalant Abuse

This text is excerpted from "A Parents' Guide to Preventing Inhalant Abuse," an undated brochure developed by the U.S. Consumer Product Safety Commission (http://www.cpcs.gov).

Inhalant Abuse Can Kill

Inhalant abuse is the deliberate inhalation or sniffing of common products found in homes and schools to obtain a "high." It can kill suddenly, and it can kill those who sniff for the first time.

Every year, young people in this country die of inhalant abuse. Hundreds also suffer severe consequences, including permanent brain damage, loss of muscle control, and destruction of the heart, blood, kidney, liver, and bone marrow.

Today more than 1,000 different products are commonly abused. The National Institute on Drug Abuse reported in 1996 that one in five American teenagers have used inhalants to get high.

Many youngsters say they begin sniffing when they're in grade school. They start because they feel these substances can't hurt them, because of peer pressure, or because of low self-esteem. Once hooked, these victims find it a tough habit to break.

What are the effects of inhalant abuse?

Sniffing can cause sickness and death. For example, victims may become nauseated, forgetful, and unable to see things clearly. Victims may lose control of their body, including the use of arms and legs. These effects can last 15 to 45 minutes after sniffing.

In addition, sniffing can severely damage many parts of the body, including the brain, heart, liver, and kidneys.

Even worse, victims can die suddenly—without any warning. "Sudden Sniffing Death" can occur during or right after sniffing. The heart begins to overwork, beating rapidly but unevenly, which can lead to cardiac arrest. Even first-time abusers have been known to die from sniffing inhalants.

What products are abused?

Ordinary household products, which can be safely used for legitimate purposes, can be problematic in the hands of an inhalant abuser. The following categories of products are reportedly abused: glues/adhesives, nail polish remover, marking pens, paint thinner, spray paint, butane lighter fluid, gasoline, propane gas, typewriter correction fluid, household cleaners, cooking sprays, deodorants, fabric protectors, whipping cream aerosols, and air conditioning coolants.

How can you tell if a young person is an inhalant abuser?

If someone is an inhalant abuser, some or all of these symptoms may be evident:

- Unusual breath odor or chemical odor on clothing.
- Slurred or disoriented speech.
- Drunk, dazed, or dizzy appearance.
- Signs of paint or other products where they wouldn't normally be, such as on the face.
- Red or runny eyes or nose.
- Spots and/or sores around the mouth.
- Nausea and/or loss of appetite.
- Chronic inhalant abusers may exhibit such symptoms as anxiety, excitability, irritability, or restlessness.
- Sitting with a pen or marker near nose.
- Constantly smelling clothing sleeves.
- Hiding rags, clothes, or empty containers of the potentially abused products in closets and other places.

Prevent Inhalant Abuse

One of the most important steps you can take is to talk with your children or other youngsters about not experimenting even a first time with inhalants. In addition, talk with your children's teachers, guidance counselors, and coaches. By discussing this problem openly and stressing the devastating consequences of inhalant abuse, you can help prevent a tragedy.

Be alert for symptoms of inhalant abuse. If you suspect there's a problem, you should consider seeking professional help. Contact a local drug rehabilitation center or other services available in your community, or seek additional information from the following:

National Inhalant Prevention Coalition
800-269-4237
Website: http://www.inhalants.org

National Drug and Alcohol Treatment Referral Service
800-662-HELP

National Clearinghouse for Alcohol and Drug Information
800-729-6686
Website: http://www.health.org

Chapter 53

Youth Violence

Chapter Contents

Section 53.1

The Angry Child

Reprinted with permission from "The Angry Child," by Jere Brophy, based on "The Aggressive Child" by Luleen S. Anderson, Ph.D, in *Children Today* (January-February 1978), published by the Children's Bureau, from ERIC (Educational Resources Information Center, U.S. Department of Health and Human Services Pub. No. (ADM) 92-0781, revised June 2000; text and additional information available online from Pediatric Development and Behavior at www.dbpeds.org.

Handling children's anger can be puzzling, draining, and distressing for adults. One of the major problems in dealing with anger in children is the angry feelings that are often stirred up in us. We need to remind ourselves that we were not always taught how to deal with anger as a fact of life during our own childhood. We were led to believe that to be angry was to be bad, and we were often made to feel guilty for expressing anger.

It will be easier to deal with children's anger if we get rid of this notion. Our goal is not to repress or destroy angry feelings in children or in ourselves but rather to accept the feelings and to help channel and direct them to constructive ends.

Parents and teachers must allow children to feel all their feelings. Adult skills can then be directed toward showing children acceptable ways of expressing their feelings. Strong feelings cannot be denied, and angry outbursts should not always be viewed as a sign of serious problems; they should be recognized and treated with respect.

To respond effectively to overly aggressive behavior in children we need to have some ideas about what may have triggered an outburst. Anger may be a defense to avoid painful feelings; it may be associated with failure, low self-esteem, and feelings of isolation; or it may be related to anxiety about situations over which the child has no control.

Angry defiance may also be associated with feelings of dependency, and anger may be associated with sadness and depression. In childhood, anger and sadness are very close to one another, and it is important to remember that much of what an adult experiences as sadness is expressed by a child as anger.

Several points are important before we go any further:

- Anger and aggression are different. Anger is a temporary emotional state caused by frustration; aggression is often an attempt to hurt a person or to destroy property.

- Anger and aggression do not have to be dirty words. We must be careful to tell the difference between behavior that indicates emotional problems and behavior that is normal.

With angry children, our actions should be motivated by the need to protect and to reach, not by a desire to punish. Show the child that you accept his or her feelings, while suggesting other ways to express the feelings. An adult might say, for example, "Let me tell you what some children would do in a situation like this." It is not enough to tell children what behaviors we find unacceptable.

We must teach them acceptable ways of coping. Also, ways must be found to communicate what we expect of them. Contrary to popular opinion, punishment is not the most effective way to communicate to children what we expect of them.

Responding to the Angry Child

Some of the following suggestions for dealing with the angry child were taken from *The Aggressive Child* by Fritz Redl and David Wineman.

- Catch the child being good. Tell the child what behaviors please you. Respond to positive efforts and reinforce good behavior. An observing and sensitive parent will find countless opportunities during the day to make such comments as, "I like the way you come in for dinner without being reminded."; "I appreciate your hanging up your clothes even though you were in a hurry to get out to play."; "You were really patient while I was on the phone."; "I'm glad you shared your snack with your sister."; "I like the way you're able to think of others."; and, "Thank you for telling the truth about what really happened."

- Similarly, teachers can positively reinforce good behavior with statements like, "I know it was difficult for you to wait your turn, and I'm pleased that you could do it."; "Thanks for sitting in your seat quietly."; "You were thoughtful in offering to help Johnny with his spelling."; "You worked hard on that project, and I admire your effort."

- Deliberately ignore inappropriate behavior that can be tolerated. This doesn't mean that you should ignore the child, just the behavior. The "ignoring" has to be planned and consistent. Even though this behavior may be tolerated, the child must recognize that it is inappropriate.

- Provide physical outlets and other alternatives. It is important for children to have opportunities for physical exercise and movement, both at home and at school.

- Manipulate the surroundings. Aggressive behavior can be encouraged by placing children in tough, tempting situations. We should try to plan the surroundings so that certain things are less apt to happen. Stop a "problem" activity and substitute, temporarily, a more desirable one. Sometimes rules and regulations, as well as physical space, may be too confining.

- Use closeness and touching. Move physically closer to the child to curb his or her angry impulse. Young children are often calmed by having an adult come close by and express interest in the child's activities. Children naturally try to involve adults in what they are doing, and the adult is often annoyed at being bothered. Very young children (and children who are emotionally deprived) seem to need much more adult involvement in their interests.

- A child about to use a toy or tool in a destructive way is sometimes easily stopped by an adult who expresses interest in having it shown to him. An outburst from an older child struggling with a difficult reading selection can be prevented by a caring adult who moves near the child to say, "Show me which words are giving you trouble."

- Be ready to show affection. Sometimes all that is needed for any angry child to regain control is a sudden hug or other impulsive show of affection. Children with serious emotional problems, however, may have trouble accepting affection.

- Ease tension through humor. Kidding the child out of a temper tantrum or outburst offers the child an opportunity to "save face." However, it is important to distinguish between face-saving humor and sarcasm, teasing, or ridicule.

- Appeal directly to the child. Tell him or her how you feel and ask for consideration. For example, a parent or a teacher may gain a child's cooperation by saying, "I know that noise you're making doesn't usually bother me, but today I've got a head-ache, so could you find something else you'd enjoy doing?"

- Explain situations. Help the child understand the cause of a stressed situation. We often fail to realize how easily young children can begin to react properly once they understand the cause of their frustration.

- Use physical restraint. Occasionally a child may lose control so completely that he has to be physically restrained or removed from the scene to prevent him from hurting himself or others. This may also "save face" for the child. Physical restraint or removal from the scene should not be viewed by the child as punishment but as a means of saying, "You can't do that." In such situations, an adult cannot afford to lose his or her temper, and unfriendly remarks by other children should not be tolerated.

- Encourage children to see their strengths as well as their weaknesses. Help them to see that they can reach their goals.

- Use promises and rewards. Promises of future pleasure can be used both to start and to stop behavior. This approach should not be compared with bribery. We must know what the child likes—what brings him pleasure—and we must deliver on our promises.

- Say, "NO!" Limits should be clearly explained and enforced. Children should be free to function within those limits.

- Tell the child that you accept his or her angry feelings, but offer other suggestions for expressing them. Teach children to put their angry feelings into words, rather than fists.

- Build a positive self-image. Encourage children to see themselves as valued and valuable people.

- Use punishment cautiously. There is a fine line between punishment that is hostile toward a child and punishment that is educational.

- Model appropriate behavior. Parents and teachers should be aware of the powerful influence of their actions on a child's or group's behavior.

- Teach children to express themselves verbally. Talking helps a child have control and thus reduces acting out behavior. Encourage the child to say, for example, "I don't like your taking my pencil. I don't feel like sharing just now."

The Role of Discipline

Good discipline includes creating an atmosphere of quiet firmness, clarity, and conscientiousness, while using reasoning. Bad discipline involves punishment which is unduly harsh and inappropriate, and it is often associated with verbal ridicule and attacks on the child's integrity.

As one fourth-grade teacher put it, "One of the most important goals we strive for as parents, educators, and mental health professionals is to help children develop respect for themselves and others." While arriving at this goal takes years of patient practice, it is a vital process in which parents, teachers, and all caring adults can play a crucial and exciting role. In order to accomplish this, we must see children as worthy human beings and be sincere in dealing with them.

Section 53.2

Fighting the Biting

From "Biters: Why They Do It and What to Do about It," © 1996 National Association for the Education of Young Children; reprinted with permission. Reviewed by David A. Cooke, M.D. May 27, 2001. The original document is available online at http://npin.org/library/1997/n00217/n00217.html.

Although biting isn't "abnormal" in the sense that one out of ten toddlers and two-year-olds does it, it is a disturbing and potentially harmful behavior that parents and educators must discourage from the very first episode. If a child bites, remain calm and think about what the child experienced just before the incident. Understanding why young children bite can help you deter this aggressive behavior and teach them positive ways to handle their feelings.

Young children may bite for different reasons, and not all will respond to the same types of intervention. Identifying the kind of biter you're dealing with will help you develop an appropriate discipline technique.

- **The experimental biter.** An infant or young child may take an experimental bite out of a mother's breast or a caregiver's shoulder. When this occurs, adults should use prompt, clear signals to communicate that children must not bite people. "No," said sharply, would be an appropriate response.

These experimental biters may simply want to touch, smell, and taste other people in order to learn more about their world. Their muscles are developing, and they need to experiment. Provide them with a variety of surfaces to play on and a colorful selection of toys to stimulate children during this stage of exploration.

This type of biter may also be motivated by teething pain. Offer children appropriate things to chew on for relief: frozen bagels, very cold, large carrots, teething biscuits, or a safe teething ring.

- **The frustrated biter.** Some biters lack the skills to cope with situations such as the desire for an adult's attention or another child's toy. Even though the child may not have intended to harm another person, adults must react with disapproval. First, tend to the victim immediately. Then explain to the biter that biting hurts others and is not allowed the caregiver's job is to keep all children safe.

You may help frustrated biters by teaching them appropriate language to show their feelings or get what they need. Give positive reinforcement when children communicate effectively. Also, watch for signs of rising frustration. Spotting potential conflict may help you intercept a potentially harmful incident.

- **The threatened biter.** Some children, feeling they are endangered, bite in self-defense. They may be overwhelmed by their surroundings, and bite as a means of regaining control. In this case, use the intervention techniques already mentioned, and assure the child that his rights and possessions are safe.

Children may become threatened by situations such as newly separated parents, the death of a grandparent, or a mother returning to the work force. The threatened biter may require additional nurturing, particularly if the danger is along the lines of physical violence at home or in the immediate neighborhood. In any case, the bond between child and caregiver should be as warm and reassuring as possible.

- **The power biter.** Some children experience a strong need for autonomy and control. As soon as they see the response they get from biting, the behavior is strongly reinforced. Give the biter choices throughout the day and reinforce positive social behavior (like sharing and saying thanks). If the biter gets attention when she is not biting, she will not have to resort to aggressive behavior to feel a sense of personal power.

Never hit or "bite back" a child for biting. This communicates that violence is an appropriate way to handle emotion. The approach should be calm and educational. A child should not experience any reward for biting—not even the "reward" of negative attention.

Parents and caregivers must cooperate to prevent children from biting. If children are permitted to demonstrate such behavior at home, there will be no chance of eliminating it in the center, program, or family child care home. Working as a team, educators and parents may identify possible reasons for a child's biting and respond accordingly. While early childhood professionals may be more familiar with positive discipline techniques, parents are experts on their own children's behavior.

Take the time to look for patterns in the biter's environment and emotional state at each episode. Does the child always bite the same individual? Is the biter simply exhausted, or hungry? Be ready to intervene immediately, but carefully. Teaching children age-appropriate ways to control themselves encourages the development of confidence and self-esteem. We can guide children towards self-control and away from biting. The key is understanding for adults and children alike.

For More Information

National Association for the Education of Young Children
1509 16ᵗʰ Street, N.W.
Washington, DC 20036-1426
Toll Free: 800-424-2460
Phone: 202-232-8777
Fax: 202-328-1846
Website: http://www.naeyc.org
E-mail: naeyc@naeyc.org

Section 53.3

Preventing Youth Violence

From: "Preventing Youth Violence," SafeUSA™, Centers for Disease Control and Prevention (CDC), updated July 2002. The full text of this document, including statistics and resources is available online at http://www.safeusa.org/youthviolence.htm. Additional information from SafeUSA is also available online at www.safeusa.org.

Violence is a learned behavior that can be changed. Parents, students, and school officials can take steps toward reducing violence in schools by responding to children's emotional and psychological needs and by implementing violence prevention programs.

To help prevent violence in schools, follow these tips adapted from the American Psychological Association's *Teach Children to Resist Violence* and from the U.S. Departments of Education and Justice's *A Guide for Safe Schools: Early Warning, Timely Response.*

For Parents

- Give your children consistent love and attention. Every child needs a strong, loving, relationship with a parent or other adult to feel safe and secure and to develop a sense of trust.

- Children learn by example, so show your children appropriate behavior by the way you act. Settle arguments with calm words, not with yelling, hitting, slapping, or spanking. If you punish children by hitting, slapping, or spanking them, you are showing them that it is okay to hit others.

- Talk with your children about the violence they see on TV, in video games, at school, at home, or in the neighborhood. Discuss why violence exists in these contexts and what the consequences of this violence are.

- Try to keep your children from seeing too much violence: limit their TV time, and screen the programs they watch. Seeing a lot of violence can lead children to behave aggressively.

- Make sure your children do not have access to guns. If you own firearms or other weapons, unload them and lock them up separately from the bullets. Never store firearms where children can find them, even if unloaded. Also, talk with your children about how dangerous weapons can be.

- Involve your children in setting rules for appropriate behavior at home; this will help them understand why the rules should be followed. Also ask your children what they think an appropriate punishment would be if a rule were broken.

- Teach your children nonaggressive ways to solve problems by discussing problems with them, asking them to consider what might happen if they use violence to solve problems, and talking about what might happen if they solve problems without violence.

- Listen to your children and respect them. They will be more likely to listen and respect others if they are listened to and treated with respect.

- Note any disturbing behaviors in your child such as angry outbursts, excessive fighting, cruelty to animals, fire-setting, lack of friends, or alcohol/drug use. These can be signs of serious problems. Don't be afraid to get help for your child if such behaviors exist, and talk with a trusted professional in the community.

For Students

To help prevent violence in schools, follow these tips adapted from the American Psychological Association and MTV's *Fight for Your Rights: Take a Stand against Violence*; the U.S. Departments of Education and Justice's *A Guide for Safe Schools: Early Warning, Timely Response*; and the *American Journal of Preventive Medicine: Youth Violence Prevention, Descriptions and Baseline Data from 13 Evaluation Projects* (Vol. 12, Number 5, Sep/Oct 1996).

- Be a role model by never physically or verbally harming, bullying, teasing, or intimidating others.

- If your friends tell you about troubling feelings or thoughts, listen well and let them know you care. Encourage them to get help from a trusted adult. If you are very concerned, talk to an adult you trust.

- When you are angry, take a few deep breaths and imagine yourself on a lake or at the beach or anywhere that makes you feel peaceful. After you are more calm, identify what is making you upset. Decide on your options for handling the problem, such as talking the problem out calmly with the people involved, avoiding the problem by staying away from certain people, or diffusing the problem by resolving to take it less seriously. After you decide what to do (or not do) and act on your decision, be sure to look back and decide if what you did helped the situation.

- Work with your school to create a process for students to safely report threats, intimidation, weapon possession, drug selling, gang activity, and vandalism.

- Help develop and participate in activities to promote understanding and respecting differences.

- Volunteer to be a mentor for younger students and/or provide tutoring for your peers.

- If you feel intensely angry, fearful, anxious, or depressed, talk about it with an adult you trust.

- Get involved in your school's violence prevention and response plan. If a plan does not exist, suggest starting one.

For School Officials

- Develop a comprehensive violence prevention plan that does not label or stigmatize children. Involve staff, parents, students, and members of the community in the creation and implementation of this plan.

- Create a school environment that is safe and responsive to all children. Students should be able to share their needs, fears, concerns, and anxieties, and also safely report threats.

- Ensure that opportunities exist for adults to spend quality personal time with children. A positive relationship with an adult who is available to provide support is one of the most critical factors in preventing school violence.

- Discuss safety issues openly. Schools can reduce the risk of violence by teaching children about the dangers of firearms as well as appropriate ways to resolve conflicts and express anger.

- Offer supervised, school-based programs, before and after school, that provide children with support and a range of options, such as counseling, tutoring, clubs, community service, and help with homework.

- Be prepared for a crisis or violent act. Provide in-service training for all faculty and staff to explain what to do in a crisis, including the evacuation procedure, communication plan, and how to contact help.

Part Seven

Additional Help and Information

Chapter 54

Glossary of Terms Related to Child Health

acute: An illness or injury that lasts for a short time and may be intense. [2]

adverse event: Any undesirable side effect that may result from a vaccination. [3]

allergic salute: A characteristic wiping or rubbing of the nose with a transverse or upward movement of the hand, as seen in children with allergic rhinitis. [1]

anaphylaxis: An immediate and severe allergic response; a shock reaction to a substance. This can result in sudden severe breathing difficulty, severe drop in blood pressure, and/or loss of consciousness. Anaphylactic shock can kill if not treated promptly. Common causes of anaphylaxis include: bee stings in people that are allergic to bees, ingestion of certain foods by people that are allergic to those foods, and drug reactions. [3]

This glossary contains terms [1] excerpted from *Stedman's Medical Dictionary, 27th Edition*, copyright © 2000 Lippincott Williams & Wilkins. All rights reserved; [2] excerpted from "Questions and Answers About Sprains and Strains," National Institute of Arthritis and Musculoskeletal and Skin Disorders, March 1999; and excerpted from [3] "Definitions of Terms Related to Immunization," National Vaccine Program Office, Centers for Disease Control and Prevention, updated April 2003.

anorexia nervosa: A mental disorder manifested by extreme fear of becoming obese and an aversion to food, usually occurring in young women and often resulting in life-threatening weight loss, accompanied by a disturbance in body image, hyperactivity, and amenorrhea. [1]

antimicrobial agents: A general term for the drugs, chemicals, or other substances that kill microbes (tiny organisms that cause disease). Among the antimicrobial agents in use today are: antibacterial drugs (kill bacteria); antiviral agents (kill viruses); antifungal agents (kill fungi); and antiparasitic drugs (kill parasites). [3]

bacteria: Plural for bacterium. Tiny microorganisms that reproduce by cell division and usually have a cell wall. Bacteria can be shaped like a sphere, rod, or spiral and can be found in virtually any environment. [3]

body mass index: A measure of body mass, defined as weight in kilograms divided by height in meters squared; a method of determining caloric nutritional status. [1]

booster: Administration of an additional vaccination to help increase or speed the immune response to a previous vaccination. [3]

bulimia nervosa: A chronic morbid disorder involving repeated and secretive episodic bouts of eating characterized by uncontrolled rapid ingestion of large quantities of food over a short period of time (binge eating), followed by self-induced vomiting, use of laxatives or diuretics, fasting, or vigorous exercise in order to prevent weight gain; often accompanied by feelings of guilt, depression, or self-disgust. [1]

child psychology: A branch of psychology the theories and applications of which focus on the cognitive and intellectual development of the child in contrast to the adult; subspecialties include developmental psychology, child clinical psychology, pediatric psychology, and pediatric neuropsychology. [1]

childhood immunizations: A series of immunizations that are given to prevent diseases that pose a threat to children. The immunizations in the United States currently include: hepatitis B, diphtheria, tetanus, acellular pertussis, *Haemophilus influenzae* type b, inactivated polio, pneumococcal conjugate, measles, mumps, rubella, varicella, and hepatitis A. [3]

chronic: An illness or injury that lasts for a long time. [2]

Columbia Mental Maturity Scale: An individually administered intelligence test that provides an estimate of the intellectual ability of children; provides mental ages ranging from 3–12 years and requires no verbal response and minimal motor response. [1]

combination vaccine: A combination of two or more vaccines (such as the diphtheria/tetanus/pertussis vaccine). Like the individual vaccines, combination vaccines are developed through scientific research. They are also tested through clinical trials for appropriateness, safety, and effectiveness before they are licensed and released for use by the public. [3]

community immunity: A concept of protecting a community against certain diseases by having a high percentage of the community's population immunized. (Sometimes referred to as "herd" immunity). Even if a few members of the community are unable to be immunized, the entire community will be indirectly protected because the disease has little opportunity for an outbreak. However, with a low percentage of population immunity, the disease would have great opportunity for an outbreak. Examples of the key role of community immunity include being vaccinated with hepatitis B, diphtheria, acellular pertussis, *Haemophilus influenzae* type b, inactivated polio, pneumococcal conjugate, measles, mumps, rubella, varicella, and hepatitis A because these are diseases that can spread through person-to-person transmission. Tetanus, on the other hand, cannot be spread through person-to-person transmission. It is transmitted through skin wounds. For example, if a person steps on a nail or sustains some kind of penetrating injury from something that has been contaminated with tetanus spores, there is significant risk for a life-threatening tetanus infection. The level of community immunity would have no impact on this risk. [3]

concretization: Inability to abstract with an overemphasis on specific details; seen in mental disorders, such as dementia and schizophrenia, and also normally in children. [1]

conduct disorder: A mental disorder of childhood or adolescence characterized by a persistent pattern of violating societal norms and the rights of others; children with the disorder may exhibit physical aggression, cruelty to animals, vandalism and robbery, along with truancy, cheating, and lying. [1]

contraindication: Any condition (especially of disease), which renders some particular line of treatment improper or undesirable. [3]

Denver Developmental Screening Test: A scale used by psychologists and pediatricians to assess the developmental, intellectual, motor, and social maturity of children at any age level from birth to adolescence. [1]

disease: Sickness; illness; an interruption, or disturbance of the bodily functions or organs, which causes or threatens pain and weakness. [3]

eating disorders: A group of mental disorders including anorexia nervosa, bulimia nervosa, pica, and rumination disorder of infancy. [1]

epidemic: An outbreak of disease that spreads within a specific region and/or country. [3] femur: The upper leg or thigh bone, which extends into the hip socket at its upper end and down to the knee at its lower end. [2]

fibula: The thin, outer bone of the leg that forms part of the ankle joint at its lower end. [2]

Goodenough draw-a-man test: A brief test for assessing an individual's level of intelligence based on how accurately drawn and how many elements are included when a child or adult is given a pencil and sheet of white paper and asked to draw a man, the best man he or she is able to draw. Also called the Goodenough Draw-A-Person test and, in its current form, the Goodenough-Harris drawing test. [1]

growing pains: Aching pains, frequently felt at night, in the limbs of children; cause is unclear, but the condition is benign. [1]

hyperactivity: General restlessness or excessive movement such as that characterizing children with attention deficit disorder or hyperkinesis. [1]

immune: A state of being protected against infectious diseases by either specific or non-specific mechanisms (such as immunization, previous natural infection, inoculation, or transfer of protective antibodies). For certain diseases, immune mothers may temporarily transfer protective antibodies to their newborns through the placenta. Protection can result from this placental transfer for up to 4–6 months. [3]

immune system: The body's very complex system (made of many organs and cells), which defends the body against infection, disease, and foreign substances. [3]

immunity: The condition of being immune or protected against infection, disease, and foreign substances. [3]

immunization: A process or procedure that increases an organism's reaction to antigens, thereby, improving its ability to resist or overcome infection. [3]

immunoglobulins: A specific protein substance, produced by plasma cells to help fight infection. [3]

incontinence: Inability to prevent the discharge of any of the excretions, especially of urine or feces. [1]

inflammation: A characteristic reaction of tissues to disease or injury; it is marked by four signs: swelling, redness, heat, and pain. [2]

inoculation: Introduction of material (such as a vaccine or bacteria) into the body's tissues. [3]

intuitive stage: In psychology, a stage of development, usually occurring between 4 and 7 years of age, in which a child's thought processes are determined by the most prominent aspects of the stimuli to which the child is exposed, rather than by some form of logical thought. [1]

joint: A junction where two bones meet. [2]

ligament: A band of tough, fibrous tissue that connects two or more bones at a joint and prevents excessive movement of the joint. [2]

live vaccine: A vaccine that contains a living, yet weakened organism or virus. [3]

measles: 1. An acute exanthematous disease, caused by measles virus (genus *Morbillivirus*), a member of the family *Paramyxoviridae*, and marked by fever and other constitutional disturbances, a catarrhal inflammation of the respiratory mucous membranes, and a generalized maculopapular eruption of a dusky red color; the eruption occurs early on the buccal mucous membrane in the form of

Koplik spots, a manifestation utilized in early diagnosis; average incubation period is from 10–12 days. Recovery is usually rapid but respiratory complications and otitis media caused by secondary bacterial infections are common. Encephalitis occurs rarely. Subacute sclerosing parencephalitis may occur later and is associated with chronic infection. [1]

microorganism: Living organisms or living things (plants or animals) so small in size that they are only visible by the aid of a microscope. [3]

multi-drug resistance: The ability to withstand many antimicrobial drugs. For example, a new strain of pathogen may be resistant to many or all of the drugs that previously worked against the disease caused by the pathogen. [3]

mumps: An acute infectious and contagious disease caused by a mumps virus of the genus Rubulavirus and characterized by fever, inflammation and swelling of the parotid gland, sometimes of other salivary glands, and occasionally by inflammation of the testis, ovary, pancreas, or meninges. [1]

muscle: Tissue composed of bundles of specialized cells that contract and produce movement when stimulated by nerve impulses. [2]

night terrors: A disorder occurring in children, in which the child awakes screaming with fright, the distress persisting for a time during a state of semiconsciousness. [1]

nocturnal enuresis: Urinary incontinence during sleep. Synonym: bed-wetting. [1]

orthopsychiatry: A cross-disciplinary science combining child psychiatry, developmental psychology, pediatrics, and family care devoted to the discovery, prevention, and treatment of mental and psychological disorders in children and adolescents. [1]

outbreak: Spread of disease, which occurs in a short period of time and in a limited geographic location (such as a neighborhood, community, school, or hospital). [3]

pandemic: An outbreak of disease that spreads throughout the world. [3]

pathogen: Bacteria, viruses, parasites, or fungi that have the capability to cause disease in humans. [3]

pediatrics: The medical specialty concerned with the study and treatment of children in health and disease during development from birth through adolescence. [1]

pedodontics: The branch of dentistry concerned with the dental care and treatment of children. [1]

pica: A perverted appetite for substances not fit as food or of no nutritional value; for example, clay, dried paint, starch, ice. [1]

play therapy: A type of therapy used with children in which they can express or reveal their problems and fantasies by playing with dolls or other toys, drawing, etc. [1]

precocious pseudopuberty: The development of pseudopuberty in very young children; commonly characterized by secretion of gonadal hormones, without stimulation of gametogenesis. [1]

quarantine: To isolate an individual who has or is suspected of having a disease, in order to prevent spreading the disease to others; alternatively, to isolate a person who does not have a disease during a disease outbreak, in order to prevent that person from catching the disease. Quarantine can be voluntary or ordered by public health officials in times of emergency. [3]

range of motion: The arc of movement of a joint from one extreme position to the other; range-of-motion exercises help increase or maintain flexibility and movement in muscles, tendons, ligaments, and joints. [2]

reality principle: The concept that the pleasure principle in personality development is modified by the demands of external reality; the principle or force that compels the growing child to adapt to the demands of external reality. [1]

rubella: An acute but mild exanthematous disease caused by rubella virus (*Rubivirus* family *Togaviridae*), with enlargement of lymph nodes, but usually with little fever or constitutional reaction; a high incidence of birth defects in children results from maternal infection during the first trimester of fetal life (congenital rubella syndrome). Synonyms: third disease, German measles, three-day measles, [1]

Stanford-Binet intelligence scale: A standardized test for the measurement of intelligence consisting of a series of questions, graded according to the intelligence of normal children at different ages, the answers to which indicate the mental age of the person tested; primarily used with children, but also contains norms for adults standardized against adult age levels rather than those of children, as formerly was the case. [1]

stature: The height of a person. [1]

stool: 1. A discharging of the bowels. 2. The matter discharged at one movement of the bowels. [1]

stuttering: A phonatory or articulatory disorder, characteristically beginning in childhood, with intense anxiety about the efficiency of oral communications, and characterized by dysfluency: hesitations, repetitions, and prolongations of sounds and syllables, interjections, broken words, circumlocutions, and words produced with excess tension. [1]

syllable-stumbling: A form of stuttering in which halting occurs at certain syllables that are difficult for the individual to enunciate. [1]

Tanner growth chart: A series of charts showing distribution of parameters of physical development, such as stature, growth curves, and skinfold thickness, for children by sex, age, and stages of puberty. [1]

Tanner stage: A stage of puberty in the Tanner growth chart, based on pubic hair growth, development of genitalia in boys, and breast development in girls. [1]

tendons: Tough, fibrous cords of tissue that connect muscle to bone. [2]

tetanus: A disease marked by painful tonic muscular contractions, caused by the neurotropic toxin (tetanospasmin) of *Clostridium tetani* acting upon the central nervous system. [1]

tibia: The thick, long bone of the lower leg (also called the shin) that forms part of the knee joint at its upper end and the ankle joint at its lower end. [2]

transitional object: An object used by many children as a substitute for a parent who is absent (usually temporarily) to help them deal with separation; typically, a blanket or stuffed toy. [1]

vaccination: Injection of a weakened or killed microorganism (bacterium or virus) given for the prevention or treatment of infectious diseases. [3]

vaccine: A product of weakened or killed microorganism (bacterium or virus) given for the prevention or treatment of infectious diseases. [3]

vaccine schedule: A chart or plan of vaccinations that are recommended for specific ages and/or circumstances. [3]

varicella: An acute contagious disease, usually occurring in children, caused by the varicella-zoster virus genus, *Varicellovirus*, a member of the family *Herpesviridae*, and marked by a sparse eruption of papules, which become vesicles and then pustules, like that of smallpox although less severe and varying in stages, usually with mild constitutional symptoms; incubation period is about 14–17 days. Synonym: chickenpox. [1]

virus: A tiny parasite that grows and reproduces in living cells. Vaccines prevent illnesses caused by the following viruses: hepatitis B, polio, measles, mumps, rubella, varicella, and hepatitis A. [3]

Wetzel grid: Chart of growth, plotting height, weight, physical fitness and related aspects of young and adolescent children during growth. [1]

Chapter 55

Suggestions for Additional Reading

Books for Parents

The books listed here represent a small sampling of the many different resources available. To make topics readily apparent, the books are listed alphabetically by title. They may be obtained through your local library or book store.

American Academy of Pediatrics Guide to Your Child's Nutrition: Making Peace at the Table and Building Healthy Eating Habits for Life
Editors: William H. Dietz and Loraine Stern
Publisher: Villard Books, 1999
ISBN: 0375754873

American Academy of Pediatrics Guide to Your Child's Symptoms: The Official, Complete Home Reference, Birth Through Adolescence
Editors: Donald Schiff and Steven P. Shelov
Publisher: Villard Books, 1997
ISBN: 0375752579

The resources on children's health and other related parenting topics listed in this chapter were compiled from many sources deemed reliable. The lists serve as starting points for further reading; they are not intended to be comprehensive or all-inclusive. Inclusion does not imply endorsement.

Child Safe: A Practical Guide for Preventing Childhood Injuries
Author: Mark A., M.D. Brandenburg
Publisher: Three Rivers Press 2000
ISBN: 060980412X

Children's Hospital Guide to Your Child's Health and Development
Editors: Alan D. Woolf, Margaret A. Kenna, and Howard C. Shane
Publisher: Perseus Publishing, 2002
ISBN: 0738207438

Common Sense Parenting: A Proven Step-by-Step Guide for Raising Responsible Kids and Creating Happy Families
Authors: Raymond V. Burke and Ronald W. Herron
Publisher: Boys Town Press, 1997
ISBN: 0938510770

Driven to Distraction: Recognizing and Coping with Attention Deficit Disorder from Childhood through Adulthood
Authors: Edward M. Hallowell and John J. Ratey
Publisher: Simon and Schuster Adult Publishing Group, 1995
ISBN: 0684801280

Guide To Your Child's Symptoms: The Official, Complete Home Reference, Birth through Adolescence
Author: Donald Schiff M.D., F.A.
Publisher: Random House, 1998
ISBN: 0375752579

Harvard Medical School Family Health Guide
Editor: Anthony L. Komaroff
Publisher: The Free Press, 1999
ISBN: 0684847035

Healing ADD: The Breakthrough Program That Allows You to See and Heal the Six Types of Attention Deficit Disorder
Authors: Daniel G. Amen and Lisa C. Routh
Publisher: Penguin Group (USA), Inc., 2001
ISBN: 039914644X

Irreducible Needs of Children: What Every Child Must Have to Grow, Learn and Flourish
Authors: T. Berry Brazelton and Stanley I. Greenspan
Publisher: Perseus Publishing, 2001
ISBN: 0738205168

Kids and Sports
Authors: Eric Small, Linda Spear, and Sheryl Swoopes
Publisher: W.W. Norton and Company, 2002
ISBN: 1557045321

Magic Trees of the Mind: How to Nurture Your Child's Intelligence, Creativity, and Healthy Emotions from Birth through Adolescence
Authors: Marian Diamond and Janet Hopson
Publisher: Dutton/Plume, 1999
ISBN: 0452278309

The Panic-Proof Parent: Creating a Safe Lifestyle for Your Family
Author: Debra Smiley Holtzman
Publisher: McGraw-Hill/Contemporary Books, 2000
ISBN: 0809223929

Parents in Charge: Setting Healthy, Loving Boundaries for You and Your Child
Author: Dana Chidekel
Publisher: Simon and Schuster Adult Publishing Group, 2002
ISBN: 0743202023

Sex and Sensibility: The Thinking Parent's Guide to Talking Sense About Sex
Author: Deborah M. Roffman
Publisher: Perseus Publishing, 2001
ISBN: 0738205206

Smart Medicine for a Healthier Child: A Practical A-To-Z Reference to Natural and Conventional Treatments for Infants and Children
Authors: Janet Zand and Robert Rountree
Publisher: Avery Penguin Putnam, 1994
ISBN: 0895295458

Successful Child: What Parents Can Do to Help Kids Turn out Well
Authors: William Sears and Martha Sears
Publisher: Little, Brown and Company, 2002
ISBN: 0316777498

Taking Care of Your Child: A Parent's Guide to Complete Medical Care, Sixth Edition
Authors: Robert H. Pantell, James Fries, and Donald Vickery
Publisher: Perseus Publishing, 2002
ISBN: 0738206016

Touchpoints: Your Child's Emotional and Behavioral Development
Author: T. Berry Brazelton
Publisher: Perseus Publishing, 1994
ISBN: 020162690X

What About the Kids? Raising Your Children Before, During, and After Divorce
Authors: Judith S. Wallerstein and Sandra Blakeslee
Publisher: Hyperion, 2003
ISBN: 0786868651

The Young Athlete: A Sports Doctor's Complete Guide for Parents
Authors: Jordan D. Metzl, M.D. and Carol Shookhoff
Publisher: Little Brown and Company, 2002
ISBN: 0316607568

Your Child's Health: The Parent's Guide to Symptoms, Emergencies, Common Illnesses, Behavior and School Problems
Author: Barton D. Schmitt
Publisher: Bantam Books, Inc., 1991
ISBN: 055335339X

Parenting and Child Health Information on the Internet

The following websites, which are listed alphabetically by organization, include a sampling the information about parenting and child health that is available on the internet. The web addresses will take you directly to the resources noted. If typing is difficult, you may wish to go to the organization's home page (usually the first part of the address, ending with .com, .org, or .gov) and use links or search features within the website.

American Academy of Child and Adolescent Psychiatry
Facts for Families: http://www.aacap.org/publications/factsfam/index.htm

American Academy of Pediatrics
You and Your Family: http://www.aap.org/family

Centers for Disease Control and Prevention (CDC)
Growth Charts: http://www.cdc.gov/growthcharts
SafeUSA™: http://www.safeusa.org

Consumer Product Safety Commission
Kid Safety: http://www.cpsc.gov/kids/kidsafety/index.html

Healthfinder®
Just for You—Parents: http://www.healthfinder.gov/justforyou/ (click on "Parents")

MedlinePlus®
Health Information: http://www.nlm.nih.gov/medlineplus

National Criminal Justice Reference Service
Parenting Resources for the 21st Century: http://www.parentingresources.ncjrs.org

Nemours Foundation, Inc.
KidsHealth: http://kidshealth.org

New York Online Access to Health
Ask NOAH about Child Health: http://www.noah-health.org/english/wellness/healthyliving/childhealth.html

Packard (David and Lucille) Foundation
The Future of Children: http://www.futureofchildren.org

U.S. Department of Health and Human Services
Families and Children: http://www.hhs.gov/children/index.shtml

Virtual Children's Hospital
http://www.vh.org/pediatric/index.html

Chapter 56

Childhood Drug Abuse Prevention, Services, and Information

African American Parents for Drug Prevention
311 Martin Luther King Drive
Cincinnati, OH 45219
Phone: 513-475-5359
Fax: 513-281-1645

Al-Anon Family Group Headquarters, Inc.
1600 Corporate Landing Parkway
Virginia Beach, VA 23454-5617
Toll free: 888-425-2666
Phone: 757-563-1600
Fax: 757-563-1655
Website: http://www.al-anon.alateen.org
E-mail: WSO@al-anon.org

Alcoholics Anonymous
475 Riverside Drive
P.O. Box 459
New York, NY 10015
Phone: 212-870-3400
Fax: 212-870-3003
Website: http://www.aa.org

American Council for Drug Education (ACDE)
164 W. 74th Street
New York, NY 10023
Toll-Free: 800-488-DRUG (800-488-3784)
Website: http://www.acde.org
E-mail: acde@phoenixhouse.org

The list of organizations in this chapter was compiled from many sources. It serves as a starting point for further research by providing a sampling of organizations; it is not all inclusive. Contact information was verified in May 2003. Inclusion does not constitute endorsement.

The Anti-Drug
White House Office of National
Drug Control Policy
Website: http://
www.theantidrug.com
Spanish-language site:
www.laantidroga.com
E-mail: ondcp@ncjrs.org

Asian American Recovery Services
965 Mission Street, Suite 325
San Francisco, CA 94103-2921
Phone: 415-541-9285
Fax: 415-541-9986
Website: http://www.aars-inc.org

Boys and Girls Clubs of America
1230 W. Peachtree Street, NW
Atlanta, GA 30309
Phone: 404-815-5700
Website: http://www.bgca.org
E-mail: info@bgca.org

Camp Fire, Inc.
4601 Madison Avenue
Kansas City, MO 64112-1278
Phone: 816-756-1950
Fax: 816-756-2650
Website: http://
www.campfireusa.org
E-mail: info@campfireusa.org

Center for Substance Abuse Prevention
5600 Fishers Lane, Rockwall II
Rockville, MD 20857
Phone: 301-443-0365
Website: http://
www.prevention.samhsa.gov
E-mail: info@samhsa.gov

Children Now
1212 Broadway, 5th Floor
Oakland, CA 94612
Phone: 510-763-2444
Fax: 510-763-1974
Website: http://
www.childrennow.org
E-mail: children@childrennow.org

Club Drugs Website
Website: http://
www.clubdrugs.org

Community Anti-Drug Coalitions of America
901 N. Pitt Street, Suite 300
Alexandria, VA 22314
Toll Free: 800-54-CADCA
Phone: 703-706-0560
Fax: 703-706-0565
Website: http://www.cadca.org
E-mail: webmaster@cadca.org
E-mail: info@cadca.org

Comprehensive Substance Abuse and Violence Prevention
1446 M. L. King Jr. Parkway
Des Moines IA 50314
Phone: 515-471-2332
Fax: 515-243-5879
Website: http://www.efr.org/sbv/
prev_services.shtml
E-mail: info@efr.org

Connect for Kids
The Benton Foundation
1625 K St., NW, 11th Floor
Washington, DC 20006
Phone: 202-638-5770
Fax: 202-638-5771
Website: www.connectforkids.org
E-mail: info@connectforkids.org

Connecticut Clearinghouse
334 Farmington Avenue
Plainville, CT 06062
Toll Free: 800-232-4424
Fax: 860-793-9813
Website: http://
www.ctclearinghouse.org
E-mail: info@ctclearinghouse.org

*Drug Enforcement
Administration (DEA)*
Information Services Section
(CPI)
2401 Jefferson Davis Highway
Alexandria, VA 22301
Phone: 202-307-1000
Website: http://www.usdoj.gov/dea

Families Anonymous
P.O. Box 3475
Culver City, CA 90231-3475
Toll-Free: 800-736-9805
Fax: 310-815-9682
Website: http://
www.familiesanonymous.org
E-mail:
famanon@FamiliesAnonymous.org

Indian Health Service
The Reyes Building
801 Thompson Avenue, Suite 400
Rockville, MD 20852-1627
Phone: 301-443-5070
Website: http://www.ihs.gov

*Indiana Prevention
Resource Center*
Indiana University
2735 E. 10th Street,
Rm. 110, Creative Arts Building
Bloomington, IN 47408-2606

*Indiana Prevention
Resource Center*, continued
Toll Free in IN: 800-346-3077
Phone: 812-855-1237
Fax: 812-855-4940
Website: http://
www.drugs.indiana.edu/
E-mail: drugprc@indiana.edu

Join Together
One Appleton Street, 4th Floor
Boston, MA 02116-5223
Phone: 617-437-1500
Fax: 617-437-9394
Website: http://
www.jointogether.org
Screening website:
www.alcoholscreening.org
E-mail: info@jointogether.org

*Leadership to Keep
Children Alcohol Free*
c/o The CDM Group
5530 Wisconsin Ave., Suite 1600
Chevy Chase, MD 20815-4305
Phone: 301-654-6740
Fax: 301-656-4012
Website:
www.alcoholfreechildren.org
E-mail:
leadership@alcoholfreechildren.org

*Mothers Against Drunk
Driving (MADD)*
511 E. John Carpenter Freeway,
Suite 700
Irving, TX 75062
Toll-Free: 800-GET-MADD
Phone: 214-744-6233
Fax: 972-869-2206
Website: http://www.madd.org
E-mail: victims@madd.org

Narcotics Anonymous
P.O. Box 9999
Van Nuys, CA 91409
Phone: 818-773-9999
Fax: 818-700-0700
Website: http://na.org
E-mail: info@na.org

National Asian Pacific American Families Against Substance Abuse (NAPAFASA)
340 East 2nd Street, Suite 409
Los Angeles, CA 90012-2818
Phone: 213-625-5795
Fax: 213-625-5796
Website: http://www.napafasa.org
E-mail: napafasa@apanet.org

National Association for Children of Alcoholics
11426 Rockville Pike, Suite 100
Rockville, MD 20852
Toll-Free: 888-554-COAS
Phone: 301-468-0985
Fax: 301-468-0987
Website: http://www.nacoa.org
E-mail: nacoa@nacoa.org

National Center on Addiction and Substance Abuse at Columbia University
633 Third Avenue, 19th Floor
New York, NY 10017-6706
Phone: 212-841-5200
Fax: 212-956-8020
Website: http://www.casacolumbia.org

National Center for Tobacco-Free Kids
1400 Eye Street, Suite 1200
Washington, DC 20005
Phone: 202-246-5469
Fax: 202-296-5427
Website: www.tobaccofreekids.org
E-mail: info@tobaccofreekids.org

National Clearinghouse for Alcohol and Drug Information (NCADI)
P.O. Box 2345
Rockville, MD 20847-2345
Toll-Free: 800-729-6686
Spanish: 877-767-8432
TTY: 800-487-4889
Phone: 301-468-2600
Website: http://www.health.org

National Council on Alcoholism and Drug Dependence
20 Exchange Place, Suite 2902
New York, NY 10005
Toll-Free: 800-NCA-CALL
Phone: 212-269-7797
Fax: 212-269-7510
Website: www.ncadd.org
E-mail: national@ncadd.org

National Crime Prevention Council
1000 Connecticut Avenue, NW
13th Floor
Washington, DC 20036
Phone: 202-466-6272
Fax: 202-296-1356
Website: www.ncpc.org

National Drug Prevention League

16 South Calvert Street
Baltimore, MD 20202
Phone: 410-385-9094
Fax: 410-385-9096
Website: http://www.ndpl.org

National Drug Strategy Network

1225 I Street NW, Suite 500
Washington, DC 20009
Phone: 202-842-2620
Website: http://www.ndsn.org
E-mail: NDSN@ndsn.org

National Families in Action

2957 Clairmont Road, Suite 150
Atlanta, GA 30329
Phone: 404-248-9676
Fax: 404-248-1312
Website: http://
www.nationalfamilies.org
E-mail: nfia@nationalfamilies.org

National Inhalant Prevention Coalition

2904 Kerbey Lane
Austin, TX 78703
Toll-Free: 800-269-4237
Phone: 512-480-8953
Fax: 512-477-3932
http://www.inhalants.org
E-mail: nipc@io.com

National Institute on Alcohol Abuse and Alcoholism (NIAAA)

6000 Executive Boulevard,
Willco Building
Bethesda, MD 20892-7003

NIAAA, continued

Phone: 301-443-3860
Fax: 301-480-1726
Website: http://
www.niaaa.nih.gov
E-mail: niaaaweb-r@exchange.nih.gov

Network International-Coalition for On-line Resources

8525 East Bonita Drive
Scottsdale, AZ 85250
Toll Free: 866-466-4267
Phone: 602-405-7750
Website: http://www.ni-cor.com
E-mail: contact@ni-cor.com

Office of National Drug Control Policy

P.O. Box 6000
Rockville, MD 20849-6000
Toll Free: 800-666-3332
Fax; 301-519-5212
Website: http://
www.whitehousedrugpolicy.gov
Alternate website: http://
www.helpyourcommunity.org
E-mail: ondcp@ncjrs.org

Office of Prevention and Youth Services Addiction, Prevention and Recovery Administration

1350 Pennsylvania Avenue, NW
Washington, DC 20004
Phone: 202-727-1000
Website: http://dchealth.dc.gov/
services/administration_offices/
apr/svc_youth.shtm

Parents. The Anti-Drug
Toll Free: 800-788-2800
White House Office of National
Drug Control Policy
Website: http://
www.theantidrug.com

Partnership for a Drug-Free America
405 Lexington Avenue
Suite 1601
New York, NY 10174
Phone: 212-922-1560
Fax: 212-922-1570
Website: http://
www.drugfreeamerica.org

Prevention Partners, Inc.
One Mustard Street, Suite 400
Rochester, NY 14609
Phone: 716-288-2800
Fax: 716-288-2847
Website: www.psquared.org
E-mail: drugslie@psquared.org

Research Institute on Addictions (RIA)
1021 Main Street
Buffalo, NY 14203
Phone: 716-887-2566
Fax: 716-887-2252
Website: http://www.ria.org
E-mail:
webmaster@ria.buffalo.edu

Substance Abuse and Mental Health Services Administration (SAMHSA)
Room 12-105 Parklawn
Building, 5600 Fishers Lane
Rockville, MD 20857

SAMHSA, continued
Phone: 301-443-4795
Fax: 301-443-0284
Website: http://www.samhsa.gov
E-mail: info@samhsa.gov

Safe and Drug-Free Schools
U.S. Department of Education
400 Maryland Avenue, SW
Washington, DC 20202
Toll-Free: 800-USA-LEARN
Website: http://www.ed.gov/
offices/OESE/index.html
E-mail:
customerservice@inet.ed.gov

Web of Addictions
Website: http://www.well.com/
user/woa

Women for Sobriety
P.O. Box 618
Quakertown, PA 18951-0618
Phone: 215-536-8026
Fax: 215-538-9026
Website: http://
www.womenforsobriety.org
E-mail: NewLife@nni.com

Youth to Youth International
700 Bryden Road
Columbus, OH 43215
Phone: 614-224-4506
Fax: 614-224-8451
Website: http://www.y2yint.com
E-mail: general@y2yint.com

Chapter 57

Education Organizations and Resources

ACCESS ERIC
2277 Research Boulevard, 6M
Rockville, MD 20850
Toll Free: 800-LET-ERIC (800-538-3742)
Phone: 301-519-5157
Fax: 301-519-6760
Website: http://www.eric.ed.gov/resources/parent/parent.html
E-mail: accesseric@accesseric.org

Activating Children Through Technology (ACTT)
Western Illinois University
Macomb Projects
27 Horrabin Hall
Macomb, IL 61455
Phone: 309-298-1634
Website: http://www.wiu.edu/users/mimacp/wiu/acct.html

American Council on Rural Special Education (ACRES)
Utah State University
2865 Old Main Hill
Logan, Utah 84322-2665
Phone: 435-797-3911
Website: http://extension.usu.edu/acres
E-mail: acres@cc.usu.edu

Association for Childhood Education International
17904 Georgia Ave., Suite 215
Olney, MD 20832
Toll-Free: 800-423-3563
Phone: 301-570-2111
Fax; 301-570-2212
Website: http://www.udel.edu/bateman/acei
E-mail: aceihq@aol.com

The list of organizations in this chapter was compiled from many sources. It serves as a starting point for further research by providing a sampling of organizations; it is not all inclusive. Contact information was verified in May 2003. Inclusion does not constitute endorsement.

CADRE (Consortium for Appropriate Dispute Resolution in Special Education) Direction Service, Inc.
P.O. Box 51360
Eugene, OR 97405-0906
Phone: 541-686-5060
Fax: 541-686-5063
TTY: 541-284-4740
Website:
www.directionservice.org/cadre
E-mail:
cadre@directionservice.org

Center for Minority Special Education (CMSE)
114 Phenix Hall
Hampton University
Hampton, VA 23668
Toll Free: 800-241-1441
Phone: 757-727-5100
Website: http://
www.hamptonu.edu/bsrc/CMSE/
index.html
E-mail: cmse@cs.hamptonu.edu

Center for the Improvement of Early Reading Achievement (CIERA)
University of Michigan School of Education
610 East University Avenue, Room 2002 SEB
Ann Arbor, MI 48109-1259
Phone: 734-647-6940
Fax: 734-615-4858
Website: http://www.ciera.org
E-mail: ciera@umich.edu

Clearinghouse for Immigrant Education (CHIME)
100 Boylston Street, Suite 737
Boston, MA 02116
Toll-Free: 800-441-7192
Phone: 617-357-8507

CH.A.D.D. (Children and Adults with Attention-Deficit/Hyperactivity Disorder)
8181 Professional Place
Suite 150
Landover, MD 20785
Toll-Free: 800-233-4050
Phone: 301-306-7070
Fax: 301-306-7090
Website: http://www.chadd.org
E-mail: national@chadd.org

Closing the Gap, Inc.
P.O. Box 68
526 Main Street
Henderson, MN 56044
Phone: 507-248-3294
Fax: 507-248-3810
Website: http://
www.closingthegap.com

Coordinated Campaign for Learning Disabilities
c/o Communications Consortium
Media Center
1200 New York Avenue, NW, Suite 300
Washington, DC 20005-1754
Toll Free: 888-478-6463
Phone: 202-326-8700
Website: http://
www.ldonline.org/ccldinfo

Council for Exceptional Children (CEC)
1110 N. Glebe Road, Suite 300
Arlington, VA 22201-5704
Toll-Free: 888-232-7733
Toll-Free TTY: 866-915-5000
Phone: 703-620-3660
Fax: 703-264-9494
CEC Website: www.cec.sped.org
Division for Learning Disabilities Website: http://www.dldcec.org
IDEA Partnerships Website: http://www.ideapractices.org
E-mail: cec@cec.sped.org

Early Childhood Research Institute on Culturally and Linguistically Appropriate Services
University of Illinois at Urbana-Champaign
61 Children's Research Center
51 Gerty Drive
Champaign, IL 61820-7498
Toll-Free: 800-583-4135
Phone: 217-333-4123
Website: http://clas.uiuc.edu
E-mail: clas@uiuc.edu

Early Head Start/Head Start Program
Information and Publication Center
1133 15th St., NW, Suite 450
Washington, DC 20002
Toll Free: 866-763-6481
Phone: 202-737-1030
Fax: 202-737-1151
Website: http://www.headstartinfo.org

ERIC Clearinghouse on Disabilities and Gifted Education
Council for Exceptional Children (CEC)
1110 N. Glebe Road, Suite 300
Arlington, VA 22201-5704
Toll-Free: 800-328-0272
Website: http://ericec.org
E-mail: ericec@cec.sped.org

ERIC Clearinghouse on Reading, English, and Communication
Indiana University
Smith Research Center
Suite 140
Bloomington, IN 47408-2698
Toll-Free: 800-759-4723
Phone: 812-855-5847
Fax: 812-856-5512
Website: http://www.Indiana.edu/ericd/~eric_rec

Even Start Family Literacy Program
U.S. Department of Education
Office of Elementary and Secondary Education
Student Achievement and School Accountability Programs
400 Independence Avenue SW
Washington, DC 20202
Phone: 202-260-0991
Fax: 202-260-7764
Website: http://www.ed.gov/offices/OESE /SASA/statecoo.html
E-mail: OESE@ed.gov

Families and Advocates Partnership for Education (FAPE)
PACER Center
8161 Normandale Blvd.
Minneapolis, MN 55437-1044
Phone: 952-838-9000
Fax: 952-838-0199
TTY: 952-838-0190
Web: http://www.fape.org
E-mail: fape@fape.org

Family Education Network
20 Park Plaza, 12th Floor
Boston, MA 02116
Phone: 617-542-6500
http://www.familyeducation.com

Federal Resource Center for Special Education
Academy for Educational Development
1875 Connecticut Ave., N.W.
Washington, DC 20009
Phone: 202-884-8215
Fax: 202-884-8443
TTY: 202-884-8200
Website: http://
www.federalresourcecenter.org/
frc

Head Start Bureau
Administration on Children, Youth and Families
U.S. Department of Health and Human Services
P.O. Box 1182
Washington, DC 20013
Website: www.acf.dhhs.gov/
programs/hsb

Home and School Institute—MegaSkills Education Center
1500 Massachusetts Ave., NW
Washington, DC 20005
Phone: 202-466-3633
Website: http://
www.megaskillshsi.org

International Dyslexia Association
Chester Building, Suite 382
8600 LaSalle Road
Baltimore, MD 21286-2044
Toll-Free: 800-222-3123
Phone: 410-296-0232
Fax: 410-321-5069
Website: http://www.interdys.org
E-mail: info@interdys.org

International Reading Association (IRA)
800 Barksdale Road
P.O. Box 8139
Newark, DE 19714-8139
Phone: 302-731-1600
Fax: 302-731-1057
Website: http://www.reading.org

LDOnline
Website: http://www.ldonline.org

Learning Disabilities Association of America
4156 Library Road
Pittsburgh, PA 15234-1349
Toll-Free: 888-300-6710
Phone: 412-341-1515
Fax: 412-344-0224
Website: http://
www.ldaamerica.org
E-mail: info@ldaamerica.org

National Alliance of Black School Educators
310 Pennsylvania Ave., SE
Washington, DC 20003
Toll-Free: 800-221-2654
Phone: 202-608-6310
Fax: 202-608-6319
Website: http://www.nabse.org

National Association for the Education of Young Children
1509 16th Street, N.W.
Washington, DC 20036-1426
Toll Free: 800-424-2460
Phone: 202-232-8777
Fax: 202-328-1846
Website: http://www.naeyc.org
E-mail: naeyc@naeyc.org

National Association of Private Special Education Centers (NAPSEC)
1522 K Street N.W., Suite 1032
Washington, DC 20005-1202
Phone: 202-408-3338
Fax: 202-408-3340
Website: http://www.napsec.com
E-mail: napsec@aol.com

National Attention Deficit Disorder Association
1788 Second Street, Suite 200
Highland Park, IL 60035
Phone: 847-432-2332
Fax: 847-432-5874
Website: http://www.add.org
E-mail: mail@add.org

National Center for Family Literacy
Waterfront Plaza
Suite 200
325 West Main Street
Louisville, KY 40202-4237
Toll-Free: 877-326-5481 (Parade Family Literacy InfoLine)
Phone: 502-584-1133
Website: http://www.famlit.org

National Center for Learning Disabilities
381 Park Avenue South
Suite 1401
New York, NY 10016
Toll-Free: 888-575-7373
Phone: 212-545-7510
Fax: 212-545-9665
Website: http://www.ld.org

National Clearinghouse for Bilingual Education (NCBE)
The George Washington University
2121 K Street NW
Suite 260
Washington, DC 20037
Toll Free: 800-321-6223
Phone: 202-467-0867
Fax: 800-531-9347; 202-467-4283
Website: http://www.ncbe.gwu.edu
E-mail: askncbe@ncbe.gwu.edu

National Clearinghouse for Comprehensive School Reform (NCCSR)
2121 K Street NW
Suite 250
Washington, DC 20037
Toll-Free: 877-766-4277
Fax: 877-308-4995
Website: http://www.goodschools.gwu.edu
E-mail: AskNCCSR@godschools.gwu.edu

National Clearinghouse for English Language Acquisition and Language Instruction Educational Programs (NCELA)
2121 K Street
Suite 260
Washington, DC 20037
Toll-Free: 800-321-6223
Phone: 202-467-0867
Fax: 800-321-9347; 202-467-4283
Website: http://www.ncela.gwu.edu
E-mail: askncela@ncela.gwu.edu

National Clearinghouse for ESL Literacy Education (NCLE)
4646 40th Street N.W.
Washington, DC 20016
Phone: 202-429-9292, ext. 200
Fax: 202-363-7204
Website: http://www.cal.org/NCLE
E-mail: ncle@cal.org

National Coalition for Parent Involvement in Education (NCPIE)
3929 Old Lee Highway
Suite 91-A
Fairfax, VA 22030-2401
Phone: 703-359-8973
Fax: 703-359-0972
Website: http://www.ncpie.org

National Congress of Parents and Teachers
330 North Wabash Avenue
Suite 2100
Chicago, IL 60611
Toll-Free: 800-307-4PTA
Phone: 312-670-6783
Fax: 312-670-6783
Website: http://www.pta.org
E-mail: info@pta.org

National Institute for Literacy (NIFL)
1775 I Street NW
Suite 730
Washington, DC 20006-2401
Phone: 202-233-2025
Fax: 202-233-2050
Website: http://www.nifl.gov

National Information Center for Educational Media
P.O. Box 8640
Albuquerque, NM 87198
Toll-Free: 800-926-8328
Website: http://www.nicem.com

National Library of Education (NLE)
400 Maryland Avenue, SW
Washington, DC 20202
Toll-Free: 800-424-1616
Phone: 202-205-4945
Fax: 202-401-0552
TTY: 202-205-7561
Website: http://www.ed.gov/NLE
E-mail: library@ed.gov

National Middle School Association
4151 Executive Parkway
Suite 300
Westerville, OH 43081
Toll-Free: 800-528-NMSA (800-528-6672)
Phone: 614-895-4730
Fax: 614-895-4750
Website: http://www.nmsa.org
E-mail: info@NMSA.org

National Resource Center for Paraprofessionals in Education and Related Services
6526 Old Main Hill
Utah State University
Logan, UT 84322-6526
Phone: 435-797-7272
Website: http://www.nrcpara.org
E-mail: info@nrcpara.org

No Child Left Behind— Parents Tool Box
U.S. Department of Education
400 Maryland Avenue SW
Washington, DC 20202
Toll-Free: 888-814-NCLB (888-814-6252)
Fax: 202-401-0689
TTY (Toll Free): 800-437-0833
Website: http://www.nochildleftbehind.gov/parents/index.html

Nonverbal Learning Disorders Association
2446 Albany Avenue
West Hartford, CT 06117
Phone: 860-570-0217
Website: http://www.nlda.org
E-mail: NLDA@nlda.org

Office of Special Education and Rehabilitative Services
U.S. Department of Education
400 Maryland Ave., SW
Washington, DC 20202
Phone: 202-205-5465
http://www.ed.gov/offices/OSERS

ProLiteracy Worldwide
1320 Jamesville Avenue
Syracuse, NY 13210
Toll Free: 888-528-2224
Phone: 315-422-9121
Fax: 315-422-6369
Website: http://www.proliteracy.org
E-mail: info@proliteracy.org

Reading Is Fundamental, Inc. (RIF)
1825 Connecticut Avenue, NW
Washington, DC 20009
Toll-Free: 877-RIF-READ (877-743-7323)
Phone: 202-673-0020
Website: http://www.rif.org
E-mail: contactus@rif.org

Schwab Learning
1650 S. Amphlett Blvd., Suite 300
San Mateo, CA 94402
Toll-Free: 800-230-0988
Phone: 650-655-2410
Fax: 650-655-2411
Website: http://
www.schwablearning.org
E-mail:
webmaster@schwablearning.org

Urban Special Education Leadership Collaborative
EDC, Inc.
55 Chapel Street
Newton, MA 02458-1060
Phone: 617-969-7100 ext. 2105
Fax: 617-969-3440
TTY: 617-964-5448
Website: http://www.edc.org/
collaborative
E-mail: collaborative@edc.org

U.S. Department of Education
400 Maryland Avenue, SW
Washington, DC 20202
Toll-Free: 800-USA-LEARN
(800-872-5327)
Fax: 202-401-0689
TTY: 800-437-0833
Website: www.ed.gov
E-mail:
customerservice@inet.ed.gov

White House Initiative on Educational Excellence for Hispanic Americans
400 Maryland Avenue, SW
Room 5E110
Washington, DC 20202-3601
Toll Free: 800-USA-Learn (800-872-5327)
Phone: 202-401-3601
Fax: 202-401-8377
Website: http://www.yic.gov/
index.html

Chapter 58

Other Child Health and Parenting Resources

Child Abuse and Domestic Violence

Child Welfare League of America
440 First Street, NW, 3rd Floor
Washington, DC 20001-2085
Phone: 202-638-2952
Fax: 202-638-4004
Website: http://www.cwla.org

Childhelp USA
15757 N. 78th Street
Scottsdale, AZ 85260
Toll-Free: 800-4-A-CHILD (800-422-4453)
Phone: 480-922-8212
Fax: 480-922-7061
Website: http://www.childhelpusa.org

Clearinghouse on Child Abuse and Neglect/Family Violence Information
330 C Street, SW
Washington, DC 20477
Toll-Free: 800-394-3366
Phone: 703-382-7576
Fax: 703-385-3206
Website: http://www.calib.com/nccanch
E-mail: nccanch@calib.com

Family Violence National Domestic Violence Hotline
Toll-Free: 800-799-SAFE (800-799-7233)
Website: http://www.ndvh.org

The list of organizations in this chapter was compiled from many sources. It serves as a starting point for further research by providing a sampling of organizations; it is not all inclusive. Contact information was verified in May 2003. Inclusion does not constitute endorsement.

National Center for Missing and Exploited Children

Charles B. Wang International
Children's Building
699 Prince Street
Alexandria, VA 22314-3175
Toll-Free: 800-843-5678
Phone: 703-274-3900
Fax: 703-274-2200
Website: http://
www.missingkids.com

National Child Abuse Hotline

Toll-Free: 800-422-4453
Website: http://
www.childhelpusa.org

National Foundation for Abused and Neglected Children

P.O. Box 1841
Chicago, IL 60660-1841
Website: http://gangfreekids.org
E-mail: nfanc@hotmail.com

National Youth Crisis Hotline

National Youth Development
Toll-Free: 800-HIT-HOME
Website: http://
www.1800hithome.com

Prevent Child Abuse America

200 S. Michigan Ave., 17th Floor
Chicago, IL 60604-2404
Toll-Free: 800-244-5373
Phone: 312-663-3520
Fax: 312-939-8962
Website: http://
www.preventchildabuse.org
E-mail:
mailbox@preventchildabuse.org

Rape Abuse and Incest National Network (RAINN)

635-B Pennsylvania Ave., SE
Washington, DC 20003
Toll-Free: 800-656-HOPE, ext. 3
Phone: 202-544-1034
Fax: 202-544-3556
Website: http://www.rainn.org
E-mail: info@rainn.org

Child Care Resources

Child Care Aware

1319 F. Street, NW, Suite 500
Washington, DC 20004-1106
Toll-Free: 800-424-2246
Fax: 202-393-1144
Website: http://
www.childcareaware.org
E-mail: info@childcareaware.org

Childcare Resource and Research Unit

Centre for Urban and
Community Studies
University of Toronto
455 Spadina Avenue, Room 305
Toronto, ON M5S 2G8 Canada
Phone: 416-978-6895
Fax: 416-971-2139
Website: http://
www.childcarecanada.org
E-mail: crru@chass.utoronto.ca

National Child Care Information Center

243 Church St., NW, 2nd Floor
Vienna, VA 22180
Toll-Free: 800-616-2242
Toll-Free TTY: 800-516-2242
Toll-Free Fax: 800-716-2242
Website: http://www.nccic.org

National Resource Center for Health and Safety in Child Care
UCHSC at Fitzsimons
Campus Mail Stop F541
P.O. Box 6508
Aurora, CO 80045-0508
Toll-Free: 800-598-KIDS
Fax: 303-724-0960
Website: http://nrc.uchsc.edu

Nation's Network of Child Care Resource and Referral
1319 F. Street, NW, Suite 500
Washington, DC 20004-1106
Phone: 202-393-5501
Fax: 202-393-1109
Website: http://www.naccrra.org
E-mail: info@naccrra.org

Child Health, General Resources

Agency for Healthcare Research and Quality Publications Clearinghouse
2101 E. Jefferson St., Suite 501
Rockville, MD 20852
Toll-Free: 800-358-9295
Phone: 301-594-1364
Website: http://www.ahrq.gov

American Academy of Family Physicians
11400 Tomahawk Creek Pkwy.
Leawood, KS 66211-2672
Toll Free: 800-274-2237
Phone: 913-906-6000
Website: http://
www.familydoctor.org
E-mail: email@familydoctor.org

American Academy of Pediatrics
141 Northwest Point Boulevard
Elk Grove Village, IL 60007-1098
Toll-Free: 888-227-1770
Phone: 847-434-4000
Fax: 847-434-8000
Website: http://www.aap.org/family
E-mail: kidsdocs@aap.org

Emergency Medical Services For Children
National Resource Center
111 Michigan Avenue, NW
Washington, DC 20010-2970
Phone: 202-884-4927
Fax: 202-884-6845
Website: http://www.ems-c.org
E-mail: information@emscnrc.com

Health Resources and Services Administration (HRSA) Information Center
Toll-Free: 888-275-4772
Website: http://
www.ask.hrsa.gov
E-mail: ask@hrsa.gov

KidsHealth
Nemours Foundation
1600 Rockland Road
Wilmington, DE 19803
Phone: 302-651-4047
Website: http://
www.kidshealth.org
E-mail: info@kidshealth.org

National Health Information Center
P.O. Box 1133
Washington, DC 20013-1133
Toll-Free: 800-336-4797
Phone: 301-565-4167
Website: www.health.gov/nhic
E-mail: info@nhic.org

Shriners Hospital
2900 Rocky Point Drive
Tampa, FL 33607-1460
Toll-Free: 800-237-5055
Phone: 813-281-0300
Website: http://
www.shrinershq.org

Virtual Children's Hospital
Website: http://www.vh.org

Zero to Three
2000 M Street NW, Suite 200
Washington, DC 20036
Toll-Free: 800-899-4301 (to request publications)
Phone: 202-638-1144
Website: http://
www.zerotothree.org

Dental Care

American Academy of Pediatric Dentistry
211 East Chicago Avenue
Suite 700
Chicago, IL 60611-2663
Phone: 312-337-2169
Fax: 312-337-6329
Website: http://aapd.org

American Dental Association
211 E. Chicago Avenue
Chicago, IL 60611
Phone: 312-440-2601
Fax: 312-440-2800
Website: http://www.ada.org
E-mail: online@ada.org

American Association of Endodontists
211 E. Chicago Ave., Suite 1100
Chicago, IL 60611-2691
Toll-free: 800-872-3636
Phone: 312-266-7255
Fax: 866-451-9020; 312-266-9867
Website: www.aae.org
E-mail: info@aae.org

National Institute of Dental and Craniofacial Research
NIDCR Public Information and Liaison Branch
45 Center Drive, MSC 6400
Bethesda, MD 20892-6400
Phone: 301-496-4261
Website: http://
www.nidcr.nih.gov
E-mail: nidcrinfo@mail.nih.gov

Disabilities/Special Needs

ADA National Access for Public Schools Project
Toll-Free: 800-893-1225, ext. 28
Website: http://
www.adaptiveenvironments.org
E-mail:
adaptive@adaptiveenvironments.org

ABLEDATA

8630 Fenton Street, Suite 930
Silver Spring, MD 20910
Toll Free: 800-227-0216
Phone: 301-608-8912
Fax: 301-608-8958
Website: http://
www.abledate.com
E-mail: abledate@macroint.com

ARCH National Respite Network and Resource Center

Chapel Hill Training-Outreach
Project
800 Eastowne Drive, Suite 105
Chapel Hill, NC 27514
Toll-Free: 800-773-5433 (National
Respite Locator Service)
Website: http://
www.archrespite.org

Disabled Sports USA

451 Hungerford Drive, Suite 100
Rockville, MD 20850
Phone: 301-217-0960
TTY: 301-217-0963
Fax: 301-217-0968
Website: http://www.dsusa.org
E-mail: Information@dsusa.org

Easter Seals—National Office

230 West Monroe St., Suite 1800
Chicago, IL 60606
Toll-Free: 800-221-6827
Phone: 312-726-6200
TTY: 312-726-4258
Website: http://www.easter-
seals.org
E-mail: info@easter-seals.org

Family Center for Technology and Disabilities

Academy for Educational
Development (AED)
1825 Connecticut Avenue, NW,
7th Floor
Washington, DC 20009-5721
Phone: 202-884-8068
Fax: 202-884-8441
Website: http://www.fctd.info
E-mail: fctd@aed.org

Family Resource Center on Disabilities

20 East Jackson Boulevard,
Room 900
Chicago, IL 60604
Toll-Free: 800-952-4199 (Illinois
only)
Phone: 312-939-3513
TDD: 312-939-3519
Fax: 312-939-7297

Institute for Health and Disability

University of Minnesota
General Pediatrics and
Adolescent Health
200 Oak Street SE, Suite 160
Minneapolis, MN 55455
Phone: 612-626-2820
Fax: 612-626-2134
Website: http://
allaboutkids.umn.edu
E-mail: instihd@tc.umn.edu

National Information Center for Children and Youth with Disabilities (NICHCY)
P.O. Box 1492
Washington, DC 20013
Toll-Free: 800-695-0285
Fax: 202-884-8441
Website: http://www.nichcy.org
E-mail: nichcy@aed.org

National Rehabilitation Information Center (NARIC)
4200 Forbes Boulevard
Suite 202
Lanham, MD 20706
Toll-Free: 800-346-2742
Phone: 301-459-5900
Website: http://www.naric.com
E-mail:
naricinfo@heitechservices.com

Parents Helping Parents: The Parent-Directed Family Resource Center for Children with Special Needs
3041 Olcott St.
Santa Clara, CA 95054
Phone: 408-727-5775
Fax: 408-727-0182
Website: http://www.php.com
E-mail: general@php.com

Immunizations

Children's Vaccine Program
PATH
1455 NW Leary Way
Seattle, WS 98107
Phone: 206-285-3500
Fax: 206-285-6619
Website: http://www.childrensvaccine.org
E-mail:
info@childrensvaccine.org

Immunization Action Coalition
1573 Selby Avenue, Suite 234
St. Paul, MN 55104
Phone: 651-647-9009
Fax: 651-647-9131
Website: http://www.immunize.org
E-mail: admin@immunize.org

Institute for Vaccine Safety at Johns Hopkins
Website: http://www.vaccinesafety.edu
E-mail: info@vaccinesafety.edu

National Immunization Program
Centers for Disease Control and Prevention
Mailstop E-05
1600 Clifton Road, NE
Atlanta, GA 30333
Toll-Free: 800-232-SHOT
Spanish: 800-232-0233
TTY: 800-243-7889
Website: http://www.cdc.gov/nip
E-mail: NIPINFO@cdc.gov

**National Network for
Immunization Information**
66 Canal Center Plaza
Suite 600
Alexandria, VA 22314
Toll Free: 877-341-6644
Fax: 703-299-0204
Website: http://
www.immunizationinfo.org
E-mail: nnii@idsociety.org

**National Vaccine
Information Center**
421-E Church Street
Vienna, VA 22180
Toll-Free: 800-909-7468
Phone: 703-938-DPT3
Fax: 703-983-5768
Website: http://
www.909shot.com

**Vaccine Adverse Event
Reporting System**
8401 Colesville Road, Suite 200
Silver Spring, MD 20910
Toll-Free: 800-822-7967
Toll Free Fax: 877-721-0366
Website: http://www.vaers.org
E-mail: info@vaers.org

Lead Information

**Childhood Lead Poisoning
Prevention Program**
National Center for
Environmental Health
Centers for Disease Control and
Prevention
NCEH Health Line: 888-232-6789
Website: www.cdc.gov/nceh/lead

**National Center for Healthy
Housing**
10227 Wincopin Circle
Suite 100
Columbia, MD 21044
Phone: 410-992-0712
Fax: 410-715-2310
Website:
www.centerforhealthyhousing.org

**National Institute of
Environmental Health
Sciences**
P.O. Box 12233
Research Triangle Park, NC
27709
Phone: 919-541-3345
TTY: 919-541-0731
Website: www.niehs.nih.gov

**National Lead Information
Center**
801 Roeder Road, Suite 600
Silver Spring, MD 20910
Toll-Free: 800-424-LEAD (800-424-5323)
Fax: 301-588-8495
Website: www.epa.gov/lead/
nlic.htm

**Office of Healthy Homes
and Lead Hazard Control**
U.S. Department of Housing and
Urban Development
451 7th Street, SW
Washington, DC
Phone: 202-708-1112
TTY: 202-708-1455
Website: www.hud.gov/offices/
lead

Mental and Emotional Health

American Academy of Child and Adolescent Psychiatry
Public Information Office
3615 Wisconsin Ave., NW
Washington, DC 20016-3007
Phone: 202-966-7300
Fax: 202-966-2891
Website: http://www.aacap.org

Anxiety Disorders Association of America
8730 Georgia Avenue, Suite 600
Silver Spring, MD 20910
Phone: 240-485-1001
Fax: 240-485-1035
Website: http://www.adaa.org
E-mail: AnxDis@adaa.org

Center for Effective Collaboration and Practice
1000 Thomas Jefferson St., N.W., Suite 400
Washington, DC 20007
Toll-Free: 888-457-1551
Toll-Free TTY: 877-334-3499
Phone: 202-944-5400
Fax: 202-944-5454
Website: http://cecp.air.org
E-mail: center@air.org

Center on Positive Behavioral Interventions and Supports
5262 University of Oregon
Eugene, OR 97403
Phone: 541-346-2505
Fax: 541-346-5689
Website: http://www.pbis.org
E-mail: pbis@oregon.uregon.edu

Child and Adolescent Bipolar Foundation
1187 Wilmette Ave., PMB #331
Wilmette, IL 60091
Phone: 847-256-8525
Fax: 847-920-9498
Website: http://www.bpkids.org
E-mail: cabf@bpkids.org

Depression and Bipolar Support Alliance
730 N. Franklin St., Suite 501
Chicago, IL 60610-7224
Toll-Free: 800-326-3632
Phone: 312-642-0049
Fax: 312-642-7243
Website: http://www.dbsalliance.org
E-mail: questions@dbsalliance.org

Federation of Families for Children's Mental Health
1101 King Street, Suite 420
Alexandria, VA 22314
Phone: 703-684-7710
Fax: 703-836-1040
Website: http://www.ffcmh.org
E-mail: ffcmh@ffcmh.com

National Alliance for the Mentally Ill (NAMI)
Colonial Place Three, 2107
Wilson Blvd., Suite 300
Arlington, VA 22201-3042
Toll-Free: 800-950-6264
Phone: 703-524-7600
TTY: 703-516-7991 or 888-344-6264
Website: http://www.nami.org
E-mail: helpline@nami.org

National Association for the Dually Diagnosed (NADD)
132 Fair Street
Kingston, NY 12401
Toll-Free: 800-331-5362
Phone: 845-331-4336
Fax: 845-331-4569
Website: http://www.thenadd.org
E-mail: info@thenadd.org

National Clearinghouse on Family Support and Children's Mental Health
Portland State University
P.O. Box 751
Portland, OR 97207-0751
Toll-Free: 800-628-1696
Phone: 503-725-4040
Fax: 503-725-4150
Website: http://www.rtc.pdx.edu/
pgClearinghouse.shtml

National Hopeline Network
Toll-Free: 800-Suicide (800-784-2433)

National Mental Health Association
2001 N. Beauregard Street
12th Floor
Alexandria, VA 22311
Toll-Free: 800-969-6642
Toll-Free TTY: 800-433-5959
Phone: 703-684-7722
Fax: 703-684-5968
Website: http://www.nmha.org
E-mail: infoctr@nmha.org

National Mental Health Information Center
P.O. Box 42557
Washington, DC 20015
Toll-Free: 800-789-2647
TTY: 301-443-9006 or 866-889-2647
Phone: 301-443-1805
Fax: 301-984-8796
Website: http://
www.mentalhealth.org
E-mail: info@mentalhealth.org

National Institute on Mental Health (NIMH)
6001 Executive Boulevard,
Room 8184
MSC 9663
Bethesda, MD 20892-9663
Toll-Free: 866-615-6464
Phone: 301-443-4513
TTY: 301-443-8431
Fax: 301-443-4279
Website: www.nimh.nih.gov
E-mail: nimhinfo@nih.gov

Nineline Crisis Hotline
Toll-Free: 800-999-9999
TTY: 800-999-9915

Obsessive Compulsive Foundation, Inc.
337 Notch Hill Road
North Branford, CT 06471
Phone: 203-315-2190
Fax: 203-315-2196
Website: http://
www.ocfoundation.org
E-mail: info@ocfoundation.org

Research and Training Center on Family Support and Children's Mental Health
Portland State University
P.O. Box 751
Portland, OR 97207-0751
Toll-Free: 800-628-1696
Phone: 503-725-4040
Website: www.rtc.pdx.edu

Minority Health

African American Family Services
2616 Nicollet Avenue South
Minneapolis, MN 55408
Toll-Free: 800-557-2190
Phone: 612-871-7878
Fax: 612-871-2567
Website: http://www.aafs.net
E-mail: contact@aafs.net

Bureau of Indian Affairs
1849 C Street, N.W.
MS-3512-MIB-OIE-23
Washington, DC 20240
Phone: 202-208-3710
Website: http://doi.gov/bureau-indian-affairs.html

Early Childhood Research Institute on Culturally and Linguistically Appropriate Services
University of Illinois at Urbana-Champaign
61 Children's Research Center
51 Gerty Drive
Champaign, IL 61821
Toll-Free: 800-583-4135
Phone: 217-333-4123
Website: http://clas.uiuc.edu
E-mail: clas@uiuc.edu

National Alliance for Hispanic Health
1501 Sixteenth Street NW
Washington DC 20036-1401
Phone: 202-387-5000
Fax: 202-797-4353
Website: http://www.hispanichealth.org
E-mail: alliance@hispanichealth.org

National Black Child Development Institute
1101 15th Street, N.W.
Suite 900
Washington, DC 20005
Phone: 202-833-2220
Fax: 202-234-1738
Website: http://www.nbcdi.org
E-mail: moreinfo@nbcdi.org

National Council of La Raza (NCLR)
1111 19th Street, N.W.
Suite 1000
Washington, DC 20036
Phone: 202-785-1670
Website: http://www.nclr.org

National Organization for People of Color Against Suicide
2999 Continental Colony Pkwy., #140
Atlanta, GA 30331
Toll-Free: 800-321-6223
Website: http://www.nopcas.com

Office of Minority Health Resource Center (OMH-RC)
Office of Minority Health, Public Health Service
U.S. Department of Health and Human Services
P.O. Box 37337
Washington, DC 20013-7337
Toll-Free: 800- 444-6472
Phone: 301-443-5224
Fax: 301-251-2160
Website: http://www.omhrc.gov
E-mail: info@omhrc.gov

Missing/Abducted/ Runaway Children

Boys/Girls Town
14100 Crawford St.
Boys Town, NE 68010
Toll-Free: 800-448-3000
Phone: 402-498-1300
Fax: 402-498-1348
Website: http://www.girlsandboystown.org
E-mail: hotline@girlsandboystown.org

Child Find of America
Toll-Free: 800-I-AM-LOST
Website: http://www.childfindofamerica.org
E-mail: childfindofamerica@aol.com

Child Find of America— Mediation
Toll-Free: 800-A-WAY-OUT
Website: http://www.childfindofamerica.org/user/capss.html

Child Quest International Sighting Line
Toll-Free: 888-818-HOPE

Covenant House Hotline
Toll-Free: 800-999-9999

National Center for Missing and Exploited Children
Charles B. Wang International Children's Building
699 Prince Street
Alexandria, VA 22314-3175
Toll-Free: 800-843-5678
Phone: 703-274-3900
Fax: 703-274-2200
Website: http://www.missingkids.com

National Referral Network for Kids in Crisis
Toll-Free: 800-KID-SAVE

National Runaway Switchboard (NRS)
3080 N. Lincoln Ave.
Chicago, IL 60657
Toll-Free: 800-621-4000
Phone: 773-880-9860
Fax: 773-929-5150
Website: http://www.nrscrisisline.org
E-mail: info@nrscrisisline.org

National Youth Crisis Hotline
Youth Developmental International
Toll-Free: 800-HIT-HOME
Website: http://www.1800hithome.com

Operation Lookout
National Center for Missing Youth
6320 Evergreen Way, Suite 201
Everett, WA 98203
Toll-Free: 800-LOOKOUT
Phone: 425-771-7335
Fax: 425-348-4411
Website: http://operationlookout.org
E-mail:
casework4@operationlookout.org

Nutrition, Weight Loss, and Eating Disorders

American Anorexia/Bulimia Association
165 West 46th Street, Suite 1108
New York, NY 10036
Phone: 212-575-6200

American Dietetic Association
120 S. Riverside Plaza, Suite 2000
Chicago, IL 60606-6995
Toll-Free: 800-877-1600
Website: http://www.eatright.org
E-mail: education@eatright.org

Food and Nutrition Information Center
U.S. Department of Agriculture
Agricultural Research Service
National Agricultural Library, Room 105
10301 Baltimore Avenue
Beltsville, MD 20705-2351
Phone: 301-504-5719
TTY: 301-504-6856
Fax: 301-504-6409
Website: http://www.nal.usda.gov/fnic
E-mail: fnic@nal.usda.gov

International Food Information Council
1100 Connecticut Avenue, NW, Suite 430
Washington, DC 20036
Phone: 202-296-6540
Fax: 202-296-6547
Website: http://ific.org
E-mail: foodinfo@ific.org

National Association of Anorexia Nervosa and Associated Disorders
P.O. Box 7
Highland Park, IL 60035
Phone: 847-831-3438
Website: http://www.altrue.net/site/anadweb
E-mail: adadadvocacy@aol.com

National Eating Disorders Association
603 Stewart Street, Suite 803
Seattle, WA 98101
Toll-Free: 800-931-2237
Phone: 206-382-3587
Website: http://www.nationaleatingdisorders.org
E-mail: info@NationalEatingDisorders.org

President's Council on Physical Fitness and Sports
Department W
200 Independence Ave., SW
Room 738-H
Washington, DC 20201-0004
Phone: 202-690-9000
Fax: 202-690-5211
Website: http://www.fitness.gov

*Weight-Control Information
Network*
1 WIN Way
Bethesda, MD 20892-3665
Toll-Free: 877-946-4627
Phone: 202-828-1025
Fax: 202-828-1028
Website: www.niddk.nih.gov/
health/nutrit/win.html
E-mail: WIN@info.niddk.nih.gov

Parenting Resources

Active Parenting
810-B Franklin Ct.
Marietta, GA 30067
Toll-Free: 800-825-0060 or 800-
235-7755
Phone: 770-429-0565
Fax: 770-429-0334
Website: http://
www.activeparenting.com
E-mail:
cservice@activeparenting.com

*Center for the Improvement
of Child Caring*
11331 Ventura Blvd., Suite 103
Studio City, CA 91604-3147
Toll-Free: 800-325-CICC
Phone: 818-980-0903
Fax: 818-753-1054
Website: http://
www.ciccparenting.org
E-mail: cicc@flash.net

*Family Resource Coalition
of America*
20 North Wacker Dr., Suite 1100
Chicago, IL 60606
Phone: 312-338-0900
Fax: 312-338-1522
Website: http://www.frca.org

*Grandparent Information
Center*
American Association of Retired
Persons (AARP)
601 E St. NW
Washington, DC 20049
Toll-Free: 800-424-3410
Fax: 202-434-6466
Website: http://www.aarp.org/
grandparents

*National Organization of
Single Mothers*
P.O. Box 68
Midland, NC 28107
Phone: 704-888-KIDS
Website: http://
www.singlemothers.org

National Parenting Center
22801 Ventura Blvd., Suite 110
Woodland Hills, CA 91367
Toll-Free: 800-753-6667
Website: http://www.tnpc.com
E-mail: ParentCtr@tnpc.com

*National Parent
Information Network*
ERIC Clearinghouse on Elementary
and Early Childhood Education
University of Illinois at Urbana-
Champaign
Children's Research Center
51 Gerty Drive
Champaign, IL 61820-7469
Toll-Free: 800-583-4135
Website: http://www.npin.org
E-mail: npin@uiuc.edu

Parent Soup
Website: http://
www.parentsoup.com

Parenthood.com
Website: http://parenthood.com

Parenting.com
Website: http://
www.parenting.com

Parenting Coalition
1025 Connecticut Avenue NW,
Suite 415
Washington, DC 20036
Phone: 202-530-0849
Fax: 202-898-1155
Website: http://
www.parentingcoalition.org
E-mail:
info@parentingcoalition.org

Parenting Resources for the 21st Century
U.S. Department of Justice
Website: http://
www.parentingresources.ncjrs.org
E-mail:
parentingresources@ncjrs.org

Parents.com
G+J Publishing USA
375 Lexington Avenue
New York, NY 10017
Phone: 212-499-2193
Website: http://www.parents.com

Parents Helping Parents, Inc.: The Family Resource Center
3041 Olcott Street
Santa Clara, CA 95054-3222
Phone: 408-727-5775
Fax: 408-727-0182
Website: http://www.php.com
E-mail: general@php.com

Parents Without Partners
1650 South Dixie Highway,
Suite 510
Boca Raton, FL ##432
Phone: 561-391-8833
Fax: 561-395-8557
Website: http://
www.parentswithoutpartners.org
E-mail: pwp@jti.net

ParentsPlace.com
Website: http://
www.parentsplace.com

ParentStages.com
Website: http://
www.parentstages.com

Responsible Single Fathers
541 Knapp NE
Grand Rapids, MI
Phone: 616-447-0798
Website: http://
www.singlefather.org
E-mail: info@singlefather.org

ToughLove International
P.O. Box 1069
Doylestown, PA 18901
Toll-Free: 800-333-1069
Phone: 215-348-7090
Fax: 215-348-9874
Website: http://
www.toughlove.org
E-mail: service@toughlove.org

Safety and Injury Prevention

American Academy of Orthopaedic Surgeons
6300 North River Road
Rosemont, IL 60018-4262
Toll-Free: 800-346-2267
Phone: 847-823-7186
Fax-on-Demand: 800-999-2939
Website: http://www.aaos.org
E-mail: custserv@aaos.org

American Association of Poison Control Centers
3201 New Mexico Avenue
Suite 330
Washington, DC 20016
Toll-Free Poisoning Emergency:
800-222-1222
Phone: 202-362-7217
Website: http://www.aapcc.org
E-mail: aapcc@poison.org

American Red Cross
431 18th Street, NW
Washington, DC 20006
Phone: 202-303-4498
Website: http://www.redcross.org

Brain Injury Association
105 North Alfred Street
Alexandria, VA 22314
Toll-Free: 800-444-6443
Phone: 703-236-6000
Fax: 703-236-6001
Website: http://www.biausa.org
E-mail:
FamilyHelpLine@biausa.org

Consumer Product Safety Commission
4330 East-West Highway
Bethesda, MD 20814-4408
Toll-Free: 800-638-2772
Phone: 301-504-6816
Fax: 301-504-0124
Website: http://www.cpsc.gov
E-mail: info@cpsc.gov

National Athletic Trainers Association
2952 Stemmons Frwy.
Dallas, TX 75247-6196
Phone: 214-637-6282
Fax: 214-637-2206
Website: http://www.nata.org

National Bicycle Safety Network
Website: http://www.cdc.gov/
ncipc/bike

National Crime Prevention Council
1000 Connecticut Avenue NW,
13th Floor
Washington, DC 20036
Phone: 202-466-6272
Website: http://www.ncpc.org

National Fire Protection Association (NFPA)
1 Batterymarch Park
Quincy, MA 02169-7471
Phone: 617-770-3000
Fax: 617-770-0700
Website: http://www.nfpa.org

National Highway Traffic Safety Administration (NHTSA)
Toll-Free: 888-327-4236 (Auto Safety Hotline)
Website: http://
www.nhtsa.dot.gov

National Program for Playground Safety
School for Health, Physical Education and Leisure Services
WRC 205
University of Northern Iowa
Cedar Falls, IA 50614-0618
Toll-Free: 800-554-PLAY (7529)
Phone: 319-273-2416
Fax: 319-273-7308
Website: http://www.uni.edu/
playground
E-mail: playgroun-
safety@uni.edu

National SAFEKIDS Campaign
1301 Pennsylvania Ave., NW,
Suite 1000
Washington, Dc 20004
Phone: 202-662-0600
Fax: 202-393-2072
Website: http://www.safekids.org

National Safety Council
1121 Spring Lake Drive
Itasca, IL 60143-3201
Toll-Free: 800-621-7619
Phone: 630-285-1121
Fax: 630-285-1315
Website: http://www.nsc.org
E-mail: info@nsc.org

National Youth Sports Safety Foundation
One Beacon Street, Suite 3333
Boston, MA 02108
Phone: 617-277-1171
Fax: 617-722-9999
Website: http://www.nyssf.org
E-mail: NYSSF@aol.com

SafeUSA™
P.O. Box 8189
Silver Springs, MD 20907-8189
Toll-Free: 888-252-7751
Website: http://www.safeusa.org

U.S. Fire Administration
16825 S. Seton Avenue
Emmittsburg, MD 21727
Phone: 301-447-1000
Website: http://
www.usfa.fema.gov

Index

Index

C

Green, M. 98n
growing pains, defined 556
growth charts, children 80–89
growth hormone deficiency, described
94–95
growth patterns, children 89–96
Guide to Web Browsing (US Department of the Interior) 493n
gum disease, described 62–63
gymnastics, injury prevention 298

H

Haemophilus influenzae
described 24
vaccine age recommendations 9,
14
halitosis, described 63
"Halloween Safety" (CDC) 265n
halloween safety tips 269–72
hallucinogens, parent/child discussions 527–28
hand washing
food safety 393–94
infections 447
hardware, defined 500
Hazardous Substances Act 264
Head Start Bureau, contact information 578
Healthfinder, Web site address 567
Health Resources and Services Administration (HRSA), contact information 585
"Healthy Sleep" (NHLBI) 474n
"Hearing Screening in Schools" (Self-Help for Hard of Hearing People,
Inc.) 46n
hearing tests, children 10–11
heat stress, prevention 310–12
helmet safety 287–89, 334–35
"Helping Your Child Become a
Reader" (Department of Education)
155n
"Helping Your Child: Tips for Parents"
(NIDDK) 353n
"Helping Your Child with
Homework" (Department of
Education) 165n

"Helping Your Preschool Child"
(Department of Education) 137n
hemolytic uremic syndrome 394
hepatitis A
described 25
foodborne illnesses 395
vaccine age recommendations *14*, *26*
hepatitis B
described 25
vaccine age recommendations 9, *14*,
26
herbal remedies, described 450
heredity
growth patterns 90–92
speech and language development
120
stuttering 123
urinary incontinence 460, 465
heroin 528
hockey, injury prevention 299
"Holiday Safety" (CDC) 265n
holiday safety tips 265–72
Home and School Institute -
MegaSkills Education Center, contact information 578
homeopathy 450
home page, defined 501
"Home Playground Safety Tips"
(CPSC) 280n
homework, overview 165–70
honey, food safety 392
hormones
growth patterns 91, 94–95
precocious puberty 94
urinary incontinence 462
"How Can Parents Protect Their Children from Foodborne Illness?"
(S.T.O.P.) 392n
"How Should Preschool and School
Children Ride Safely" (NHTSA)
323n
"How to Care for Minor Wounds:
Cuts, Scrapes, and Abrasions"
(D'Alessandro; Huth) 217n
"How to Encourage Children to Wear
Their Glasses" (American Optometric Association) 41n
"How to Give Medicine to Children"
(Williams) 441n

610

Health Reference Series
COMPLETE CATALOG

Adolescent Health Sourcebook

Basic Consumer Health Information about Common Medical, Mental, and Emotional Concerns in Adolescents, Including Facts about Acne, Body Piercing, Mononucleosis, Nutrition, Eating Disorders, Stress, Depression, Behavior Problems, Peer Pressure, Violence, Gangs, Drug Use, Puberty, Sexuality, Pregnancy, Learning Disabilities, and More

Along with a Glossary of Terms and Other Resources for Further Help and Information

Edited by Chad T. Kimball. 658 pages. 2002. 0-7808-0248-9. $78.

"It is written in clear, nontechnical language aimed at general readers. . . . Recommended for public libraries, community colleges, and other agencies serving health care consumers."
— *American Reference Books Annual, 2003*

"Recommended for school and public libraries. Parents and professionals dealing with teens will appreciate the easy-to-follow format and the clearly written text. This could become a 'must have' for every high school teacher." — *E-Streams, Jan '03*

"A good starting point for information related to common medical, mental, and emotional concerns of adolescents." — *School Library Journal, Nov '02*

"This book provides accurate information in an easy to access format. It addresses topics that parents and caregivers might not be aware of and provides practical, useable information." — *Doody's Health Sciences Book Review Journal, Sep-Oct '02*

"Recommended reference source."
— *Booklist, American Library Association, Sep '02*

AIDS Sourcebook, 3rd Edition

Basic Consumer Health Information about Acquired Immune Deficiency Syndrome (AIDS) and Human Immunodeficiency Virus (HIV) Infection, Including Facts about Transmission, Prevention, Diagnosis, Treatment, Opportunistic Infections, and Other Complications, with a Section for Women and Children, Including Details about Associated Gynecological Concerns, Pregnancy, and Pediatric Care

Along with Updated Statistical Information, Reports on Current Research Initiatives, a Glossary, and Directories of Internet, Hotline, and Other Resources

Edited by Dawn D. Matthews. 664 pages. 2003. 0-7808-0631-X. $78.

ALSO AVAILABLE: *AIDS Sourcebook, 1st Edition.* Edited by Karen Bellenir and Peter D. Dresser. 831 pages. 1995. 0-7808-0031-1. $78.

AIDS Sourcebook, 2nd Edition. Edited by Karen Bellenir. 751 pages. 1999. 0-7808-0225-X. $78.

"Highly recommended."
— *American Reference Books Annual, 2000*

"Excellent sourcebook. This continues to be a highly recommended book. There is no other book that provides as much information as this book provides."
— *AIDS Book Review Journal, Dec-Jan 2000*

"Recommended reference source."
— *Booklist, American Library Association, Dec '99*

"A solid text for college-level health libraries."
— *The Bookwatch, Aug '99*

Cited in *Reference Sources for Small and Medium-Sized Libraries, American Library Association, 1999*

Alcoholism Sourcebook

Basic Consumer Health Information about the Physical and Mental Consequences of Alcohol Abuse, Including Liver Disease, Pancreatitis, Wernicke-Korsakoff Syndrome (Alcoholic Dementia), Fetal Alcohol Syndrome, Heart Disease, Kidney Disorders, Gastrointestinal Problems, and Immune System Compromise and Featuring Facts about Addiction, Detoxification, Alcohol Withdrawal, Recovery, and the Maintenance of Sobriety

Along with a Glossary and Directories of Resources for Further Help and Information

Edited by Karen Bellenir. 613 pages. 2000. 0-7808-0325-6. $78.

"This title is one of the few reference works on alcoholism for general readers. For some readers this will be a welcome complement to the many self-help books on the market. Recommended for collections serving general readers and consumer health collections."
— *E-Streams, Mar '01*

"This book is an excellent choice for public and academic libraries."
— *American Reference Books Annual, 2001*

"Recommended reference source."
— *Booklist, American Library Association, Dec '00*

"Presents a wealth of information on alcohol use and abuse and its effects on the body and mind, treatment, and prevention." — *SciTech Book News, Dec '00*

"Important new health guide which packs in the latest consumer information about the problems of alcoholism." — *Reviewer's Bookwatch, Nov '00*

SEE ALSO *Drug Abuse Sourcebook, Substance Abuse Sourcebook*

625

Allergies Sourcebook, 2nd Edition

Basic Consumer Health Information about Allergic Disorders, Triggers, Reactions, and Related Symptoms, Including Anaphylaxis, Rhinitis, Sinusitis, Asthma, Dermatitis, Conjunctivitis, and Multiple Chemical Sensitivity

Along with Tips on Diagnosis, Prevention, and Treatment, Statistical Data, a Glossary, and a Directory of Sources for Further Help and Information

Edited by Annemarie S. Muth. 598 pages. 2002. 0-7808-0376-0. $78.

ALSO AVAILABLE: *Allergies Sourcebook, 1st Edition.* Edited by Allan R. Cook. 611 pages. 1997. 0-7808-0036-2. $78.

"This book brings a great deal of useful material together.... This is an excellent addition to public and consumer health library collections."
— *American Reference Books Annual, 2003*

"This second edition would be useful to laypersons with little or advanced knowledge of the subject matter. This book would also serve as a resource for nursing and other health care professions students. It would be useful in public, academic, and hospital libraries with consumer health collections." — *E-Streams, Jul '02*

Alternative Medicine Sourcebook, 2nd Edition

Basic Consumer Health Information about Alternative and Complementary Medical Practices, Including Acupuncture, Chiropractic, Herbal Medicine, Homeopathy, Naturopathic Medicine, Mind-Body Interventions, Ayurveda, and Other Non-Western Medical Traditions

Along with Facts about such Specific Therapies as Massage Therapy, Aromatherapy, Qigong, Hypnosis, Prayer, Dance, and Art Therapies, a Glossary, and Resources for Further Information

Edited by Dawn D. Matthews. 618 pages. 2002. 0-7808-0605-0. $78.

ALSO AVAILABLE: *Alternative Medicine Sourcebook, 1st Edition.* Edited by Allan R. Cook. 737 pages. 1999. 0-7808-0200-4. $78.

"Recommended for public, high school, and academic libraries that have consumer health collections. Hospital libraries that also serve the public will find this to be a useful resource." — *E-Streams, Feb '03*

"Recommended reference source."
— *Booklist, American Library Association, Jan '03*

"An important alternate health reference."
— *MBR Bookwatch, Oct '02*

"A great addition to the reference collection of every type of library." — *American Reference Books Annual, 2000*

Alzheimer's Disease Sourcebook, 3rd Edition

Basic Consumer Health Information about Alzheimer's Disease, Other Dementias, and Related Disorders, Including Multi-Infarct Dementia, AIDS Dementia Complex, Dementia with Lewy Bodies, Huntington's Disease, Wernicke-Korsakoff Syndrome (Alcohol-Reated Dementia), Delirium, and Confusional States

Along with Information for People Newly Diagnosed with Alzheimer's Disease and Caregivers, Reports Detailing Current Research Efforts in Prevention, Diagnosis, and Treatment, Facts about Long-Term Care Issues, and Listings of Sources for Additional Information

Edited by Karen Bellenir. 645 pages. 2003. 0-7808-0666-2. $78.

ALSO AVAILABLE: *Alzheimer's, Stroke & 29 Other Neurological Disorders Sourcebook, 1st Edition.* Edited by Frank E. Bair. 579 pages. 1993. 1-55888-748-2. $78.

ALSO AVAILABLE: *Alzheimer's Disease Sourcebook, 2nd Edition.* Edited by Karen Bellenir. 524 pages. 1999. 0-7808-0223-3. $78.

"Provides a wealth of useful information not otherwise available in one place. This resource is recommended for all types of libraries."
— *American Reference Books Annual, 2000*

"Recommended reference source."
— *Booklist, American Library Association, Oct '99*

SEE ALSO Brain Disorders Sourcebook

Arthritis Sourcebook

Basic Consumer Health Information about Specific Forms of Arthritis and Related Disorders, Including Rheumatoid Arthritis, Osteoarthritis, Gout, Polymyalgia Rheumatica, Psoriatic Arthritis, Spondyloarthropathies, Juvenile Rheumatoid Arthritis, and Juvenile Ankylosing Spondylitis

Along with Information about Medical, Surgical, and Alternative Treatment Options, and Including Strategies for Coping with Pain, Fatigue, and Stress

Edited by Allan R. Cook. 550 pages. 1998. 0-7808-0201-2. $78.

"... accessible to the layperson."
— *Reference and Research Book News, Feb '99*

Asthma Sourcebook

Basic Consumer Health Information about Asthma, Including Symptoms, Traditional and Nontraditional Remedies, Treatment Advances, Quality-of-Life Aids, Medical Research Updates, and the Role of Allergies, Exercise, Age, the Environment, and Genetics in the Development of Asthma

Along with Statistical Data, a Glossary, and Directories of Support Groups, and Other Resources for Further Information

Edited by Annemarie S. Muth. 628 pages. 2000. 0-7808-0381-7. $78.

"A worthwhile reference acquisition for public libraries and academic medical libraries whose readers desire a quick introduction to the wide range of asthma information." —*Choice, Association of College & Research Libraries, Jun '01*

"Recommended reference source."
—*Booklist, American Library Association, Feb '01*

"Highly recommended." —*The Bookwatch, Jan '01*

"There is much good information for patients and their families who deal with asthma daily."
—*American Medical Writers Association Journal, Winter '01*

"This informative text is recommended for consumer health collections in public, secondary school, and community college libraries and the libraries of universities with a large undergraduate population."
—*American Reference Books Annual, 2001*

■

Attention Deficit Disorder Sourcebook

Basic Consumer Health Information about Attention Deficit/Hyperactivity Disorder in Children and Adults, Including Facts about Causes, Symptoms, Diagnostic Criteria, and Treatment Options Such as Medications, Behavior Therapy, Coaching, and Homeopathy

Along with Reports on Current Research Initiatives, Legal Issues, and Government Regulations, and Featuring a Glossary of Related Terms, Internet Resources, and a List of Additional Reading Material

Edited by Dawn D. Matthews. 470 pages. 2002. 0-7808-0624-7. $78.

"Recommended reference source."
—*Booklist, American Library Association, Jan '03*

"This book is recommended for all school libraries and the reference or consumer health sections of public libraries." —*American Reference Books Annual, 2003*

■

Back & Neck Disorders Sourcebook

Basic Information about Disorders and Injuries of the Spinal Cord and Vertebrae, Including Facts on Chiropractic Treatment, Surgical Interventions, Paralysis, and Rehabilitation

Along with Advice for Preventing Back Trouble

Edited by Karen Bellenir. 548 pages. 1997. 0-7808-0202-0. $78.

"The strength of this work is its basic, easy-to-read format. Recommended."
—*Reference and User Services Quarterly, American Library Association, Winter '97*

Blood & Circulatory Disorders Sourcebook

Basic Information about Blood and Its Components, Anemias, Leukemias, Bleeding Disorders, and Circulatory Disorders, Including Aplastic Anemia, Thalassemia, Sickle-Cell Disease, Hemochromatosis, Hemophilia, Von Willebrand Disease, and Vascular Diseases

Along with a Special Section on Blood Transfusions and Blood Supply Safety, a Glossary, and Source Listings for Further Help and Information

Edited by Karen Bellenir and Linda M. Shin. 554 pages. 1998. 0-7808-0203-9. $78.

"Recommended reference source."
—*Booklist, American Library Association, Feb '99*

"An important reference sourcebook written in simple language for everyday, non-technical users. "
—*Reviewer's Bookwatch, Jan '99*

■

Brain Disorders Sourcebook

Basic Consumer Health Information about Strokes, Epilepsy, Amyotrophic Lateral Sclerosis (ALS/Lou Gehrig's Disease), Parkinson's Disease, Brain Tumors, Cerebral Palsy, Headache, Tourette Syndrome, and More

Along with Statistical Data, Treatment and Rehabilitation Options, Coping Strategies, Reports on Current Research Initiatives, a Glossary, and Resource Listings for Additional Help and Information

Edited by Karen Bellenir. 481 pages. 1999. 0-7808-0229-2. $78.

"Belongs on the shelves of any library with a consumer health collection." —*E-Streams, Mar '00*

"Recommended reference source."
—*Booklist, American Library Association, Oct '99*

SEE ALSO *Alzheimer's Disease Sourcebook*

■

Breast Cancer Sourcebook

Basic Consumer Health Information about Breast Cancer, Including Diagnostic Methods, Treatment Options, Alternative Therapies, Self-Help Information, Related Health Concerns, Statistical and Demographic Data, and Facts for Men with Breast Cancer

Along with Reports on Current Research Initiatives, a Glossary of Related Medical Terms, and a Directory of Sources for Further Help and Information

Edited by Edward J. Prucha and Karen Bellenir. 580 pages. 2001. 0-7808-0244-6. $78.

"It would be a useful reference book in a library or on loan to women in a support group."
—*Cancer Forum, Mar '03*

"Recommended reference source."
—*Booklist, American Library Association, Jan '02*

"This reference source is highly recommended. It is quite informative, comprehensive and detailed in nature, and yet it offers practical advice in easy-to-read language. It could be thought of as the 'bible' of breast cancer for the consumer." — *E-Streams, Jan '02*

"The broad range of topics covered in lay language make the *Breast Cancer Sourcebook* an excellent addition to public and consumer health library collections." — *American Reference Books Annual 2002*

"From the pros and cons of different screening methods and results to treatment options, *Breast Cancer Sourcebook* provides the latest information on the subject." — *Library Bookwatch, Dec '01*

"This thoroughgoing, very readable reference covers all aspects of breast health and cancer.... Readers will find much to consider here. Recommended for all public and patient health collections." — *Library Journal, Sep '01*

SEE ALSO Cancer Sourcebook for Women, Women's Health Concerns Sourcebook

■

Breastfeeding Sourcebook

Basic Consumer Health Information about the Benefits of Breastmilk, Preparing to Breastfeed, Breastfeeding as a Baby Grows, Nutrition, and More, Including Information on Special Situations and Concerns Such as Mastitis, Illness, Medications, Allergies, Multiple Births, Prematurity, Special Needs, and Adoption

Along with a Glossary and Resources for Additional Help and Information

Edited by Jenni Lynn Colson. 388 pages. 2002. 0-7808-0332-9. $78.

SEE ALSO Pregnancy & Birth Sourcebook

"Particularly useful is the information about professional lactation services and chapters on breastfeeding when returning to work.... *Breastfeeding Sourcebook* will be useful for public libraries, consumer health libraries, and technical schools offering nurse assistant training, especially in areas where Internet access is problematic." — *American Reference Books Annual, 2003*

■

Burns Sourcebook

Basic Consumer Health Information about Various Types of Burns and Scalds, Including Flame, Heat, Cold, Electrical, Chemical, and Sun Burns

Along with Information on Short-Term and Long-Term Treatments, Tissue Reconstruction, Plastic Surgery, Prevention Suggestions, and First Aid

Edited by Allan R. Cook. 604 pages. 1999. 0-7808-0204-7. $78.

"This is an exceptional addition to the series and is highly recommended for all consumer health collections, hospital libraries, and academic medical centers." — *E-Streams, Mar '00*

"This key reference guide is an invaluable addition to all health care and public libraries in confronting this ongoing health issue." — *American Reference Books Annual, 2000*

"Recommended reference source." — *Booklist, American Library Association, Dec '99*

SEE ALSO Skin Disorders Sourcebook

■

Cancer Sourcebook, 4th Edition

Basic Consumer Health Information about Major Forms and Stages of Cancer, Featuring Facts about Head and Neck Cancers, Lung Cancers, Gastrointestinal Cancers, Genitourinary Cancers, Lymphomas, Blood Cell Cancers, Endocrine Cancers, Skin Cancers, Bone Cancers, Sarcomas, and Others, and Including Information about Cancer Treatments and Therapies, Identifying and Reducing Cancer Risks, and Strategies for Coping with Cancer and the Side Effects of Treatment

Along with a Cancer Glossary, Statistical and Demographic Data, and a Directory of Sources for Additional Help and Information

Edited by Karen Bellenir. 1,119 pages. 2003. 0-7808-0633-6. $78.

ALSO AVAILABLE: Cancer Sourcebook, 1st Edition. Edited by Frank E. Bair. 932 pages. 1990. 1-55888-888-8. $78.

New Cancer Sourcebook, 2nd Edition. Edited by Allan R. Cook. 1,313 pages. 1996. 0-7808-0041-9. $78.

Cancer Sourcebook, 3rd Edition. Edited by Edward J. Prucha. 1,069 pages. 2000. 0-7808-0227-6. $78.

"This title is recommended for health sciences and public libraries with consumer health collections." — *E-Streams, Feb '01*

"... can be effectively used by cancer patients and their families who are looking for answers in a language they can understand. Public and hospital libraries should have it on their shelves." — *American Reference Books Annual, 2001*

"Recommended reference source." — *Booklist, American Library Association, Dec '00*

Cited in *Reference Sources for Small and Medium-Sized Libraries, American Library Association, 1999*

"The amount of factual and useful information is extensive. The writing is very clear, geared to general readers. Recommended for all levels." — *Choice, Association of College & Research Libraries, Jan '97*

SEE ALSO Breast Cancer Sourcebook, Cancer Sourcebook for Women, Pediatric Cancer Sourcebook, Prostate Cancer Sourcebook

Cancer Sourcebook for Women, 2nd Edition

Basic Consumer Health Information about Gynecologic Cancers and Related Concerns, Including Cervical Cancer, Endometrial Cancer, Gestational Trophoblastic Tumor, Ovarian Cancer, Uterine Cancer, Vaginal Cancer, Vulvar Cancer, Breast Cancer, and Common Non-Cancerous Uterine Conditions, with Facts about Cancer Risk Factors, Screening and Prevention, Treatment Options, and Reports on Current Research Initiatives

Along with a Glossary of Cancer Terms and a Directory of Resources for Additional Help and Information

Edited by Karen Bellenir. 604 pages. 2002. 0-7808-0226-8. $78.

ALSO AVAILABLE: *Cancer Sourcebook for Women, 1st Edition.* Edited by Allan R. Cook and Peter D. Dresser. 524 pages. 1996. 0-7808-0076-1. $78.

"An excellent addition to collections in public, consumer health, and women's health libraries."
— *American Reference Books Annual, 2003*

"Overall, the information is excellent, and complex topics are clearly explained. As a reference book for the consumer it is a valuable resource to assist them to make informed decisions about cancer and its treatments." — *Cancer Forum, Nov '02*

"Highly recommended for academic and medical reference collections." — *Library Bookwatch, Sep '02*

"This is a highly recommended book for any public or consumer library, being reader friendly and containing accurate and helpful information."
— *E-Streams, Aug '02*

"Recommended reference source."
— *Booklist, American Library Association, Jul '02*

SEE ALSO *Breast Cancer Sourcebook, Women's Health Concerns Sourcebook*

Cardiovascular Diseases & Disorders Sourcebook, 1st Edition

SEE *Heart Diseases & Disorders Sourcebook, 2nd Edition*

Caregiving Sourcebook

Basic Consumer Health Information for Caregivers, Including a Profile of Caregivers, Caregiving Responsibilities and Concerns, Tips for Specific Conditions, Care Environments, and the Effects of Caregiving

Along with Facts about Legal Issues, Financial Information, and Future Planning, a Glossary, and a Listing of Additional Resources

Edited by Joyce Brennfleck Shannon. 600 pages. 2001. 0-7808-0331-0. $78.

"Essential for most collections."
— *Library Journal, Apr 1, 2002*

"An ideal addition to the reference collection of any public library. Health sciences information professionals may also want to acquire the *Caregiving Sourcebook* for their hospital or academic library for use as a ready reference tool by health care workers interested in aging and caregiving." — *E-Streams, Jan '02*

"Recommended reference source."
— *Booklist, American Library Association, Oct '01*

Childhood Diseases & Disorders Sourcebook

Basic Consumer Health Information about Medical Problems Often Encountered in Pre-Adolescent Children, Including Respiratory Tract Ailments, Ear Infections, Sore Throats, Disorders of the Skin and Scalp, Digestive and Genitourinary Diseases, Infectious Diseases, Inflammatory Disorders, Chronic Physical and Developmental Disorders, Allergies, and More

Along with Information about Diagnostic Tests, Common Childhood Surgeries, and Frequently Used Medications, with a Glossary of Important Terms and Resource Directory

Edited by Chad T. Kimball. 662 pages. 2003. 0-7808-0458-9. $78.

Colds, Flu & Other Common Ailments Sourcebook

Basic Consumer Health Information about Common Ailments and Injuries, Including Colds, Coughs, the Flu, Sinus Problems, Headaches, Fever, Nausea and Vomiting, Menstrual Cramps, Diarrhea, Constipation, Hemorrhoids, Back Pain, Dandruff, Dry and Itchy Skin, Cuts, Scrapes, Sprains, Bruises, and More

Along with Information about Prevention, Self-Care, Choosing a Doctor, Over-the-Counter Medications, Folk Remedies, and Alternative Therapies, and Including a Glossary of Important Terms and a Directory of Resources for Further Help and Information

Edited by Chad T. Kimball. 638 pages. 2001. 0-7808-0435-X. $78.

"A good starting point for research on common illnesses. It will be a useful addition to public and consumer health library collections."
— *American Reference Books Annual 2002*

"Will prove valuable to any library seeking to maintain a current, comprehensive reference collection of health resources. . . . Excellent reference."
— *The Bookwatch, Aug '01*

"Recommended reference source."
— *Booklist, American Library Association, July '01*

Communication Disorders Sourcebook

Basic Information about Deafness and Hearing Loss, Speech and Language Disorders, Voice Disorders, Balance and Vestibular Disorders, and Disorders of Smell, Taste, and Touch

Edited by Linda M. Ross. 533 pages. 1996. 0-7808-0077-X. $78.

"This is skillfully edited and is a welcome resource for the layperson. It should be found in every public and medical library." —*Booklist Health Sciences Supplement, American Library Association, Oct '97*

Congenital Disorders Sourcebook

Basic Information about Disorders Acquired during Gestation, Including Spina Bifida, Hydrocephalus, Cerebral Palsy, Heart Defects, Craniofacial Abnormalities, Fetal Alcohol Syndrome, and More

Along with Current Treatment Options and Statistical Data

Edited by Karen Bellenir. 607 pages. 1997. 0-7808-0205-5. $78.

"Recommended reference source." —*Booklist, American Library Association, Oct '97*

SEE ALSO Pregnancy & Birth Sourcebook

Consumer Issues in Health Care Sourcebook

Basic Information about Health Care Fundamentals and Related Consumer Issues, Including Exams and Screening Tests, Physician Specialties, Choosing a Doctor, Using Prescription and Over-the-Counter Medications Safely, Avoiding Health Scams, Managing Common Health Risks in the Home, Care Options for Chronically or Terminally Ill Patients, and a List of Resources for Obtaining Help and Further Information

Edited by Karen Bellenir. 618 pages. 1998. 0-7808-0221-7. $78.

"Both public and academic libraries will want to have a copy in their collection for readers who are interested in self-education on health issues." —*American Reference Books Annual, 2000*

"The editor has researched the literature from government agencies and others, saving readers the time and effort of having to do the research themselves. Recommended for public libraries." —*Reference and User Services Quarterly, American Library Association, Spring '99*

"Recommended reference source." —*Booklist, American Library Association, Dec '98*

Contagious & Non-Contagious Infectious Diseases Sourcebook

Basic Information about Contagious Diseases like Measles, Polio, Hepatitis B, and Infectious Mononucleosis, and Non-Contagious Infectious Diseases like Tetanus and Toxic Shock Syndrome, and Diseases Occurring as Secondary Infections Such as Shingles and Reye Syndrome

Along with Vaccination, Prevention, and Treatment Information, and a Section Describing Emerging Infectious Disease Threats

Edited by Karen Bellenir and Peter D. Dresser. 566 pages. 1996. 0-7808-0075-3. $78.

Death & Dying Sourcebook

Basic Consumer Health Information for the Layperson about End-of-Life Care and Related Ethical and Legal Issues, Including Chief Causes of Death, Autopsies, Pain Management for the Terminally Ill, Life Support Systems, Insurance, Euthanasia, Assisted Suicide, Hospice Programs, Living Wills, Funeral Planning, Counseling, Mourning, Organ Donation, and Physician Training

Along with Statistical Data, a Glossary, and Listings of Sources for Further Help and Information

Edited by Annemarie S. Muth. 641 pages. 1999. 0-7808-0230-6. $78.

"Public libraries, medical libraries, and academic libraries will all find this sourcebook a useful addition to their collections." —*American Reference Books Annual, 2001*

"An extremely useful resource for those concerned with death and dying in the United States." —*Respiratory Care, Nov '00*

"Recommended reference source." —*Booklist, American Library Association, Aug '00*

"This book is a definite must for all those involved in end-of-life care." —*Doody's Review Service, 2000*

Dental Care & Oral Health Sourcebook, 2nd Edition

Basic Consumer Health Information about Dental Care, Including Oral Hygiene, Dental Visits, Pain Management, Cavities, Crowns, Bridges, Dental Implants, and Fillings, and Other Oral Health Concerns, Such as Gum Disease, Bad Breath, Dry Mouth, Genetic and Developmental Abnormalities, Oral Cancers, Orthodontics, and Temporomandibular Disorders

Along with Updates on Current Research in Oral Health, a Glossary, a Directory of Dental and Oral Health Organizations, and Resources for People with Dental and Oral Health Disorders

Edited by Amy L. Sutton. 609 pages. 2003. 0-7808-0634-4. $78.

Depression Sourcebook

Basic Consumer Health Information about Unipolar Depression, Bipolar Disorder, Postpartum Depression, Seasonal Affective Disorder, and Other Types of Depression in Children, Adolescents, Women, Men, the Elderly, and Other Selected Populations

Along with Facts about Causes, Risk Factors, Diagnostic Criteria, Treatment Options, Coping Strategies, Suicide Prevention, a Glossary, and a Directory of Sources for Additional Help and Information

Edited by Karen Belleni. 602 pages. 2002. 0-7808-0611-5. $78.

Diabetes Sourcebook, 3rd Edition

Basic Consumer Health Information about Type 1 Diabetes (Insulin-Dependent or Juvenile-Onset Diabetes), Type 2 Diabetes (Noninsulin-Dependent or Adult-Onset Diabetes), Gestational Diabetes, Impaired Glucose Tolerance (IGT), and Related Complications, Such as Amputation, Eye Disease, Gum Disease, Nerve Damage, and End-Stage Renal Disease, Including Facts about Insulin, Oral Diabetes Medications, Blood Sugar Testing, and the Role of Exercise and Nutrition in the Control of Diabetes

Along with a Glossary and Resources for Further Help and Information

Edited by Dawn D. Matthews. 622 pages. 2003. 0-7808-0629-8. $78.

ALSO AVAILABLE: Diabetes Sourcebook, 1st Edition. Edited by Karen Bellenir and Peter D. Dresser. 827 pages. 1994. 1-55888-751-2. $78.

Diabetes Sourcebook, 2nd Edition. Edited by Karen Bellenir. 688 pages. 1998. 0-7808-0224-1. $78.

Diet & Nutrition Sourcebook, 2nd Edition

Basic Consumer Health Information about Dietary Guidelines, Recommended Daily Intake Values, Vitamins, Minerals, Fiber, Fat, Weight Control, Dietary Supplements, and Food Additives

Along with Special Sections on Nutrition Needs throughout Life and Nutrition for People with Such Specific Medical Concerns as Allergies, High Blood Cholesterol, Hypertension, Diabetes, Celiac Disease, Seizure Disorders, Phenylketonuria (PKU), Cancer, and Eating Disorders, and Including Reports on Current Nutrition Research and Source Listings for Additional Help and Information

Edited by Karen Bellenir. 650 pages. 1999. 0-7808-0228-4. $78.

ALSO AVAILABLE: Diet & Nutrition Sourcebook, 1st Edition. Edited by Dan R. Harris. 662 pages. 1996. 0-7808-0084-2. $78.

SEE ALSO Digestive Diseases & Disorders Sourcebook, Eating Disorders Sourcebook, Gastrointestinal Diseases & Disorders Sourcebook, Vegetarian Sourcebook

Digestive Diseases & Disorders Sourcebook

Basic Consumer Health Information about Diseases and Disorders that Impact the Upper and Lower Digestive System, Including Celiac Disease, Constipation,

Crohn's Disease, Cyclic Vomiting Syndrome, Diarrhea, Diverticulosis and Diverticulitis, Gallstones, Heartburn, Hemorrhoids, Hernias, Indigestion (Dyspepsia), Irritable Bowel Syndrome, Lactose Intolerance, Ulcers, and More

Along with Information about Medications and Other Treatments, Tips for Maintaining a Healthy Digestive Tract, a Glossary, and Directory of Digestive Diseases Organizations

Edited by Karen Bellenir. 335 pages. 2000. 0-7808-0327-2. $78.

"This title would be an excellent addition to all public or patient-research libraries."
—American Reference Books Annual, 2001

"This title is recommended for public, hospital, and health sciences libraries with consumer health collections."
—E-Streams, Jul-Aug '00

"Recommended reference source."
—Booklist, American Library Association, May '00

SEE ALSO *Diet & Nutrition Sourcebook, Eating Disorders Sourcebook, Gastrointestinal Diseases & Disorders Sourcebook*

Disabilities Sourcebook

Basic Consumer Health Information about Physical and Psychiatric Disabilities, Including Descriptions of Major Causes of Disability, Assistive and Adaptive Aids, Workplace Issues, and Accessibility Concerns

Along with Information about the Americans with Disabilities Act, a Glossary, and Resources for Additional Help and Information

Edited by Dawn D. Matthews. 616 pages. 2000. 0-7808-0389-2. $78.

"It is a must for libraries with a consumer health section."
— American Reference Books Annual 2002

"A much needed addition to the Omnigraphics *Health Reference Series*. A current reference work to provide people with disabilities, their families, caregivers or those who work with them, a broad range of information in one volume, has not been available until now. . . . It is recommended for all public and academic library reference collections."
— E-Streams, May '01

"An excellent source book in easy-to-read format covering many current topics; highly recommended for all libraries."
— Choice, Association of College and Research Libraries, Jan '01

"Recommended reference source."
—Booklist, American Library Association, Jul '00

Domestic Violence & Child Abuse Sourcebook

Basic Consumer Health Information about Spousal/ Partner, Child, Sibling, Parent, and Elder Abuse, Covering Physical, Emotional, and Sexual Abuse, Teen Dating Violence, and Stalking; Includes Information

about Hotlines, Safe Houses, Safety Plans, and Other Resources for Support and Assistance, Community Initiatives, and Reports on Current Directions in Research and Treatment

Along with a Glossary, Sources for Further Reading, and Governmental and Non-Governmental Organizations Contact Information

Edited by Helene Henderson. 1,064 pages. 2001. 0-7808-0235-7. $78.

"Interested lay persons should find the book extremely beneficial. . . . A copy of *Domestic Violence and Child Abuse Sourcebook* should be in every public library in the United States."
— Social Science & Medicine, No. 56, 2003

"This is important information. The Web has many resources but this sourcebook fills an important societal need. I am not aware of any other resources of this type."
— Doody's Review Service, Sep '01

"Recommended for all libraries, scholars, and practitioners."
— Choice, Association of College & Research Libraries, Jul '01

"Recommended reference source."
— Booklist, American Library Association, Apr '01

"Important pick for college-level health reference libraries."
— The Bookwatch, Mar '01

"Because this problem is so widespread and because this book includes a lot of issues within one volume, this work is recommended for all public libraries."
— American Reference Books Annual, 2001

Drug Abuse Sourcebook

Basic Consumer Health Information about Illicit Substances of Abuse and the Diversion of Prescription Medications, Including Depressants, Hallucinogens, Inhalants, Marijuana, Narcotics, Stimulants, and Anabolic Steroids

Along with Facts about Related Health Risks, Treatment Issues, and Substance Abuse Prevention Programs, a Glossary of Terms, Statistical Data, and Directories of Hotline Services, Self-Help Groups, and Organizations Able to Provide Further Information

Edited by Karen Bellenir. 629 pages. 2000. 0-7808-0242-X. $78.

"Containing a wealth of information . . . . This resource belongs in libraries that serve a lower-division undergraduate or community college clientele as well as the general public."
— Choice, Association of College and Research Libraries, Jun '01

"Recommended reference source."
— Booklist, American Library Association, Feb '01

"Highly recommended." *— The Bookwatch, Jan '01*

"Even though there is a plethora of books on drug abuse, this volume is recommended for school, public, and college libraries."
—American Reference Books Annual, 2001

SEE ALSO *Alcoholism Sourcebook, Substance Abuse Sourcebook*

Ear, Nose & Throat Disorders Sourcebook

Basic Information about Disorders of the Ears, Nose, Sinus Cavities, Pharynx, and Larynx, Including Ear Infections, Tinnitus, Vestibular Disorders, Allergic and Non-Allergic Rhinitis, Sore Throats, Tonsillitis, and Cancers That Affect the Ears, Nose, Sinuses, and Throat

Along with Reports on Current Research Initiatives, a Glossary of Related Medical Terms, and a Directory of Sources for Further Help and Information

Edited by Karen Bellenir and Linda M. Shin. 576 pages. 1998. 0-7808-0206-3. $78.

"Overall, this sourcebook is helpful for the consumer seeking information on ENT issues. It is recommended for public libraries."
— *American Reference Books Annual, 1999*

"Recommended reference source."
— *Booklist, American Library Association, Dec '98*

■

Eating Disorders Sourcebook

Basic Consumer Health Information about Eating Disorders, Including Information about Anorexia Nervosa, Bulimia Nervosa, Binge Eating, Body Dysmorphic Disorder, Pica, Laxative Abuse, and Night Eating Syndrome

Along with Information about Causes, Adverse Effects, and Treatment and Prevention Issues, and Featuring a Section on Concerns Specific to Children and Adolescents, a Glossary, and Resources for Further Help and Information

Edited by Dawn D. Matthews. 322 pages. 2001. 0-7808-0335-3. $78.

"Recommended for health science libraries that are open to the public, as well as hospital libraries. This book is a good resource for the consumer who is concerned about eating disorders." — *E-Streams, Mar '02*

"This volume is another convenient collection of excerpted articles. Recommended for school and public library patrons; lower-division undergraduates; and two-year technical program students." — *Choice, Association of College & Research Libraries, Jan '02*

"Recommended reference source." — *Booklist, American Library Association, Oct '01*

SEE ALSO *Diet & Nutrition Sourcebook, Digestive Diseases & Disorders Sourcebook, Gastrointestinal Diseases & Disorders Sourcebook*

■

Emergency Medical Services Sourcebook

Basic Consumer Health Information about Preventing, Preparing for, and Managing Emergency Situations, When and Who to Call for Help, What to Expect in the Emergency Room, the Emergency Medical Team, Patient Issues, and Current Topics in Emergency Medicine

Along with Statistical Data, a Glossary, and Sources of Additional Help and Information

Edited by Jenni Lynn Colson. 494 pages. 2002. 0-7808-0420-1. $78.

"Handy and convenient for home, public, school, and college libraries. Recommended."
— *Choice, Association of College and Research Libraries, Apr '03*

"This reference can provide the consumer with answers to most questions about emergency care in the United States, or it will direct them to a resource where the answer can be found."
— *American Reference Books Annual, 2003*

"Recommended reference source."
— *Booklist, American Library Association, Feb '03*

■

Endocrine & Metabolic Disorders Sourcebook

Basic Information for the Layperson about Pancreatic and Insulin-Related Disorders Such as Pancreatitis, Diabetes, and Hypoglycemia; Adrenal Gland Disorders Such as Cushing's Syndrome, Addison's Disease, and Congenital Adrenal Hyperplasia; Pituitary Gland Disorders Such as Growth Hormone Deficiency, Acromegaly, and Pituitary Tumors; Thyroid Disorders Such as Hypothyroidism, Graves' Disease, Hashimoto's Disease, and Goiter; Hyperparathyroidism; and Other Diseases and Syndromes of Hormone Imbalance or Metabolic Dysfunction

Along with Reports on Current Research Initiatives

Edited by Linda M. Shin. 574 pages. 1998. 0-7808-0207-1. $78.

"Omnigraphics has produced another needed resource for health information consumers."
— *American Reference Books Annual, 2000*

"Recommended reference source."
— *Booklist, American Library Association, Dec '98*

■

Environmental Health Sourcebook, 2nd Edition

Basic Consumer Health Information about the Environment and Its Effect on Human Health, Including the Effects of Air Pollution, Water Pollution, Hazardous Chemicals, Food Hazards, Radiation Hazards, Biological Agents, Household Hazards, Such as Radon, Asbestos, Carbon Monoxide, and Mold, and Information about Associated Diseases and Disorders, Including Cancer, Allergies, Respiratory Problems, and Skin Disorders

Along with Information about Environmental Concerns for Specific Populations, a Glossary of Related Terms, and Resources for Further Help and Information

Edited by Dawn D. Matthews. 673 pages. 2003. 0-7808-0632-8. $78.

ALSO AVAILABLE: *Environmentally Induced Disorders Sourcebook, 1st Edition.* Edited by Allan R. Cook. 620 pages. 1997. 0-7808-0083-4. $78.

■

Environmentally Induced Disorders Sourcebook, 1st Edition

SEE *Environmental Health Sourcebook, 2nd Edition*

■

Ethnic Diseases Sourcebook

Basic Consumer Health Information for Ethnic and Racial Minority Groups in the United States, Including General Health Indicators and Behaviors, Ethnic Diseases, Genetic Testing, the Impact of Chronic Diseases, Women's Health, Mental Health Issues, and Preventive Health Care Services

Along with a Glossary and a Listing of Additional Resources

Edited by Joyce Brennfleck Shannon. 664 pages. 2001. 0-7808-0336-1. $78.

■

Eye Care Sourcebook, 2nd Edition

Basic Consumer Health Information about Eye Care and Eye Disorders, Including Facts about the Diag-

nosis, Prevention, and Treatment of Common Refractive Problems Such as Myopia, Hyperopia, Astigmatism, and Presbyopia, and Eye Diseases, Including Glaucoma, Cataract, Age-Related Macular Degeneration, and Diabetic Retinopathy

Along with a Section on Vision Correction and Refractive Surgeries, Including LASIK and LASEK, a Glossary, and Directories of Resources for Additional Help and Information

Edited by Amy L. Sutton. 543 pages. 2003. 0-7808-0635-2. $78.

ALSO AVAILABLE: *Ophthalmic Disorders Sourcebook, 1st Edition.* Edited by Linda M. Ross. 631 pages. 1996. 0-7808-0081-8. $78.

■

Family Planning Sourcebook

Basic Consumer Health Information about Planning for Pregnancy and Contraception, Including Traditional Methods, Barrier Methods, Hormonal Methods, Permanent Methods, Future Methods, Emergency Contraception, and Birth Control Choices for Women at Each Stage of Life

Along with Statistics, a Glossary, and Sources of Additional Information

Edited by Amy Marcaccio Keyzer. 520 pages. 2001. 0-7808-0379-5. $78.

SEE ALSO *Pregnancy & Birth Sourcebook*

■

Fitness & Exercise Sourcebook, 2nd Edition

Basic Consumer Health Information about the Fundamentals of Fitness and Exercise, Including How to Begin and Maintain a Fitness Program, Fitness as a Lifestyle, the Link between Fitness and Diet, Advice for Specific Groups of People, Exercise as It Relates to Specific Medical Conditions, and Recent Research in Fitness and Exercise

Along with a Glossary of Important Terms and Resources for Additional Help and Information

Edited by Kristen M. Gledhill. 646 pages. 2001. 0-7808-0334-5. $78.

ALSO AVAILABLE: *Fitness & Exercise Sourcebook, 1st Edition.* Edited by Dan R. Harris. 663 pages. 1996. 0-7808-0186-5. $78.

"This work is recommended for all general reference collections."
— *American Reference Books Annual 2002*

"Highly recommended for public, consumer, and school grades fourth through college."
—*E-Streams, Nov '01*

"Recommended reference source."   — *Booklist, American Library Association, Oct '01*

"The information appears quite comprehensive and is considered reliable. . . . This second edition is a welcomed addition to the series."
—*Doody's Review Service, Sep '01*

"This reference is a valuable choice for those who desire a broad source of information on exercise, fitness, and chronic-disease prevention through a healthy lifestyle."   —*American Medical Writers Association Journal, Fall '01*

"Will prove valuable to any library seeking to maintain a current, comprehensive reference collection of health resources. . . . Excellent reference."
— *The Bookwatch, Aug '01*

■

Food & Animal Borne Diseases Sourcebook

Basic Information about Diseases That Can Be Spread to Humans through the Ingestion of Contaminated Food or Water or by Contact with Infected Animals and Insects, Such as Botulism, E. Coli, Hepatitis A, Trichinosis, Lyme Disease, and Rabies

Along with Information Regarding Prevention and Treatment Methods, and Including a Special Section for International Travelers Describing Diseases Such as Cholera, Malaria, Travelers' Diarrhea, and Yellow Fever, and Offering Recommendations for Avoiding Illness

Edited by Karen Bellenir and Peter D. Dresser. 535 pages. 1995. 0-7808-0033-8. $78.

"Targeting general readers and providing them with a single, comprehensive source of information on selected topics, this book continues, with the excellent caliber of its predecessors, to catalog topical information on health matters of general interest. Readable and thorough, this valuable resource is highly recommended for all libraries."
— *Academic Library Book Review, Summer '96*

"A comprehensive collection of authoritative information."   — *Emergency Medical Services, Oct '95*

■

Food Safety Sourcebook

Basic Consumer Health Information about the Safe Handling of Meat, Poultry, Seafood, Eggs, Fruit Juices, and Other Food Items, and Facts about Pesticides, Drinking Water, Food Safety Overseas, and the Onset, Duration, and Symptoms of Foodborne Illnesses,

Including Types of Pathogenic Bacteria, Parasitic Protozoa, Worms, Viruses, and Natural Toxins

Along with the Role of the Consumer, the Food Handler, and the Government in Food Safety; a Glossary, and Resources for Additional Help and Information

Edited by Dawn D. Matthews. 339 pages. 1999. 0-7808-0326-4. $78.

"This book is recommended for public libraries and universities with home economic and food science programs."   —*E-Streams, Nov '00*

"Recommended reference source."
—*Booklist, American Library Association, May '00*

"This book takes the complex issues of food safety and foodborne pathogens and presents them in an easily understood manner. [It does] an excellent job of covering a large and often confusing topic."
—*American Reference Books Annual, 2000*

■

Forensic Medicine Sourcebook

Basic Consumer Information for the Layperson about Forensic Medicine, Including Crime Scene Investigation, Evidence Collection and Analysis, Expert Testimony, Computer-Aided Criminal Identification, Digital Imaging in the Courtroom, DNA Profiling, Accident Reconstruction, Autopsies, Ballistics, Drugs and Explosives Detection, Latent Fingerprints, Product Tampering, and Questioned Document Examination

Along with Statistical Data, a Glossary of Forensics Terminology, and Listings of Sources for Further Help and Information

Edited by Annemarie S. Muth. 574 pages. 1999. 0-7808-0232-2. $78.

"Given the expected widespread interest in its content and its easy to read style, this book is recommended for most public and all college and university libraries."
— *E-Streams, Feb '01*

"Recommended for public libraries."
—*Reference & User Services Quarterly, American Library Association, Spring 2000*

"Recommended reference source."
—*Booklist, American Library Association, Feb '00*

"A wealth of information, useful statistics, references are up-to-date and extremely complete. This wonderful collection of data will help students who are interested in a career in any type of forensic field. It is a great resource for attorneys who need information about types of expert witnesses needed in a particular case. It also offers useful information for fiction and nonfiction writers whose work involves a crime. A fascinating compilation. All levels."   — *Choice, Association of College and Research Libraries, Jan 2000*

"There are several items that make this book attractive to consumers who are seeking certain forensic data. . . . This is a useful current source for those seeking general forensic medical answers."
—*American Reference Books Annual, 2000*

Gastrointestinal Diseases & Disorders Sourcebook

Basic Information about Gastroesophageal Reflux Disease (Heartburn), Ulcers, Diverticulosis, Irritable Bowel Syndrome, Crohn's Disease, Ulcerative Colitis, Diarrhea, Constipation, Lactose Intolerance, Hemorrhoids, Hepatitis, Cirrhosis, and Other Digestive Problems, Featuring Statistics, Descriptions of Symptoms, and Current Treatment Methods of Interest for Persons Living with Upper and Lower Gastrointestinal Maladies

Edited by Linda M. Ross. 413 pages. 1996. 0-7808-0078-8. $78.

". . . very readable form. The successful editorial work that brought this material together into a useful and understandable reference makes accessible to all readers information that can help them more effectively understand and obtain help for digestive tract problems."
— *Choice, Association of College & Research Libraries, Feb '97*

SEE ALSO Diet & Nutrition Sourcebook, Digestive Diseases & Disorders, Eating Disorders Sourcebook

■

Genetic Disorders Sourcebook, 2nd Edition

Basic Consumer Health Information about Hereditary Diseases and Disorders, Including Cystic Fibrosis, Down Syndrome, Hemophilia, Huntington's Disease, Sickle Cell Anemia, and More; Facts about Genes, Gene Research and Therapy, Genetic Screening, Ethics of Gene Testing, Genetic Counseling, and Advice on Coping and Caring

Along with a Glossary of Genetic Terminology and a Resource List for Help, Support, and Further Information

Edited by Kathy Massimini. 768 pages. 2001. 0-7808-0241-1. $78.

ALSO AVAILABLE: Genetic Disorders Sourcebook, 1st Edition. Edited by Karen Bellenir. 642 pages. 1996. 0-7808-0034-6. $78.

"Recommended for public libraries and medical and hospital libraries with consumer health collections."
— *E-Streams, May '01*

"Recommended reference source."
— *Booklist, American Library Association, Apr '01*

"Important pick for college-level health reference libraries." — *The Bookwatch, Mar '01*

"Provides essential medical information to both the general public and those diagnosed with a serious or fatal genetic disease or disorder." — *Choice, Association of College and Research Libraries, Jan '97*

Head Trauma Sourcebook

Basic Information for the Layperson about Open-Head and Closed-Head Injuries, Treatment Advances, Recovery, and Rehabilitation

Along with Reports on Current Research Initiatives

Edited by Karen Bellenir. 414 pages. 1997. 0-7808-0208-X. $78.

■

Headache Sourcebook

Basic Consumer Health Information about Migraine, Tension, Cluster, Rebound and Other Types of Headaches, with Facts about the Cause and Prevention of Headaches, the Effects of Stress and the Environment, Headaches during Pregnancy and Menopause, and Childhood Headaches

Along with a Glossary and Other Resources for Additional Help and Information

Edited by Dawn D. Matthews. 362 pages. 2002. 0-7808-0337-X. $78.

"Highly recommended for academic and medical reference collections." — *Library Bookwatch, Sep '02*

■

Health Insurance Sourcebook

Basic Information about Managed Care Organizations, Traditional Fee-for-Service Insurance, Insurance Portability and Pre-Existing Conditions Clauses, Medicare, Medicaid, Social Security, and Military Health Care

Along with Information about Insurance Fraud

Edited by Wendy Wilcox. 530 pages. 1997. 0-7808-0222-5. $78.

"Particularly useful because it brings much of this information together in one volume. This book will be a handy reference source in the health sciences library, hospital library, college and university library, and medium to large public library."
— *Medical Reference Services Quarterly, Fall '98*

Awarded "Books of the Year Award"
— *American Journal of Nursing, 1997*

"The layout of the book is particularly helpful as it provides easy access to reference material. A most useful addition to the vast amount of information about health insurance. The use of data from U.S. government agencies is most commendable. Useful in a library or learning center for healthcare professional students."
— *Doody's Health Sciences Book Reviews, Nov '97*

■

Health Reference Series Cumulative Index 1999

A Comprehensive Index to the Individual Volumes of the Health Reference Series, Including a Subject Index, Name Index, Organization Index, and Publication Index

Along with a Master List of Acronyms and Abbreviations

Edited by Edward J. Prucha, Anne Holmes, and Robert Rudnick. 990 pages. 2000. 0-7808-0382-5. $78.

"This volume will be most helpful in libraries that have a relatively complete collection of the Health Reference Series." —American Reference Books Annual, 2001

"Essential for collections that hold any of the numerous *Health Reference Series* titles." —Choice, Association of College and Research Libraries, Nov '00

■

Healthy Aging Sourcebook

Basic Consumer Health Information about Maintaining Health through the Aging Process, Including Advice on Nutrition, Exercise, and Sleep, Help in Making Decisions about Midlife Issues and Retirement, and Guidance Concerning Practical and Informed Choices in Health Consumerism

Along with Data Concerning the Theories of Aging, Different Experiences in Aging by Minority Groups, and Facts about Aging Now and Aging in the Future; and Featuring a Glossary, a Guide to Consumer Help, Additional Suggested Reading, and Practical Resource Directory

Edited by Jenifer Swanson. 536 pages. 1999. 0-7808-0390-6. $78.

"Recommended reference source." —Booklist, American Library Association, Feb '00

SEE ALSO *Physical & Mental Issues in Aging Sourcebook*

■

Healthy Children Sourcebook

Basic Consumer Health Information about the Physical and Mental Development of Children between the Ages of 3 and 12, Including Routine Health Care, Preventative Health Services, Safety and First Aid, Healthy Sleep, Dental Care, Nutrition, and Fitness, and Featuring Parenting Tips on Such Topics as Bedwetting, Choosing Day Care, Monitoring TV and Other Media, and Establishing a Foundation for Substance Abuse Prevention

Along with a Glossary of Commonly Used Pediatric Terms and Resources for Additional Help and Information.

Edited by Chad T. Kimball. 647 pages. 2003. 0-7808-0247-0. $78.

■

Healthy Heart Sourcebook for Women

Basic Consumer Health Information about Cardiac Issues Specific to Women, Including Facts about Major Risk Factors and Prevention, Treatment and Control Strategies, and Important Dietary Issues

Along with a Special Section Regarding the Pros and Cons of Hormone Replacement Therapy and Its Impact on Heart Health, and Additional Help, Including Recipes, a Glossary, and a Directory of Resources

Edited by Dawn D. Matthews. 336 pages. 2000. 0-7808-0329-9. $78.

"A good reference source and recommended for all public, academic, medical, and hospital libraries." —Medical Reference Services Quarterly, Summer '01

"Because of the lack of information specific to women on this topic, this book is recommended for public libraries and consumer libraries." —American Reference Books Annual, 2001

"Contains very important information about coronary artery disease that all women should know. The information is current and presented in an easy-to-read format. The book will make a good addition to any library." —American Medical Writers Association Journal, Summer '00

"Important, basic reference." —Reviewer's Bookwatch, Jul '00

SEE ALSO *Heart Diseases & Disorders Sourcebook, Women's Health Concerns Sourcebook*

■

Heart Diseases & Disorders Sourcebook, 2nd Edition

Basic Consumer Health Information about Heart Attacks, Angina, Rhythm Disorders, Heart Failure, Valve Disease, Congenital Heart Disorders, and More, Including Descriptions of Surgical Procedures and Other Interventions, Medications, Cardiac Rehabilitation, Risk Identification, and Prevention Tips

Along with Statistical Data, Reports on Current Research Initiatives, a Glossary of Cardiovascular Terms, and Resource Directory

Edited by Karen Bellenir. 612 pages. 2000. 0-7808-0238-1. $78.

ALSO AVAILABLE: *Cardiovascular Diseases & Disorders Sourcebook, 1st Edition.* Edited by Karen Bellenir and Peter D. Dresser. 683 pages. 1995. 0-7808-0032-X. $78.

"This work stands out as an imminently accessible resource for the general public. It is recommended for the reference and circulating shelves of school, public, and academic libraries." —American Reference Books Annual, 2001

"Recommended reference source." —Booklist, American Library Association, Dec '00

"Provides comprehensive coverage of matters related to the heart. This title is recommended for health sciences and public libraries with consumer health collections." —E-Streams, Oct '00

SEE ALSO *Healthy Heart Sourcebook for Women*

■

Household Safety Sourcebook

Basic Consumer Health Information about Household Safety, Including Information about Poisons, Chemicals, Fire, and Water Hazards in the Home

Along with Advice about the Safe Use of Home Maintenance Equipment, Choosing Toys and Nursery Furni-

ture, Holiday and Recreation Safety, a Glossary, and Resources for Further Help and Information

Edited by Dawn D. Matthews. 606 pages. 2002. 0-7808-0338-8. $78.

"This work will be useful in public libraries with large consumer health and wellness departments."
— American Reference Books Annual, 2003

"As a sourcebook on household safety this book meets its mark. It is encyclopedic in scope and covers a wide range of safety issues that are commonly seen in the home." — E-Streams, Jul '02

■

Immune System Disorders Sourcebook

Basic Information about Lupus, Multiple Sclerosis, Guillain-Barré Syndrome, Chronic Granulomatous Disease, and More

Along with Statistical and Demographic Data and Reports on Current Research Initiatives

Edited by Allan R. Cook. 608 pages. 1997. 0-7808-0209-8. $78.

■

Infant & Toddler Health Sourcebook

Basic Consumer Health Information about the Physical and Mental Development of Newborns, Infants, and Toddlers, Including Neonatal Concerns, Nutrition Recommendations, Immunization Schedules, Common Pediatric Disorders, Assessments and Milestones, Safety Tips, and Advice for Parents and Other Caregivers

Along with a Glossary of Terms and Resource Listings for Additional Help

Edited by Jenifer Swanson. 585 pages. 2000. 0-7808-0246-2. $78.

"As a reference for the general public, this would be useful in any library." — E-Streams, May '01

"Recommended reference source."
— Booklist, American Library Association, Feb '01

"This is a good source for general use."
— American Reference Books Annual, 2001

■

Injury & Trauma Sourcebook

Basic Consumer Health Information about the Impact of Injury, the Diagnosis and Treatment of Common and Traumatic Injuries, Emergency Care, and Specific Injuries Related to Home, Community, Workplace, Transportation, and Recreation

Along with Guidelines for Injury Prevention, a Glossary, and a Directory of Additional Resources

Edited by Joyce Brennfleck Shannon. 696 pages. 2002. 0-7808-0421-X. $78.

"This publication is the most comprehensive work of its kind about injury and trauma."
— American Reference Books Annual, 2003

"This sourcebook provides concise, easily readable, basic health information about injuries. . . . This book is well organized and an easy to use reference resource suitable for hospital, health sciences and public libraries with consumer health collections."
— E-Streams, Nov '02

"Practitioners should be aware of guides such as this in order to facilitate their use by patients and their families." — Doody's Health Sciences
Book Review Journal, Sep-Oct '02

"Recommended reference source."
— Booklist, American Library Association, Sep '02

"Highly recommended for academic and medical reference collections." — Library Bookwatch, Sep '02

■

Kidney & Urinary Tract Diseases & Disorders Sourcebook

Basic Information about Kidney Stones, Urinary Incontinence, Bladder Disease, End Stage Renal Disease, Dialysis, and More

Along with Statistical and Demographic Data and Reports on Current Research Initiatives

Edited by Linda M. Ross. 602 pages. 1997. 0-7808-0079-6. $78.

■

Learning Disabilities Sourcebook, 2nd Edition

Basic Consumer Health Information about Learning Disabilities, Including Dyslexia, Developmental Speech and Language Disabilities, Non-Verbal Learning Disorders, Developmental Arithmetic Disorder, Developmental Writing Disorder, and Other Conditions That Impede Learning Such as Attention Deficit/ Hyperactivity Disorder, Brain Injury, Hearing Impairment, Klinefelter Syndrome, Dyspraxia, and Tourette Syndrome

Along with Facts about Educational Issues and Assistive Technology, Coping Strategies, a Glossary of Related Terms, and Resources for Further Help and Information

Edited by Dawn D. Matthews. 621 pages. 2003. 0-7808-0626-3. $78.

ALSO AVAILABLE: Learning Disabilities Sourcebook, 1st Edition. Edited by Linda M. Shin. 579 pages. 1998. 0-7808-0210-1. $78.

"Teachers as well as consumers will find this an essential guide to understanding various syndromes and their latest treatments. [An] invaluable reference for public and school library collections alike."
— Library Bookwatch, Apr '03

Named "Outstanding Reference Book of 1999."
— New York Public Library, Feb 2000

"An excellent candidate for inclusion in a public library reference section. It's a great source of information. Teachers will also find the book useful. Definitely worth reading."
— Journal of Adolescent & Adult Literacy, Feb 2000

"Readable . . . provides a solid base of information regarding successful techniques used with individuals who have learning disabilities, as well as practical suggestions for educators and family members. Clear language, concise descriptions, and pertinent information for contacting multiple resources add to the strength of this book as a useful tool."
— *Choice, Association of College and Research Libraries, Feb '99*

"Recommended reference source."
— *Booklist, American Library Association, Sep '98*

"A useful resource for libraries and for those who don't have the time to identify and locate the individual publications." — *Disability Resources Monthly, Sep '98*

■

Leukemia Sourcebook

Basic Consumer Health Information about Adult and Childhood Leukemias, Including Acute Lymphocytic Leukemia (ALL), Chronic Lymphocytic Leukemia (CLL), Acute Myelogenous Leukemia (AML), Chronic Myelogenous Leukemia (CML), and Hairy Cell Leukemia, and Treatments Such as Chemotherapy, Radiation Therapy, Peripheral Blood Stem Cell and Marrow Transplantation, and Immunotherapy

Along with Tips for Life During and After Treatment, a Glossary, and Directories of Additional Resources

Edited by Joyce Brennfleck Shannon. 587 pages. 2003. 0-7808-0627-1. $78.

■

Liver Disorders Sourcebook

Basic Consumer Health Information about the Liver and How It Works; Liver Diseases, Including Cancer, Cirrhosis, Hepatitis, and Toxic and Drug Related Diseases; Tips for Maintaining a Healthy Liver; Laboratory Tests, Radiology Tests, and Facts about Liver Transplantation

Along with a Section on Support Groups, a Glossary, and Resource Listings

Edited by Joyce Brennfleck Shannon. 591 pages. 2000. 0-7808-0383-3. $78.

"A valuable resource."
— *American Reference Books Annual, 2001*

"This title is recommended for health sciences and public libraries with consumer health collections."
— *E-Streams, Oct '00*

"Recommended reference source."
— *Booklist, American Library Association, Jun '00*

■

Lung Disorders Sourcebook

Basic Consumer Health Information about Emphysema, Pneumonia, Tuberculosis, Asthma, Cystic Fibrosis, and Other Lung Disorders, Including Facts about Diagnostic Procedures, Treatment Strategies, Disease Prevention Efforts, and Such Risk Factors as Smoking, Air Pollution, and Exposure to Asbestos, Radon, and Other Agents

Along with a Glossary and Resources for Additional Help and Information

Edited by Dawn D. Matthews. 678 pages. 2002. 0-7808-0339-6. $78.

"This title is a great addition for public and school libraries because it provides concise health information on the lungs."
— *American Reference Books Annual, 2003*

"Highly recommended for academic and medical reference collections." — *Library Bookwatch, Sep '02*

■

Medical Tests Sourcebook

Basic Consumer Health Information about Medical Tests, Including Periodic Health Exams, General Screening Tests, Tests You Can Do at Home, Findings of the U.S. Preventive Services Task Force, X-ray and Radiology Tests, Electrical Tests, Tests of Blood and Other Body Fluids and Tissues, Scope Tests, Lung Tests, Genetic Tests, Pregnancy Tests, Newborn Screening Tests, Sexually Transmitted Disease Tests, and Computer Aided Diagnoses

Along with a Section on Paying for Medical Tests, a Glossary, and Resource Listings

Edited by Joyce Brennfleck Shannon. 691 pages. 1999. 0-7808-0243-8. $78.

"Recommended for hospital and health sciences libraries with consumer health collections."
— *E-Streams, Mar '00*

"This is an overall excellent reference with a wealth of general knowledge that may aid those who are reluctant to get vital tests performed."
— *Today's Librarian, Jan 2000*

"A valuable reference guide."
— *American Reference Books Annual, 2000*

■

Men's Health Concerns Sourcebook

Basic Information about Health Issues That Affect Men, Featuring Facts about the Top Causes of Death in Men, Including Heart Disease, Stroke, Cancers, Prostate Disorders, Chronic Obstructive Pulmonary Disease, Pneumonia and Influenza, Human Immunodeficiency Virus and Acquired Immune Deficiency Syndrome, Diabetes Mellitus, Stress, Suicide, Accidents and Homicides; and Facts about Common Concerns for Men, Including Impotence, Contraception, Circumcision, Sleep Disorders, Snoring, Hair Loss, Diet, Nutrition, Exercise, Kidney and Urological Disorders, and Backaches

Edited by Allan R. Cook. 738 pages. 1998. 0-7808-0212-8. $78.

"This comprehensive resource and the series are highly recommended."
— *American Reference Books Annual, 2000*

"Recommended reference source."
— *Booklist, American Library Association, Dec '98*

Mental Health Disorders Sourcebook, 2nd Edition

Basic Consumer Health Information about Anxiety Disorders, Depression and Other Mood Disorders, Eating Disorders, Personality Disorders, Schizophrenia, and More, Including Disease Descriptions, Treatment Options, and Reports on Current Research Initiatives

Along with Statistical Data, Tips for Maintaining Mental Health, a Glossary, and Directory of Sources for Additional Help and Information

Edited by Karen Bellenir. 605 pages. 2000. 0-7808-0240-3. $78.

ALSO AVAILABLE: *Mental Health Disorders Sourcebook, 1st Edition. Edited by Karen Bellenir. 548 pages. 1995. 0-7808-0040-0. $78.*

"Well organized and well written."
—*American Reference Books Annual, 2001*

"Recommended reference source."
—*Booklist, American Library Association, Jun '00*

Mental Retardation Sourcebook

Basic Consumer Health Information about Mental Retardation and Its Causes, Including Down Syndrome, Fetal Alcohol Syndrome, Fragile X Syndrome, Genetic Conditions, Injury, and Environmental Sources

Along with Preventive Strategies, Parenting Issues, Educational Implications, Health Care Needs, Employment and Economic Matters, Legal Issues, a Glossary, and a Resource Listing for Additional Help and Information

Edited by Joyce Brennfleck Shannon. 642 pages. 2000. 0-7808-0377-9. $78.

"Public libraries will find the book useful for reference and as a beginning research point for students, parents, and caregivers."
—*American Reference Books Annual, 2001*

"The strength of this work is that it compiles many basic fact sheets and addresses for further information in one volume. It is intended and suitable for the general public. This sourcebook is relevant to any collection providing health information to the general public."
—*E-Streams, Nov '00*

"From preventing retardation to parenting and family challenges, this covers health, social and legal issues and will prove an invaluable overview."
—*Reviewer's Bookwatch, Jul '00*

Movement Disorders Sourcebook

Basic Consumer Health Information about Neurological Movement Disorders, Including Essential Tremor, Parkinson's Disease, Dystonia, Cerebral Palsy, Huntington's Disease, Myasthenia Gravis, Multiple Sclerosis, and Other Early-Onset and Adult-Onset Movement Disorders, Their Symptoms and Causes, Diagnostic Tests, and Treatments

Along with Mobility and Assistive Technology Information, a Glossary, and a Directory of Additional Resources

Edited by Joyce Brennfleck Shannon. 655 pages. 2003. 0-7808-0628-X. $78.

Obesity Sourcebook

Basic Consumer Health Information about Diseases and Other Problems Associated with Obesity, and Including Facts about Risk Factors, Prevention Issues, and Management Approaches

Along with Statistical and Demographic Data, Information about Special Populations, Research Updates, a Glossary, and Source Listings for Further Help and Information

Edited by Wilma Caldwell and Chad T. Kimball. 376 pages. 2001. 0-7808-0333-7. $78.

"The book synthesizes the reliable medical literature on obesity into one easy-to-read and useful resource for the general public."
— *American Reference Books Annual 2002*

"This is a very useful resource book for the lay public."
—*Doody's Review Service, Nov '01*

"Well suited for the health reference collection of a public library or an academic health science library that serves the general population." —*E-Streams, Sep '01*

"Recommended reference source."
—*Booklist, American Library Association, Apr '01*

" Recommended pick both for specialty health library collections and any general consumer health reference collection." — *The Bookwatch, Apr '01*

Ophthalmic Disorders Sourcebook, 1st Edition

SEE Eye Care Sourcebook, 2nd Edition

Oral Health Sourcebook

SEE Dental Care & Oral Health Sourcebook, 2nd Edition

Osteoporosis Sourcebook

Basic Consumer Health Information about Primary and Secondary Osteoporosis and Juvenile Osteoporosis and Related Conditions, Including Fibrous Dysplasia, Gaucher Disease, Hyperthyroidism, Hypophosphatasia, Myeloma, Osteopetrosis, Osteogenesis Imperfecta, and Paget's Disease

Along with Information about Risk Factors, Treatments, Traditional and Non-Traditional Pain Management, a Glossary of Related Terms, and a Directory of Resources

Edited by Allan R. Cook. 584 pages. 2001. 0-7808-0239-X. $78.

"This would be a book to be kept in a staff or patient library. The targeted audience is the layperson, but the therapist who needs a quick bit of information on a particular topic will also find the book useful."
— *Physical Therapy, Jan '02*

"This resource is recommended as a great reference source for public, health, and academic libraries, and is another triumph for the editors of Omnigraphics."
— *American Reference Books Annual 2002*

"Recommended for all public libraries and general health collections, especially those supporting patient education or consumer health programs."
— *E-Streams, Nov '01*

"Will prove valuable to any library seeking to maintain a current, comprehensive reference collection of health resources. . . . From prevention to treatment and associated conditions, this provides an excellent survey."
— *The Bookwatch, Aug '01*

"Recommended reference source."
— *Booklist, American Library Association, July '01*

SEE ALSO *Women's Health Concerns Sourcebook*

■

Pain Sourcebook, 2nd Edition

Basic Consumer Health Information about Specific Forms of Acute and Chronic Pain, Including Muscle and Skeletal Pain, Nerve Pain, Cancer Pain, and Disorders Characterized by Pain, Such as Fibromyalgia, Shingles, Angina, Arthritis, and Headaches

Along with Information about Pain Medications and Management Techniques, Complementary and Alternative Pain Relief Options, Tips for People Living with Chronic Pain, a Glossary, and a Directory of Sources for Further Information

Edited by Karen Bellenir. 670 pages. 2002. 0-7808-0612-3. $78.

ALSO AVAILABLE: *Pain Sourcebook, 1st Edition.* Edited by Allan R. Cook. 667 pages. 1997. 0-7808-0213-6. $78.

"A source of valuable information. . . . This book offers help to nonmedical people who need information about pain and pain management. It is also an excellent reference for those who participate in patient education."
— *Doody's Review Service, Sep '02*

"The text is readable, easily understood, and well indexed. This excellent volume belongs in all patient education libraries, consumer health sections of public libraries, and many personal collections."
— *American Reference Books Annual, 1999*

"A beneficial reference." — *Booklist Health Sciences Supplement, American Library Association, Oct '98*

"The information is basic in terms of scholarship and is appropriate for general readers. Written in journalistic style . . . intended for non-professionals. Quite thorough in its coverage of different pain conditions and summarizes the latest clinical information regarding pain treatment." — *Choice, Association of College and Research Libraries, Jun '98*

"Recommended reference source."
— *Booklist, American Library Association, Mar '98*

Pediatric Cancer Sourcebook

Basic Consumer Health Information about Leukemias, Brain Tumors, Sarcomas, Lymphomas, and Other Cancers in Infants, Children, and Adolescents, Including Descriptions of Cancers, Treatments, and Coping Strategies

Along with Suggestions for Parents, Caregivers, and Concerned Relatives, a Glossary of Cancer Terms, and Resource Listings

Edited by Edward J. Prucha. 587 pages. 1999. 0-7808-0245-4. $78.

"An excellent source of information. Recommended for public, hospital, and health science libraries with consumer health collections." — *E-Streams, Jun '00*

"Recommended reference source."
— *Booklist, American Library Association, Feb '00*

"A valuable addition to all libraries specializing in health services and many public libraries."
— *American Reference Books Annual, 2000*

■

Physical & Mental Issues in Aging Sourcebook

Basic Consumer Health Information on Physical and Mental Disorders Associated with the Aging Process, Including Concerns about Cardiovascular Disease, Pulmonary Disease, Oral Health, Digestive Disorders, Musculoskeletal and Skin Disorders, Metabolic Changes, Sexual and Reproductive Issues, and Changes in Vision, Hearing, and Other Senses

Along with Data about Longevity and Causes of Death, Information on Acute and Chronic Pain, Descriptions of Mental Concerns, a Glossary of Terms, and Resource Listings for Additional Help

Edited by Jenifer Swanson. 660 pages. 1999. 0-7808-0233-0. $78.

"This is a treasure of health information for the layperson." — *Choice Health Sciences Supplement, Association of College & Research Libraries, May 2000*

"Recommended for public libraries."
— *American Reference Books Annual, 2000*

"Recommended reference source."
— *Booklist, American Library Association, Oct '99*

SEE ALSO *Healthy Aging Sourcebook*

■

Podiatry Sourcebook

Basic Consumer Health Information about Foot Conditions, Diseases, and Injuries, Including Bunions, Corns, Calluses, Athlete's Foot, Plantar Warts, Hammertoes and Clawtoes, Clubfoot, Heel Pain, Gout, and More

Along with Facts about Foot Care, Disease Prevention, Foot Safety, Choosing a Foot Care Specialist, a Glossary of Terms, and Resource Listings for Additional Information

Edited by M. Lisa Weatherford. 380 pages. 2001. 0-7808-0215-2. $78.

"There is a lot of information presented here on a topic that is usually only covered sparingly in most larger comprehensive medical encyclopedias."

—*American Reference Books Annual 2002*

Pregnancy & Birth Sourcebook

Basic Information about Planning for Pregnancy, Maternal Health, Fetal Growth and Development, Labor and Delivery, Postpartum and Perinatal Care, Pregnancy in Mothers with Special Concerns, and Disorders of Pregnancy, Including Genetic Counseling, Nutrition and Exercise, Obstetrical Tests, Pregnancy Discomfort, Multiple Births, Cesarean Sections, Medical Testing of Newborns, Breastfeeding, Gestational Diabetes, and Ectopic Pregnancy

Edited by Heather E. Aldred. 737 pages. 1997. 0-7808-0216-0. $78.

"A well-organized handbook. Recommended."

—*Choice, Association of College and Research Libraries, Apr '98*

"Recommended reference source."

—*Booklist, American Library Association, Mar '98*

"Recommended for public libraries."

—*American Reference Books Annual, 1998*

SEE ALSO *Congenital Disorders Sourcebook, Family Planning Sourcebook*

Prostate Cancer Sourcebook

Basic Consumer Health Information about Prostate Cancer, Including Information about the Associated Risk Factors, Detection, Diagnosis, and Treatment of Prostate Cancer

Along with Information on Non-Malignant Prostate Conditions, and Featuring a Section Listing Support and Treatment Centers and a Glossary of Related Terms

Edited by Dawn D. Matthews. 358 pages. 2001. 0-7808-0324-8. $78.

"Recommended reference source."

—*Booklist, American Library Association, Jan '02*

"A valuable resource for health care consumers seeking information on the subject. . . . All text is written in a clear, easy-to-understand language that avoids technical jargon. Any library that collects consumer health resources would strengthen their collection with the addition of the *Prostate Cancer Sourcebook*."

—*American Reference Books Annual 2002*

Public Health Sourcebook

Basic Information about Government Health Agencies, Including National Health Statistics and Trends, Healthy People 2000 Program Goals and Objectives, the Centers for Disease Control and Prevention, the

Food and Drug Administration, and the National Institutes of Health

Along with Full Contact Information for Each Agency

Edited by Wendy Wilcox. 698 pages. 1998. 0-7808-0220-9. $78.

"Recommended reference source."

—*Booklist, American Library Association, Sep '98*

"This consumer guide provides welcome assistance in navigating the maze of federal health agencies and their data on public health concerns."

—*SciTech Book News, Sep '98*

Reconstructive & Cosmetic Surgery Sourcebook

Basic Consumer Health Information on Cosmetic and Reconstructive Plastic Surgery, Including Statistical Information about Different Surgical Procedures, Things to Consider Prior to Surgery, Plastic Surgery Techniques and Tools, Emotional and Psychological Considerations, and Procedure-Specific Information

Along with a Glossary of Terms and a Listing of Resources for Additional Help and Information

Edited by M. Lisa Weatherford. 374 pages. 2001. 0-7808-0214-4. $78.

"An excellent reference that addresses cosmetic and medically necessary reconstructive surgeries. . . . The style of the prose is calm and reassuring, discussing the many positive outcomes now available due to advances in surgical techniques."

—*American Reference Books Annual 2002*

"Recommended for health science libraries that are open to the public, as well as hospital libraries that are open to the patients. This book is a good resource for the consumer interested in plastic surgery."

—*E-Streams, Dec '01*

"Recommended reference source."

—*Booklist, American Library Association, July '01*

Rehabilitation Sourcebook

Basic Consumer Health Information about Rehabilitation for People Recovering from Heart Surgery, Spinal Cord Injury, Stroke, Orthopedic Impairments, Amputation, Pulmonary Impairments, Traumatic Injury, and More, Including Physical Therapy, Occupational Therapy, Speech/ Language Therapy, Massage Therapy, Dance Therapy, Art Therapy, and Recreational Therapy

Along with Information on Assistive and Adaptive Devices, a Glossary, and Resources for Additional Help and Information

Edited by Dawn D. Matthews. 531 pages. 1999. 0-7808-0236-5. $78.

"This is an excellent resource for public library reference and health collections."

—*American Reference Books Annual, 2001*

"Recommended reference source."

—*Booklist, American Library Association, May '00*

Respiratory Diseases & Disorders Sourcebook

Basic Information about Respiratory Diseases and Disorders, Including Asthma, Cystic Fibrosis, Pneumonia, the Common Cold, Influenza, and Others, Featuring Facts about the Respiratory System, Statistical and Demographic Data, Treatments, Self-Help Management Suggestions, and Current Research Initiatives

Edited by Allan R. Cook and Peter D. Dresser. 771 pages. 1995. 0-7808-0037-0. $78.

"Designed for the layperson and for patients and their families coping with respiratory illness. . . . an extensive array of information on diagnosis, treatment, management, and prevention of respiratory illnesses for the general reader." — *Choice, Association of College and Research Libraries, Jun '96*

"A highly recommended text for all collections. It is a comforting reminder of the power of knowledge that good books carry between their covers." — *Academic Library Book Review, Spring '96*

"A comprehensive collection of authoritative information presented in a nontechnical, humanitarian style for patients, families, and caregivers." — *Association of Operating Room Nurses, Sep/Oct '95*

SEE ALSO Lung Disorders Sourcebook

■

Sexually Transmitted Diseases Sourcebook, 2nd Edition

Basic Consumer Health Information about Sexually Transmitted Diseases, Including Information on the Diagnosis and Treatment of Chlamydia, Gonorrhea, Hepatitis, Herpes, HIV, Mononucleosis, Syphilis, and Others

Along with Information on Prevention, Such as Condom Use, Vaccines, and STD Education; And Featuring a Section on Issues Related to Youth and Adolescents, a Glossary, and Resources for Additional Help and Information

Edited by Dawn D. Matthews. 538 pages. 2001. 0-7808-0249-7. $78.

ALSO AVAILABLE: Sexually Transmitted Diseases Sourcebook, 1st Edition. Edited by Linda M. Ross. 550 pages. 1997. 0-7808-0217-9. $78.

"Recommended for consumer health collections in public libraries, and secondary school and community college libraries." — *American Reference Books Annual 2002*

"Every school and public library should have a copy of this comprehensive and user-friendly reference book." — *Choice, Association of College & Research Libraries, Sep '01*

"This is a highly recommended book. This is an especially important book for all school and public libraries." — *AIDS Book Review Journal, Jul-Aug '01*

"Recommended reference source." — *Booklist, American Library Association, Apr '01*

"Recommended pick both for specialty health library collections and any general consumer health reference collection." — *The Bookwatch, Apr '01*

■

Skin Disorders Sourcebook

Basic Information about Common Skin and Scalp Conditions Caused by Aging, Allergies, Immune Reactions, Sun Exposure, Infectious Organisms, Parasites, Cosmetics, and Skin Traumas, Including Abrasions, Cuts, and Pressure Sores

Along with Information on Prevention and Treatment

Edited by Allan R. Cook. 647 pages. 1997. 0-7808-0080-X. $78.

". . . comprehensive, easily read reference book." — *Doody's Health Sciences Book Reviews, Oct '97*

SEE ALSO Burns Sourcebook

■

Sleep Disorders Sourcebook

Basic Consumer Health Information about Sleep and Its Disorders, Including Insomnia, Sleepwalking, Sleep Apnea, Restless Leg Syndrome, and Narcolepsy

Along with Data about Shiftwork and Its Effects, Information on the Societal Costs of Sleep Deprivation, Descriptions of Treatment Options, a Glossary of Terms, and Resource Listings for Additional Help

Edited by Jenifer Swanson. 439 pages. 1998. 0-7808-0234-9. $78.

"This text will complement any home or medical library. It is user-friendly and ideal for the adult reader." — *American Reference Books Annual, 2000*

"A useful resource that provides accurate, relevant, and accessible information on sleep to the general public. Health care providers who deal with sleep disorders patients may also find it helpful in being prepared to answer some of the questions patients ask." — *Respiratory Care, Jul '99*

"Recommended reference source." — *Booklist, American Library Association, Feb '99*

■

Sports Injuries Sourcebook, 2nd Edition

Basic Consumer Health Information about the Diagnosis, Treatment, and Rehabilitation of Common Sports-Related Injuries in Children and Adults

Along with Suggestions for Conditioning and Training, Information and Prevention Tips for Injuries Frequently Associated with Specific Sports and Special Populations, a Glossary, and a Directory of Additional Resources

Edited by Joyce Brennfleck Shannon. 614 pages. 2002. 0-7808-0604-2. $78.

ALSO AVAILABLE: Sports Injuries Sourcebook, 1st Edition. Edited by Heather E. Aldred. 624 pages. 1999. 0-7808-0218-7. $78.

"This is an excellent reference for consumers and it is recommended for public, community college, and undergraduate libraries."
— *American Reference Books Annual, 2003*

"Recommended reference source."
— *Booklist, American Library Association, Feb '03*

Stress-Related Disorders Sourcebook

Basic Consumer Health Information about Stress and Stress-Related Disorders, Including Stress Origins and Signals, Environmental Stress at Work and Home, Mental and Emotional Stress Associated with Depression, Post-Traumatic Stress Disorder, Panic Disorder, Suicide, and the Physical Effects of Stress on the Cardiovascular, Immune, and Nervous Systems

Along with Stress Management Techniques, a Glossary, and a Listing of Additional Resources

Edited by Joyce Brennfleck Shannon. 610 pages. 2002. 0-7808-0560-7. $78.

"Well written for a general readership, the *Stress-Related Disorders Sourcebook* is a useful addition to the health reference literature."
— *American Reference Books Annual, 2003*

"I am impressed by the amount of information. It offers a thorough overview of the causes and consequences of stress for the layperson. . . . A well-done and thorough reference guide for professionals and nonprofessionals alike." — *Doody's Review Service, Dec '02*

Stroke Sourcebook

Basic Consumer Health Information about Stroke, Including Ischemic, Hemorrhagic, Transient Ischemic Attack (TIA), and Pediatric Stroke, Stroke Triggers and Risks, Diagnostic Tests, Treatments, and Rehabilitation Information

Along with Stroke Prevention Guidelines, Legal and Financial Information, a Glossary, and a Directory of Additional Resources

Edited by Joyce Brennfleck Shannon. 606 pages. 2003. 0-7808-0630-1. $78.

Substance Abuse Sourcebook

Basic Health-Related Information about the Abuse of Legal and Illegal Substances Such as Alcohol, Tobacco, Prescription Drugs, Marijuana, Cocaine, and Heroin; and Including Facts about Substance Abuse Prevention Strategies, Intervention Methods, Treatment and Recovery Programs, and a Section Addressing the Special Problems Related to Substance Abuse during Pregnancy

Edited by Karen Bellenir. 573 pages. 1996. 0-7808-0038-9. $78.

"A valuable addition to any health reference section. Highly recommended."

— *The Book Report, Mar/Apr '97*

". . . a comprehensive collection of substance abuse information that's both highly readable and compact. Families and caregivers of substance abusers will find the information enlightening and helpful, while teachers, social workers and journalists should benefit from the concise format. Recommended."
— *Drug Abuse Update, Winter '96/'97*

SEE ALSO Alcoholism Sourcebook, Drug Abuse Sourcebook

Surgery Sourcebook

Basic Consumer Health Information about Inpatient and Outpatient Surgeries, Including Cardiac, Vascular, Orthopedic, Ocular, Reconstructive, Cosmetic, Gynecologic, and Ear, Nose, and Throat Procedures and More

Along with Information about Operating Room Policies and Instruments, Laser Surgery Techniques, Hospital Errors, Statistical Data, a Glossary, and Listings of Sources for Further Help and Information

Edited by Annemarie S. Muth and Karen Bellenir. 596 pages. 2002. 0-7808-0380-9. $78.

"Invaluable reference for public and school library collections alike." — *Library Bookwatch, Apr '03*

Transplantation Sourcebook

Basic Consumer Health Information about Organ and Tissue Transplantation, Including Physical and Financial Preparations, Procedures and Issues Relating to Specific Solid Organ and Tissue Transplants, Rehabilitation, Pediatric Transplant Information, the Future of Transplantation, and Organ and Tissue Donation

Along with a Glossary and Listings of Additional Resources

Edited by Joyce Brennfleck Shannon. 628 pages. 2002. 0-7808-0322-1. $78.

"Along with these advances [in transplantation technology] have come a number of daunting questions for potential transplant patients, their families, and their health care providers. This reference text is the best single tool to address many of these questions. . . . It will be a much-needed addition to the reference collections in health care, academic, and large public libraries."
— *American Reference Books Annual, 2003*

"Recommended for libraries with an interest in offering consumer health information." — *E-Streams, Jul '02*

"This is a unique and valuable resource for patients facing transplantation and their families."
— *Doody's Review Service, Jun '02*

Traveler's Health Sourcebook

Basic Consumer Health Information for Travelers, Including Physical and Medical Preparations, Transportation Health and Safety, Essential Information about Food and Water, Sun Exposure, Insect and Snake Bites, Camping and Wilderness Medicine, and Travel with Physical or Medical Disabilities

Along with International Travel Tips, Vaccination Recommendations, Geographical Health Issues, Disease Risks, a Glossary, and a Listing of Additional Resources

Edited by Joyce Brennfleck Shannon. 613 pages. 2000. 0-7808-0384-1. $78.

"Recommended reference source."
—Booklist, American Library Association, Feb '01

"This book is recommended for any public library, any travel collection, and especially any collection for the physically disabled."
—American Reference Books Annual, 2001

◼

Vegetarian Sourcebook

Basic Consumer Health Information about Vegetarian Diets, Lifestyle, and Philosophy, Including Definitions of Vegetarianism and Veganism, Tips about Adopting Vegetarianism, Creating a Vegetarian Pantry, and Meeting Nutritional Needs of Vegetarians, with Facts Regarding Vegetarianism's Effect on Pregnant and Lactating Women, Children, Athletes, and Senior Citizens

Along with a Glossary of Commonly Used Vegetarian Terms and Resources for Additional Help and Information

Edited by Chad T. Kimball. 360 pages. 2002. 0-7808-0439-2. $78.

"Organizes into one concise volume the answers to the most common questions concerning vegetarian diets and lifestyles. This title is recommended for public and secondary school libraries." *— E-Streams, Apr '03*

"Invaluable reference for public and school library collections alike." *— Library Bookwatch, Apr '03*

"The articles in this volume are easy to read and come from authoritative sources. The book does not necessarily support the vegetarian diet but instead provides the pros and cons of this important decision. The *Vegetarian Sourcebook* is recommended for public libraries and consumer health libraries."
—American Reference Books Annual, 2003

◼

Women's Health Concerns Sourcebook

Basic Information about Health Issues That Affect Women, Featuring Facts about Menstruation and Other Gynecological Concerns, Including Endometriosis, Fibroids, Menopause, and Vaginitis; Reproductive Concerns, Including Birth Control, Infertility, and Abortion; and Facts about Additional Physical, Emotional, and Mental Health Concerns Prevalent among Women Such as Osteoporosis, Urinary Tract Disorders, Eating Disorders, and Depression

Along with Tips for Maintaining a Healthy Lifestyle

Edited by Heather E. Aldred. 567 pages. 1997. 0-7808-0219-5. $78.

"Handy compilation. There is an impressive range of diseases, devices, disorders, procedures, and other phys-

ical and emotional issues covered . . . well organized, illustrated, and indexed." *—Choice, Association of College and Research Libraries, Jan '98*

SEE ALSO *Breast Cancer Sourcebook, Cancer Sourcebook for Women, Healthy Heart Sourcebook for Women, Osteoporosis Sourcebook*

◼

Workplace Health & Safety Sourcebook

Basic Consumer Health Information about Workplace Health and Safety, Including the Effect of Workplace Hazards on the Lungs, Skin, Heart, Ears, Eyes, Brain, Reproductive Organs, Musculoskeletal System, and Other Organs and Body Parts

Along with Information about Occupational Cancer, Personal Protective Equipment, Toxic and Hazardous Chemicals, Child Labor, Stress, and Workplace Violence

Edited by Chad T. Kimball. 626 pages. 2000. 0-7808-0231-4. $78.

"As a reference for the general public, this would be useful in any library." *—E-Streams, Jun '01*

"Provides helpful information for primary care physicians and other caregivers interested in occupational medicine. . . . General readers; professionals."
— Choice, Association of College & Research Libraries, May '01

"Recommended reference source."
—Booklist, American Library Association, Feb '01

"Highly recommended." *—The Bookwatch, Jan '01*

◼

Worldwide Health Sourcebook

Basic Information about Global Health Issues, Including Malnutrition, Reproductive Health, Disease Dispersion and Prevention, Emerging Diseases, Risky Health Behaviors, and the Leading Causes of Death

Along with Global Health Concerns for Children, Women, and the Elderly, Mental Health Issues, Research and Technology Advancements, and Economic, Environmental, and Political Health Implications, a Glossary, and a Resource Listing for Additional Help and Information

Edited by Joyce Brennfleck Shannon. 614 pages. 2001. 0-7808-0330-2. $78.

"Named an Outstanding Academic Title."
—Choice, Association of College & Research Libraries, Jan '02

"Yet another handy but also unique compilation in the extensive Health Reference Series, this is a useful work because many of the international publications reprinted or excerpted are not readily available. Highly recommended." *—Choice, Association of College & Research Libraries, Nov '01*

"Recommended reference source."
—Booklist, American Library Association, Oct '01

Teen Health Series

*Helping Young Adults Understand, Manage,
and Avoid Serious Illness*

Diet Information for Teens
Health Tips about Diet and Nutrition

*Including Facts about Nutrients, Dietary Guidelines,
Breakfasts, School Lunches, Snacks, Party Food, Weight
Control, Eating Disorders, and More*

Edited by Karen Bellenir. 399 pages. 2001. 0-7808-0441-4. $58.

"Full of helpful insights and facts throughout the book.
. . . An excellent resource to be placed in public libraries
or even in personal collections."
—American Reference Books Annual 2002

"Recommended for middle and high school libraries
and media centers as well as academic libraries that
educate future teachers of teenagers. It is also a suitable
addition to health science libraries that serve patrons
who are interested in teen health promotion and education."
—E-Streams, Oct '01

"This comprehensive book would be beneficial to collections that need information about nutrition, dietary
guidelines, meal planning, and weight control. . . . This
reference is so easy to use that its purchase is recommended."
—The Book Report, Sep-Oct '01

"This book is written in an easy to understand format
describing issues that many teens face every day, and
then provides thoughtful explanations so that teens can
make informed decisions. This is an interesting book
that provides important facts and information for
today's teens."
*—Doody's Health Sciences
Book Review Journal, Jul-Aug '01*

"A comprehensive compendium of diet and nutrition.
The information is presented in a straightforward,
plain-spoken manner. This title will be useful to those
working on reports on a variety of topics, as well as to
general readers concerned about their dietary health."
— School Library Journal, Jun '01

Drug Information for Teens
Health Tips about the Physical and Mental Effects of Substance Abuse

*Including Facts about Alcohol, Anabolic Steroids, Club
Drugs, Cocaine, Depressants, Hallucinogens, Herbal
Products, Inhalants, Marijuana, Narcotics, Stimulants,
Tobacco, and More*

Edited by Karen Bellenir. 452 pages. 2002. 0-7808-0444-9. $58.

"The chapters are quick to make a connection to their
teenage reading audience. The prose is straightforward
and the book lends itself to spot reading. It should be
useful both for practical information and for research,
and it is suitable for public and school libraries."
— American Reference Books Annual, 2003

"Recommended reference source."
—Booklist, American Library Association, Feb '03

"This is an excellent resource for teens and their parents. Education about drugs and substances is key to
discouraging teen drug abuse and this book provides
this much needed information in a way that is interesting and factual."
—Doody's Review Service, Dec '02

Mental Health Information for Teens
Health Tips about Mental Health and Mental Illness

*Including Facts about Anxiety, Depression, Suicide,
Eating Disorders, Obsessive-Compulsive Disorders,
Panic Attacks, Phobias, Schizophrenia, and More*

Edited by Karen Bellenir. 406 pages. 2001. 0-7808-0442-2. $58.

"In both language and approach, this user-friendly entry
in the *Teen Health Series* is on target for teens needing
information on mental health concerns." *— Booklist,
American Library Association, Jan '02*

"Readers will find the material accessible and informative, with the shaded notes, facts, and embedded glossary insets adding appropriately to the already interesting and succinct presentation."
—School Library Journal, Jan '02

"This title is highly recommended for any library that
serves adolescents and parents/caregivers of adolescents."
—E-Streams, Jan '02

"Recommended for high school libraries and young
adult collections in public libraries. Both health professionals and teenagers will find this book useful."
—American Reference Books Annual 2002

"This is a nice book written to enlighten the society,
primarily teenagers, about common teen mental health
issues. It is highly recommended to teachers and parents as well as adolescents."
—Doody's Review Service, Dec '01

Sexual Health Information for Teens
Health Tips about Sexual Development, Human Reproduction, and Sexually Transmitted Diseases

*Including Facts about Puberty, Reproductive Health,
Chlamydia, Human Papillomavirus, Pelvic Inflam-*

matory Disease, Herpes, AIDS, Contraception, Pregnancy, and More

Edited by Deborah A. Stanley. 391 pages. 2003. 0-7808-0445-7. $58.

Skin Health Information For Teens
Health Tips about Dermatological Concerns and Skin Cancer Risks

Including Facts about Acne, Warts, Hives, and Other Conditions and Lifestyle Choices, Such as Tanning, Tattooing, and Piercing, That Affect the Skin, Nails, Scalp, and Hair

Edited by Robert Aquinas McNally. 430 pages. 2003. 0-7808-0446-5. $58.

Sports Injuries Information For Teens
Health Tips about Sports Injuries and Injury Protection

Including Facts about Specific Injuries, Emergency Treatment, Rehabilitation, Sports Safety, Competition Stress, Fitness, Sports Nutrition, Steroid Risks, and More

Edited by Joyce Brennfleck Shannon. 425 pages. 2003. 0-7808-0447-3. $58.

Health Reference Series